Foliated spaces look locally like products, but their global structure is generally not a product, and tangential differential operators are correspondingly more complex. In the 1980s, Alain Connes founded what is now known as noncommutative geometry and topology. One of the first results was his generalization of the Atiyah-Singer index theorem to compute the analytic index associated with a tangential (pseudo)-differential operator and an invariant transverse measure on a foliated manifold, in terms of topological data on the manifold and the operator.

This book presents a complete proof of this beautiful result, generalized to foliated spaces (not just manifolds). It includes the necessary background from analysis, geometry, and topology. This second edition has improved exposition, an updated bibliography, an index, and additional material covering developments and applications since the first edition came out, including the confirmation of the Gap Labeling Conjecture of Jean Bellissard.

Mathematical Sciences Research Institute Publications

9

Global Analysis on Foliated Spaces

Mathematical Sciences Research Institute Publications

1 Freed/Uhlenbeck: *Instantons and Four-Manifolds*, second edition
2 Chern (ed.): *Seminar on Nonlinear Partial Differential Equations*
3 Lepowsky/Mandelstam/Singer (eds.): *Vertex Operators in Mathematics and Physics*
4 Kac (ed.): *Infinite Dimensional Groups with Applications*
5 Blackadar: *K-Theory for Operator Algebras*, second edition
6 Moore (ed.): *Group Representations, Ergodic Theory, Operator Algebras, and Mathematical Physics*
7 Chorin/Majda (eds.): *Wave Motion: Theory, Modelling, and Computation*
8 Gersten (ed.): *Essays in Group Theory*
9 Moore/Schochet: *Global Analysis on Foliated Spaces*, second edition
10–11 Drasin/Earle/Gehring/Kra/Marden (eds.): *Holomorphic Functions and Moduli*
12–13 Ni/Peletier/Serrin (eds.): *Nonlinear Diffusion Equations and Their Equilibrium States*
14 Goodman/de la Harpe/Jones: *Coxeter Graphs and Towers of Algebras*
15 Hochster/Huneke/Sally (eds.): *Commutative Algebra*
16 Ihara/Ribet/Serre (eds.): *Galois Groups over* $\mathbb{Q}$
17 Concus/Finn/Hoffman (eds.): *Geometric Analysis and Computer Graphics*
18 Bryant/Chern/Gardner/Goldschmidt/Griffiths: *Exterior Differential Systems*
19 Alperin (ed.): *Arboreal Group Theory*
20 Dazord/Weinstein (eds.): *Symplectic Geometry, Groupoids, and Integrable Systems*
21 Moschovakis (ed.): *Logic from Computer Science*
22 Ratiu (ed.): *The Geometry of Hamiltonian Systems*
23 Baumslag/Miller (eds.): *Algorithms and Classification in Combinatorial Group Theory*
24 Montgomery/Small (eds.): *Noncommutative Rings*
25 Akbulut/King: *Topology of Real Algebraic Sets*
26 Judah/Just/Woodin (eds.): *Set Theory of the Continuum*
27 Carlsson/Cohen/Hsiang/Jones (eds.): *Algebraic Topology and Its Applications*
28 Clemens/Kollár (eds.): *Current Topics in Complex Algebraic Geometry*
29 Nowakowski (ed.): *Games of No Chance*
30 Grove/Petersen (eds.): *Comparison Geometry*
31 Levy (ed.): *Flavors of Geometry*
32 Cecil/Chern (eds.): *Tight and Taut Submanifolds*
33 Axler/McCarthy/Sarason (eds.): *Holomorphic Spaces*
34 Ball/Milman (eds.): *Convex Geometric Analysis*
35 Levy (ed.): *The Eightfold Way*
36 Gavosto/Krantz/McCallum (eds.): *Contemporary Issues in Mathematics Education*
37 Schneider/Siu (eds.): *Several Complex Variables*
38 Billera/Björner/Green/Simion/Stanley (eds.): *New Perspectives in Geometric Combinatorics*
39 Haskell/Pillay/Steinhorn (eds.): *Model Theory, Algebra, and Geometry*
40 Bleher/Its (eds.): *Random Matrix Models and Their Applications*
41 Schneps (ed.): *Galois Groups and Fundamental Groups*
42 Nowakowski (ed.): *More Games of No Chance*
43 Montgomery/Schneider (eds.): *New Directions in Hopf Algebras*
44 Buhler/Stevenhagen (eds.): *Algorithmic Number Theory*
45 Jensen/Ledet/Yui: *Generic Polynomials: Constructive Aspects of the Inverse Galois Problem*
46 Rockmore/Healy (eds.): *Modern Signal Processing*
47 Uhlmann (ed.): *Inside Out: Inverse Problems and Applications*
48 Gross/Kotiuga: *Electromagnetic Theory and Computation: A Topological Approach*
49 Darmon/Zhang (eds.): *Heegner Points and Rankin L-Series*
50 Bao/Bryant/Chern/Shen (eds.): *A Sampler of Riemann–Finsler Geometry*
51 Avramov/Green/Huneke/Smith/Sturmfels (eds.): *Trends in Commutative Algebra*
52 Goodman/Pach/Welzl (eds.): *Combinatorial and Computational Geometry*

Volumes 1–4, 6–8 and 10–27 are published by Springer-Verlag

Global Analysis on Foliated Spaces

Second Edition

Calvin C. Moore
University of California, Berkeley

Claude L. Schochet
Wayne State University

CAMBRIDGE
UNIVERSITY PRESS

Calvin C. Moore: Mathematics Department, Evans Hall, University of California, Berkeley, CA 94720, United States ccmoore@math.berkeley.edu

Claude L. Schochet: Mathematics Department, Wayne State University, 656 W. Kirby, Detroit, MI 48202, United States claude@math.wayne.edu

Silvio Levy (*Series Editor*): Mathematical Sciences Research Institute, 17 Gauss Way, Berkeley, CA 94720, United States levy@msri.org

The Mathematical Sciences Research Institute wishes to acknowledge support by the National Science Foundation. This material is based upon work supported by NSF Grant 9810361.

CAMBRIDGE
UNIVERSITY PRESS

Shaftesbury Road, Cambridge CB2 8EA, United Kingdom

One Liberty Plaza, 20th Floor, New York, NY 10006, USA

477 Williamstown Road, Port Melbourne, VIC 3207, Australia

314–321, 3rd Floor, Plot 3, Splendor Forum, Jasola District Centre, New Delhi – 110025, India

103 Penang Road, #05–06/07, Visioncrest Commercial, Singapore 238467

Cambridge University Press is part of Cambridge University Press & Assessment, a department of the University of Cambridge.

We share the University's mission to contribute to society through the pursuit of education, learning and research at the highest international levels of excellence.

www.cambridge.org
Information on this title: www.cambridge.org/9780521613057

First published 2006

A catalogue record for this publication is available from the British Library

Library of Congress Cataloging-in-Publication data

Moore, C. C. (Calvin C.), 1936–
Global analysis on foliated spaces / Calvin C. Moore, Claude L. Schochet – 2nd ed.
p. cm. – (Mathematical Sciences Research Institute publications ; 9)
Includes bibliographical references and index.
ISBN-13: 978-0-521-61305-7 (pbk.) ISBN-10: 0-521-61305-1 (pbk.)
1. Global analysis (Mathematics) 2. Foliations (Mathematics) I. Schochet, Claude, 1944–
II. Title. III. Series.

QA614.M65 2006
514′.74–dc22 2005054277

ISBN 978-0-521-61305-7 Paperback

To Doris and Rivka

Contents

Preface to the Second Edition

A lot has happened in the realm of foliated spaces and their operator algebras since 1988, when this book first appeared. We are pleased that, as we had hoped, this book has served as an introduction to the subject and a reference for researchers and students.

Our colleagues have convinced us that there is merit in issuing a second edition of our work, so that a new generation of students may have access to its contents. Cambridge University Press was amenable to the idea, so we (slowly) went to work.

We have taken the opportunity of a new edition to make a number of changes and additions to the book:

(1) We have corrected a few minor errors, filled some gaps, and made many changes to improve the exposition.

(2) We have added updates at the end of each chapter as well as occasional footnotes in which we discuss some of the relevant mathematical developments since 1988. This discussion is understandably brief. We do try to point the reader to the papers where the results themselves appear.

(3) We have enlarged the bibliography correspondingly.

(4) We have added a new appendix; it is a reprint of a *Mathematical Reviews* Featured Review by the second author on the Gap Labeling Theorem. We felt this was appropriate since it illustrates a very interesting and important application of the Index Theorem.

(5) We have added an index to the book.

(6) MSRI has provided for the resetting of the book in LaTeX and for the redrafting of all the art.

As originally formulated, the Connes' Index Theorem [1979] applied to foliated manifolds. The version presented here is valid for foliated spaces, a category that is strictly larger than foliated manifolds and laminations obtained from manifolds. It turns out that this extra generality is crucial for some of the applications of the Index Theorem in the past few years. For instance, the

Gap Labeling results discussed in Appendix D require this extra generality. We discuss this in some detail at the end of Chapter VIII.

We acknowledge with gratitude the help that we have received from Jean Bellissard, Alberto Candel, Larry Conlon, Steve Hurder, Jerry Kaminker, Masoud Khalkhali, Paul Muhly, and especially our friend and editor *par excellence* Silvio Levy in the preparation of this edition. The second author is grateful to Baruch Solel and the faculty of the Technion for a sabbatical year at a critical time. We are grateful to the editors of *Mathematical Reviews* for permission to reproduce the Featured Review on the Gap Labeling Theorem as Appendix D of this work.

Finally, we can but repeat the final paragraph of the preface of the first edition: *We owe a profound debt to Alain Connes, whose work on the index theorem aroused our own interest in the subject. This work would not exist had we not been so stimulated by his results to try to understand them better.*

Preface to the First Edition

This book grew out of lectures and the lecture notes generated therefrom by the first named author at UC Berkeley in 1980 and by the second named author at UCLA, also in 1980. We were motivated to develop these notes more fully by the urgings of our colleagues and friends and by the desire to make the general subject and the work of Alain Connes in particular more readily accessible to the mathematical public. The book develops a variety of aspects of analysis and geometry on foliated spaces which should be useful in many contexts. These strands are then brought together to provide a context and to expose Connes' index theorem for foliated spaces [Connes 1979], a theorem which asserts the equality of the analytic and the topological index (two real numbers) which are associated to a tangentially elliptic operator. The exposition, we believe, serves an additional purpose of preparing the way towards the more general index theorem of Connes and Skandalis [1981; 1984]. This index theorem describes the abstract index class in $K_0(C_r^*(G(M)))$, the index group of the C^*-algebra of the foliated space, and is necessarily substantially more abstract, while the tools used here are relatively elementary and straightforward, and are based on the heat equation method.

We must thank several people who have aided us in the preparation of this book. The origins of this book are embedded in lectures and seminars at Berkeley and UCLA (respectively) and we wish to acknowledge the patience and assistance of our colleagues there, particularly Bill Arveson, Ed Effros, Marc Rieffel and Masamichi Takesaki. More recently, we have benefitted from conversations and help from Ron Douglas, Peter Gilkey, Jane Hawkins, Steve Hurder, Jerry Kaminker, John Roe, Jon Rosenberg, Bert Schreiber, George Skandalis, Michael Taylor, and Bob Zimmer.

We owe a profound debt to Alain Connes, whose work on the index theorem aroused our own interest in the subject. This work would not exist had we not been so stimulated by his results to try to understand them better.

Introduction

Global analysis has as its primary focus the interplay between the local analysis and the global geometry and topology of a manifold. This is seen classically in the Gauss–Bonnet theorem and its generalizations, which culminate in the Atiyah–Singer Index Theorem [Atiyah and Singer 1968a]. This places constraints on the solutions of elliptic systems of partial differential equations in terms of the Fredholm index of the associated elliptic operator and characteristic differential forms which are related to global topological properties of the manifold.

The Atiyah–Singer Index Theorem has been generalized in several directions, notably by Atiyah and Singer themselves [1971] to an index theorem for families. The typical setting here is given by a family of elliptic operators $P = \{P_b\}$ on the total space of a fibre bundle $F \to M \to B$, where P_b is defined on the Hilbert space $L^2(p^{-1}(b), \mathrm{dvol}(F))$. In this case there is an abstract index class $\mathrm{ind}(P) \in K^0(B)$. Once the problem is properly formulated it turns out that no further deep analytic information is needed in order to identify the class. These theorems and their equivariant counterparts have been enormously useful in topology, geometry, physics, and in representation theory.

A smooth manifold M^n with an integrable p-dimensional subbundle F of its tangent bundle TM may be partitioned into p-dimensional manifolds called *leaves* such that the restriction of F to the leaf is just the tangent bundle of the leaf. This structure is called a *foliation* of M. Locally a foliation has the form $\mathbb{R}^p \times N$, with leaves of the form $\mathbb{R}^p \times \{n\}$. Locally, then, a foliation is a fibre bundle. However the same leaf may pass through a given coordinate patch infinitely often. So globally the situation is much more complicated.

Foliations arise in the study of flows and dynamics, in group representations, automorphic forms, groups acting on spaces (continuously or even measurably), and in situations not easily modeled in classical algebraic topology. For instance, a diffeomorphism acting ergodically on a manifold M yields a one-dimensional foliation on $M \times_{\mathbb{Z}} \mathbb{R}$ with almost all leaves dense. The space of leaves of a foliation in these cases is not decent topologically (every point is dense in the example above) or even measure-theoretically (the space may not be a standard

Borel space). Foliations carry interesting differential operators, such as signature operators along the leaves. Following the Atiyah–Singer pattern, one might hope that there would be an analytic index class of the type

$$\mathrm{ind}\{P\} = \text{ Average } \mathrm{ind}(P_x).$$

There are two difficulties. First of all, leaves of compact foliations need not be compact, so an elliptic operator on a leaf may well have infinite-dimensional kernel or cokernel, and thus "$\mathrm{ind}(P_x)$" makes no sense. This problem aside, the fact that the space of leaves may not be even a standard Borel space suggests strongly that there is no way to average over it. There was thus no analytic index to try to compute for foliations.

Alain Connes saw his way through these difficulties. He realized that the "space of leaves" of a foliation should be a noncommutative space — that is, a C^*-algebra $C_r^*(G(M))$. In the case of a foliated fibre bundle this algebra is stably isomorphic to the algebra of continuous functions on the base space. This suggests $K_0(C_r^*(G(M)))$ as a home for an abstract index $\mathrm{ind}(P)$ for tangentially elliptic operators.

Next Connes realized that in the fibre bundle case there is an invariant transverse measure ν which corresponds to the volume measure on B. So we must assume given some invariant transverse measure in general. These may not exist. If one exists it may not be unique up to scale. An invariant transverse measure ν gives rise to a trace ϕ_ν on $C_r^*(G(M))$ and thus a real number

$$\mathrm{ind}_\nu(P) = \phi_\nu(\mathrm{ind}(P)) \in \mathbb{R}$$

which Connes declared to be the *analytic index*. Actually we are cheating here; the most basic definition of the analytic index is in terms of locally traceable operators as we shall explain below and in Chapters I and IV. With an analytic index to compute, Connes computed it.

Connes Index Theorem. *Let M be a compact smooth manifold with an oriented foliation and let ν be an invariant transverse measure with associated Ruelle–Sullivan current C_ν. Let P be a tangentially elliptic pseudodifferential operator. Then*

$$\mathrm{ind}_\nu(P) = \big\langle \mathrm{ch}(P)\,\mathrm{Td}(M), [C_\nu] \big\rangle.$$

Connes' theorem is very satisfying. Its proof involves a tour of many areas of modern mathematics. We decided to write an exposition of this theorem and to use it as a centerpiece to discuss this region of mathematics. Along the way we realized that the setting of *foliated spaces* (local picture $\mathbb{R}^p \times N$ with N not necessarily Euclidean) was at once simpler pedagogically and yielded a somewhat more general theorem, since foliated spaces which are not manifolds occur with some frequency.

The local picture of a foliated space is a topological space of the form $L \times N$, where L is a copy of $\mathbb{R}^p$ and N is a separable metric space, not necessarily a manifold.

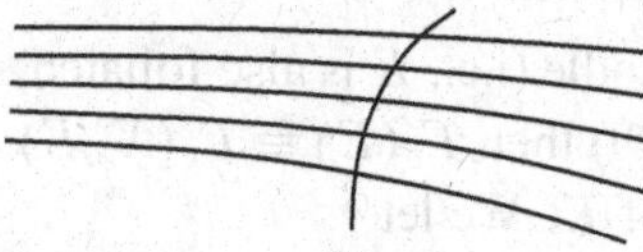

A *tangentially smooth* function

$$f : L \times N \to \mathbb{R}$$

is a continuous function with the following properties:

(1) For each $n \in N$, the function $f(\cdot, n) : L \to \mathbb{R}$ is smooth.

(2) All partial derivatives of f in the L directions are continuous on $L \times N$.

This notion extends naturally to tangentially smooth functions

$$f : L_1 \times N_1 \to L_2 \times N_2.$$

Definition. A *foliated space* X of dimension p is a separable metrizable space equipped with a regular foliated atlas $\mathcal{U} = \{(U_\alpha, \varphi_\alpha)\}$ such that, whenever U_α and U_β intersect, the composition

$$\varphi_\alpha(U_\alpha \cap U_\beta) \xrightarrow{\varphi_\alpha^{-1}} U_\alpha \cap U_\beta \xrightarrow{\varphi_\beta} \varphi_\beta(U_\alpha \cap U_\beta)$$

is tangentially smooth. A *tangentially smooth* function $f : X_1 \to X_2$ of foliated spaces is a continuous function such that if $U_i \subset X_i$ are foliated charts with associated maps

$$\varphi_i : U_i \longrightarrow L_i \times N_i$$

then the composition

$$\varphi_1(U_1 \cap f^{-1}(U_2)) \xrightarrow{\varphi_1^{-1}} U_1 \cap f^{-1}(U_2) \xrightarrow{f} f(U_1) \cap U_2 \xrightarrow{\varphi_2} L_2 \times N_2$$

is tangentially smooth.

This guarantees that the leaves in each coordinate patch coalesce to form leaves ℓ in X which are smooth p-manifolds, and that there is a natural vector bundle $FX \to X$ of dimension p which restricts to the tangent bundle of each leaf.

Any foliated manifold is a foliated space. There are interesting examples of foliated spaces which are not foliated manifolds. For instance, a solenoid is a foliated space with leaves of dimension 1 and with N_i homeomorphic to Cantor sets. If M^n is a manifold which is foliated by leaves of dimension p and if N is a transversal of M^n then any subset of N determines a foliated subspace of M simply by taking those leaves of M^n which meet the subset. This includes the laminations of much current interest in low-dimensional topology, and it includes the topological spaces that arise in the study of quasicrystals and tilings of Euclidean space. Finally, X may well be infinite-dimensional: take $\prod_1^\infty S^1$ foliated by lines corresponding to algebraically independent irrational rotations. Then $\{1\} \times \prod_2^\infty S^1$ is transversal![1]

If $E \xrightarrow{\pi} X$ is a foliated bundle (i.e., E is also foliated, π takes leaves to leaves, and π is tangentially smooth) then $\Gamma_\tau(E) \equiv \Gamma_\tau(X, E)$ denotes continuous tangentially smooth sections of E. We let

$$\Omega_\tau^k(X) = \Gamma_\tau(\Lambda^k F^*)$$

and define the *tangential cohomology* groups of a foliated space by

$$H_\tau^k(X) = H^k(\Omega_\tau^*(X)),$$

where $d : \Omega_\tau^k(X) \to \Omega_\tau^{k+1}(X)$ is the analogue of the de Rham differential obtained by differentiating in the leaf directions. Similar (but not the same) groups have been studied by many authors. Tangential cohomology groups are based upon forms which are *continuous* transversely (even if X is a foliated manifold.) It turns out that this small point has some major consequences. The groups may be described as

$$H_\tau^k(X) = H^k(X : \mathcal{R}_\tau),$$

where $\mathcal{R}_\tau$ is the sheaf of germs of continuous functions which are constant along leaves. The tangential cohomology groups are functors from foliated spaces and leaf-preserving tangentially smooth maps to graded commutative $\mathbb{R}$-algebras. They vanish for $k > p$. There is the usual apparatus of long exact sequences, suspension isomorphisms, and a Thom isomorphism for oriented k-plane bundles.

The groups $H_\tau^*(X)$ have a natural topology and are not necessarily Hausdorff; we let

$$\bar{H}_\tau^k(X) = H_\tau^k(X)/\overline{\{0\}}$$

denote the maximal Hausdorff quotient. For example, if X is the torus $S^1 \times S^1$ foliated by an irrational flow, $H_\tau^1(X)$ has infinite dimension but $\bar{H}_\tau^1(X) \cong \mathbb{R}$. The parallel between de Rham theory and tangential cohomology theory extends to the existence of characteristic classes. Given a tangentially smooth vector bundle $E \to X$ we construct tangential connections, curvature forms, and Chern classes.

Next we recall the construction of the groupoid of a foliated space; the idea is due to Ehresmann, Thom and Reeb and was elaborated upon by Winkelnkemper. A foliated space X has a natural equivalence relation: $x \sim y$ if and only if x

[1] This paragraph appeared in the first edition. Since then there has been an explosion of interest in laminations. (Nowadays some authors use the word *lamination* as a synonym for *foliated space*.) The books [Candel and Conlon 2000; 2003] contain a host of examples and references.

and y are on the same leaf. The resulting space $\mathcal{R}(X) \subset X \times X$ is not a well-behaved topological space. The holonomy groupoid $G(X)$ of a foliated space is designed to by-pass this difficulty. It contains holonomy data not given by $\mathcal{R}(X)$; holonomy is essential for diffeomorphism and structural questions about the foliated space. The *holonomy groupoid* $G(X)$ consists of triples $(x, y, [\alpha])$, where x and y lie on the same leaf ℓ of X, α is a path from x to y in ℓ, and $[\alpha]$ denotes the holonomy class of the path α. The map $G(X) \to \mathcal{R}(X)$ is simply $(x, y, [\alpha]) \to (x, y)$. The preimages of (x, y) correspond to holonomy classes of maps from x to y. The space $G(X)$ is a (possibly non-Hausdorff) foliated space. If N is a complete transversal (meaning that N is Borel and for each leaf ℓ the intersection $N \cap \ell$ is nonempty and at most countable), G_N^N is the subgroupoid of $G(X)$ consisting of triples $(x, y, [\alpha])$ with $x, y \in N$. In a sense which we make precise, G_N^N is a good discrete model for $G(X)$.

We turn next to a study of differential and pseudodifferential operators on X. Suppose that E_0 and E_1 are foliated bundles over X and

$$D : \Gamma_\tau(E_0) \to \Gamma_\tau(E_1).$$

The operator D is said to be *tangential* if D restricts to

$$D_\ell : \Gamma(E_0 \mid_\ell) \to \Gamma(E_1 \mid_\ell)$$

for each ℓ, and D is *tangentially elliptic* if each operator D_ℓ is an elliptic operator. If D is a tangential, tangentially elliptic operator then Ker D_ℓ and Ker D_ℓ^* consist of smooth functions on l. These spaces may well be infinite-dimensional, and hence expressions such as

$$\dim \text{Ker } D_\ell - \dim \text{Ker } D_\ell^*$$

make no sense. However there is some additional structure at our disposal, for Ker D_ℓ and Ker D_ℓ^* are $C^\infty(\ell)$-modules. We shall show that these spaces are for each ℓ *locally* finite-dimensional in a sense that we now describe.

Let Y be a locally compact space endowed with a measure (in the application to index theory $Y = \ell$ is a leaf and the measure is a volume measure) and suppose that T is a positive operator on $L^2(Y, E)$ for some bundle E over Y. Then

$$\text{Trace}(f^{1/2}Tf^{1/2}) = \text{Trace}(T^{1/2}fT^{1/2})$$

for every bounded positive function f. We define a measure μ_T by

$$\text{Trace}(f^{1/2}TF^{1/2}) = \int_Y f \, d\mu_T$$

and declare T to be *locally traceable* with local trace μ_T if, for some family $\{Y_i\}$ of compact sets with union Y, we have

$$\mu_T(Y_i) < \infty.$$

If

$$T = \sum \lambda_i T_i$$

with each T_i locally traceable, T is locally traceable with local trace $\mu_T = \sum \lambda_i \mu_{T_i}$. We identify a closed subspace $V \subset L^2(Y, E)$ with the orthogonal projection onto it and say that the subspace is *locally finite-dimensional* if the projection is locally traceable. Any closed subspace of $L^2(Y, E)$ that consists entirely of continuous functions is easily seen to be locally finite-dimensional.

If Y is a C^∞ manifold and D is an elliptic pseudodifferential operator on Y then DD^* and D^*D are locally traceable so Ker D and Ker D^* are locally finite-dimensional. The *local index* of D is defined to be

$$\iota_D = \mu_{\text{Ker } D} - \mu_{\text{Ker } D^*}.$$

If Y is a compact manifold then $\int_Y \iota_D = \text{ind}(D)$, the classical Fredholm index.

The notion of locally traceable operator makes it possible to discuss the index of an elliptic operator on a noncompact manifold. As we observed previously, if D is a tangential, tangentially elliptic operator on a compact foliated space X then D_ℓ is an elliptic operator on the leaf ℓ and its local index

$$\iota_{D_\ell} = \mu_{\text{Ker } D_\ell} - \mu_{\text{Ker } D_\ell^*}$$

does make sense as a (signed) Radon measure on ℓ. Write $\iota_D^x = \iota_{D_\ell}$ for each $x \in \ell$. Then $\iota_D = \{\iota_D^x\}$ is a *tangential measure*; that is, a family of Radon measures supported on leaves of X with suitable invariance properties (see Definition 4.11). We regard ι_D as the abstract analytic index of D. If the foliation bundle F is oriented then a tangential measure determines a class in $\overline{H}_\tau^p(X)$. The task of an index theorem is to identify that class.

To proceed further along these lines and as they are of substantial independent interest, we introduce transverse measures. For this we move temporarily to a measure-theoretic context. Suppose that $(X, \mathcal{R})$ is a standard Borel equivalence relation. We assume that there is a complete Borel transversal; that is, a Borel set which meets all equivalences classes and where the intersection with each class is denumerable. This condition holds easily in the setting of foliated spaces. Assume further that we are given a one-cocycle $\Delta \in Z^1(\mathcal{R}, \mathbb{R}^*)$. A *transverse measure* of modulus Δ is a measure ν on the σ-ring of all Borel transversals which is σ-finite on each transversal and such that $\nu|_T$ is quasi-invariant with modulus $\Delta|_T$ for the countable equivalence relation $\mathcal{R} \cap (T \times T)$ for each transversal T. If $\Delta \equiv 1$ then ν is an *invariant* transverse measure. For example, if X is the total space of a fibration $\ell \to X \to B$ foliated with fibres as leaves then an invariant transverse measure on X is precisely a σ-finite measure on B.

Recall that a tangential measure λ is an assignment $\ell \mapsto \lambda_\ell$ of a measure to each leaf (or class of $\mathcal{R}$) which satisfies suitable Borel smoothness properties (see Definition 4.11). For example, if D is a tangential, tangentially elliptic operator on X then the local index ι_D is a tangential measure. If we choose a coherent family of volume measures for each leaf ℓ then these coalesce to a tangential measure.

Given a tangential measure λ and an invariant transverse measure ν, we describe an integration process that produces a measure $\lambda\, d\nu$ on X and a number $\int \lambda\, d\nu$ obtained by taking the total mass of the measure. Choose a complete transversal N. There is a Borel map $\sigma : X \to N$ with $\sigma(x) \sim x$. Regard X as fibring measure-theoretically over N, and let λ_n be the restriction of λ_ℓ to the set $\sigma^{-1}(n)$, which is contained in the leaf where n lies. Then $\int_N \lambda_n\, d\nu(n) = \lambda\, d\nu$ is a measure on X. This integration process is related to the pairing of currents with foliation cycles in [Sullivan 1976].

How many invariant transverse measures are there? Let $MT(X)$ be the vector space of Radon invariant transverse measures. The construction above provides a pairing

$$MT(X) \times \Omega_\tau^p(X) \to \mathbb{R}$$

and hence a Ruelle–Sullivan map

$$MT(X) \to \mathrm{Hom}_{\mathrm{cont}}(H_\tau^p(X), \mathbb{R}) \cong H_p^\tau(X).$$

We prove a Riesz representation theorem: this map is an isomorphism. For example, if X is foliated by points then $H_\tau^0(X) = C(X)$ and an invariant transverse measure is just a measure, so our result reduces to the usual Riesz representation theorem. We see also that X has no invariant transverse measure if and only if $\overline{H}_\tau^p(X) = 0$.

With this machinery in hand we can state and prove the remarkable index theorem of A. Connes. Let D be a tangential, tangentially elliptic pseudodifferential operator on a compact oriented foliated space of leaf dimension p. As described above, we obtain the analytic index of D as a tangential measure ι_D. For any invariant transverse measure ν the real number $\int_X \iota_D\, d\nu$ is the analytic ν-index $\mathrm{ind}_\nu(D)$ defined by Connes. The Connes index theorem states that for any invariant transverse measure ν,

$$\int \iota_D\, d\nu = \int \iota_D^{\mathrm{top}}\, d\nu,$$

where

$$\iota_D^{\mathrm{top}} = \pm[\Phi_\tau^{-1}\,\mathrm{ch}_\tau(D)]\,\mathrm{Td}_\tau(X)$$

is the topological index of the symbol of D. (See Chapter V for definitions). Using the Riesz representation theorem we reformulate Connes' theorem to read

$$[\iota_D] = [\iota_D^{\mathrm{top}}] \in \overline{H}_\tau^p(X)$$

which, as is evident, does not involve invariant transverse measures. Of course if X has no invariant transverse measures then $\overline{H}_\tau^p(X) = 0$ and $\iota_D \in \overline{\{0\}}$.

There is a stronger form of the index theorem for foliated manifolds which is due to Connes and Skandalis. To state it we need to introduce the reduced C^*-algebra of the foliated space. The compactly supported tangentially smooth functions on $G(X)$ form a $*$-algebra under convolution. (If $G(X)$ is not Hausdorff then a modification is required.) For each leaf G^x of $G(X)$ with its natural volume measure there is a natural regular representation of this $*$-algebra on $\mathcal{B}(L^2(G^x))$. Complete the $*$-algebra with respect to these representations and one obtains $C_r^*(G(X))$. This algebra enters into index theory because there is a natural pseudodifferential operator extension

$$0 \to C_r^*(G(X)) \longrightarrow \bar{\mathcal{P}}^0 \xrightarrow{\ \sigma\ } \Gamma(S^*F, \operatorname{End}(E)) \to 0$$

and hence the tangential principal symbol of D yields an element of

$$K_0(C_r^*(G(X))).$$

Connes and Skandalis [Connes and Skandalis 1984] identify this element and thereby obtain a sharper form of the index theorem which is useful in the Type III situation. Even in the presence of an invariant transverse measure, if the symbol of an operator D has finite order in $K_0(C_r^*(X))$ then $[\iota_D] = 0$ in $H_\tau^p(X)$.

We conclude this introduction with a brief summary of the contents of each chapter.

I. Locally Traceable Operators

Given an operator T on $L^2(Y, E)$ for a locally compact space Y, we explain the concept of local traceability and we construct the local trace μ_T of T. The local index ι_D of an elliptic operator on a noncompact manifold is one motivating example. We also discuss several situations outside the realm of foliations where locally traceable operators shed some light. In particular, we interpret the formal degree of a representation of a unimodular locally compact group in these terms.

II. Foliated Spaces

Here we set forth the topological foundations of our study. We give many examples of foliated spaces and construct tangentially smooth partitions of unity. Then follow smoothing results which enable us, for instance, to assume freely that bundles over our spaces are tangentially smooth. It is perhaps worth noting that $K^0(X)$ coincides with the subgroup generated by tangentially smooth bundles. Next we explain holonomy and, following Winkelnkemper, introduce the holonomy groupoid of a foliated space. We consider the relationship between $G(X)$ and its discrete model G_N^N and determine the structure of G_N^N in several examples.

III. Tangential Cohomology

In this chapter we define the tangential cohomology groups $H_\tau^*(X)$ as the cohomology of the de Rham complex $\Gamma_\tau(\Lambda^* F^*)$ and equivalently as the cohomology of X with coefficients in the sheaf of germs of continuous functions on X which are constant along leaves. There is an analogous compactly supported theory $H_{\tau c}^*(X)$ and an analogous tangential vertical theory $H_{\tau v}^*(E)$ on bundles. We develop the properties parallel to the expected properties from de Rham theory. There is a Mayer–Vietoris sequence (for open subsets) and a Künneth isomorphism

$$H_\tau^*(X) \otimes H^*(M) \xrightarrow{\cong} H_\tau^*(X \times M)$$

provided that M is a manifold foliated as one leaf and $X \times M$ is foliated with leaves $\ell \times M$. We establish a Thom isomorphism theorem (3.30) of the type

$$\Phi : H_\tau^k(X) \xrightarrow{\cong} H_{\tau v}^{n+k}(E)$$

for an oriented tangentially smooth n-plane bundle $E \to X$. Finally we indicate the definition of tangential homology theory. In an appendix we rephrase these constructions in terms of Lie algebra cohomology.

IV. Transverse Measures

We develop here the general theory of groupoids, both in the measurable and topological contexts, in order to give a proper home to transverse measures. The prime examples are $G(X)$ and G_N^N, of course. We introduce transverse measures and their elementary properties. The proper integrands for transverse measures are tangential measures, as we have previously explained in the foliation context. We carefully explain the integration process

$$(\lambda, \nu) \mapsto \lambda\, d\nu \mapsto \int \lambda\, d\nu$$

and indicate the necessary boundedness results. Specializing to topological groupoids and continuous Radon tangential measures, we recount the Ruelle–Sullivan construction of the current $C_\nu \in \Omega_p^\tau(X)$ associated to the transverse measure ν. The current is a cycle if and only if ν is an invariant transverse measure.

Next we relate the space of invariant transverse measures $MT(X)$ on X to invariant measures on a complete transversal N. Finally we establish the Riesz representation theorem: if X is a compact oriented foliated space with leaf dimension p then the Ruelle–Sullivan map

$$MT(X) \longrightarrow \mathrm{Hom}_{\mathrm{cont}}(H_\tau^p(X), \mathbb{R})$$

is an isomorphism. One useful consequence of this result is that a linear functional F on $MT(X)$ is representable as $F(\nu) = \int \omega \, d\nu$ for some $\omega \in H_\tau^p(X)$ if and only if the functional is continuous in the weak topology on $MT(X)$.

V. Characteristic Classes

This chapter contains the Chern–Weil development of tangential characteristic classes. This comes down to carefully generalizing the usual constructions of connections, curvature, and their classes. This results in tangential Chern classes $c_n^\tau \in H_\tau^{2n}(X)$, tangential Pontryagin classes $p_n^\tau \in H_\tau^{4n}(X)$, and a tangential Euler class, as well as the now classical universal combinations of these. We construct these classes at the level of forms, so that, for a fixed tangential Riemannian connection, the topological index is a uniquely defined form. We verify the necessary properties of the tangential Chern character and the tangential Todd genus which relates the K-theory and tangential cohomology Thom isomorphisms.

VI. Operator Algebras

Each foliated space has an associated C^*-algebra $C_r^*(G(X))$ introduced by A. Connes. In this chapter we present its basic properties. Central to our treatment is the Hilsum–Skandalis isomorphism

$$C_r^*(G(X)) \cong C_r^*(G_N^N) \otimes \mathcal{K},$$

which shows that, at the level of C^*-algebras, the foliated space "fibres" over a complete transversal N. The C^*-algebra $C_r^*(G_N^N)$ is the C^*-algebra of the discrete model G_N^N of $G(X)$. An invariant transverse measure ν induces a trace ϕ_ν on $C_r^*(G(X))$, and one then may construct the von Neumann algebra $W^*(G(X), \tilde{\mu})$. The analogous splitting

$$W^*(G(X), \tilde{\mu}) \cong W^*(G_N^N, \tilde{\mu}) \otimes \mathcal{B}(\mathcal{H})$$

at the von Neumann algebra level *is* expected, of course. In the ergodic setting this corresponds to the usual decomposition of a II_∞ factor into the tensor product of II_1 and I_∞ factors. We conclude with a brief introduction to K-theory and the construction of a partial Chern character $c : K_0(C_r^*(G)) \to \overline{H}_\tau^p(X)$.

VII. Pseudodifferential Operators

The usual theory of pseudodifferential operators takes place on a smooth manifold. In this chapter we "parametrize" the theory to the setting of foliated spaces. This involves constructing the pseudodifferential operator algebra and its closure, defining the tangential principal symbol, and showing that the analytic index class ι_D depends only upon the homotopy class of the principal symbol. We construct the pseudodifferential operator extension which has the form

$$0 \to C_r^*(X) \to \bar{\mathcal{P}}^0 \to \Gamma(S^*F, \operatorname{End}(E)) \to 0.$$

We introduce the analytic and topological index at this point. Both depend upon the principal symbol of the operator, and this dependence is carefully explained. We show how the partial Chern character and the tangential Chern character (respectively) are used to obtain cohomology classes in $\overline{H}_\tau^p(X)$; the Connes Theorem is the assertion that these classes agree.

Turning to tangential differential operators, we introduce bounded geometry and finite propagation techniques to demonstrate that ι_D is well-defined. We establish the McKean–Singer formula: for $t > 0$,

$$\operatorname{ind}_\nu(D) = \phi_\nu([e^{-tD^*D}] - [e^{-tDD^*}]) = \phi_\nu^s(e^{-t\hat{D}}),$$

where $\hat{D}$ is an associated self-adjoint superoperator and ϕ_ν^s is the supertrace. Next we prove that as $t \to 0$ there is an asymptotic expansion

$$\phi_\nu^s(e^{-t\hat{D}}) \sim \sum_{j \geq -p} t^{j/2p} \int_X \lambda_j(\hat{D})\, d\nu,$$

where each $\lambda_j(\hat{D})$ is a signed tangential measure independent of t. As $\operatorname{ind}_\nu(D)$ is independent of t, it is immediate that

$$\operatorname{ind}_\nu(D) = \int \omega_D(g, E)\, d\nu,$$

where ω_D is a tangentially smooth p-form which depends on the bundle E of D and upon the tangential Riemannian metric.

VIII. The Index Theorem

If D is a tangential, tangentially elliptic pseudodifferential operator on a compact foliated space with oriented foliation bundle of dimension p, then we have defined the analytic index ι_D and the topological index ι_D^{top} as tangential measures. We establish the Connes index theorem which asserts that for any invariant transverse measure ν,

$$\int \iota_D\, d\nu = \int \iota_D^{\text{top}}\, d\nu.$$

We reformulate this result, in light of the Riesz representation theorem, as

$$[\iota_D] = [\iota_D^{\text{top}}] \in \overline{H}_\tau^p(X).$$

Chapter VIII is devoted to the proof of the index theorem. We verify the theorem for tangential twisted signature operators and then argue on topological grounds that this suffices.

Appendices

There are four appendices to the book; each applies the index theorem in concrete situations and so demonstrates some possible uses of the theorem. The first appendix, by Steven Hurder, develops some interesting examples and applications of the theorem to the case when the leaves of the foliation have a complex structure. The second appendix, by the authors and Robert J. Zimmer, explores the use of the index theorem to demonstrate the existence of square-integrable harmonic forms on certain noncompact manifolds. The third appendix, by Robert J. Zimmer, discusses the application of some of the Gromov–Lawson ideas regarding the existence of a tangential metric which has positive scalar curvature along the leaves. The fourth appendix is a reprint of a featured review from *Mathematical Reviews* on the Gap Labeling Theorem recently established using techniques from this book. These provide a complement to the general development.

CHAPTER I

Locally Traceable Operators

Our object in this chapter is to develop the notion of what we call locally traceable operators — or, more or less equivalently, the notion of locally finite-dimensional subspaces relative to an abelian von Neumann algebra $\mathcal{A}$. The underlying idea here is that certain operators, although not of trace class in the usual sense, are of trace class when suitably localized relative to $\mathcal{A}$. The trace, or perhaps better, the *local* trace of such an operator is not any longer a number, but is rather a measure on a measurable space X associated to the situation with $\mathcal{A} = L^\infty(X)$. This measure is in general infinite but σ-finite, and it will be finite precisely when the operator in question is of trace class in the usual sense, and then its total mass will be the usual trace of the operator. Heuristically, the local trace, as a measure, will tell us how the total trace — infinite in amount — is distributed over the space X. Once we have the notion of a locally traceable operator, and hence the notion of locally finite-dimensional subspaces, one can define then the local index of certain operators. This will be the difference of local dimensions of the kernel and cokernel, and will therefore be, as the difference of two σ-finite measures, a σ-finite signed measure on X. One has to be slightly careful about expressions such as $\infty - \infty$ that arise, but this is a minor matter and can be avoided easily by restricting consideration to sets of finite measure. These ideas are developed to some extent in [Atiyah 1976] for a very similar purpose to what we have in mind here, and we are pleased to acknowledge our gratitude to him.

To be more formal and more exact about this notion, we consider a separable Hilbert space H with an abelian von Neumann algebra $\mathcal{A}$ inside of $\mathcal{B}(H)$, the algebra of all bounded operators on H. (We could dispense in part with this separability hypothesis, but it would make life unnecessarily difficult; all the examples and applications we have in mind are separable.) For example, suppose that X is a standard Borel space (see [Arveson 1976] and [Zimmer 1984, Appendix A] for definitions and properties of such spaces). It is a fact that X is isomorphic to either the unit interval $[0, 1]$ with the usual σ-field of Borel sets or is a countable set with every subset a Borel set; see [Arveson 1976] for details. Now let μ be a σ-finite measure on X and let H_n be a fixed n-dimensional Hilbert space where $n = 1, 2, \ldots, \infty$. Then $H = L^2(X, \mu, H_n)$, the set of equivalence classes of square-integrable H_n-valued functions on X, is a separable Hilbert space. The algebra $L^\infty(X, \mu)$ of equivalence classes of bounded measurable functions acts as a von Neumann algebra on H. We recall that an H_n-valued function f on X is measurable if $(f(\cdot), \xi)$ is measurable for each fixed ξ on H_n and square integrability means that $|f(\cdot)|^2$ is integrable.

This example is almost the most general such example of an abelian von Neumann algebra acting on a separable Hilbert space. Indeed, let us choose standard measure spaces (X_n, μ_n), one for each $n = 1, 2, \ldots, \infty$, with the understanding that some X_n's may be the void set and so will not contribute anything; then form

$$H^{(n)} = L^2(X_n, \mu_n, H_n)$$

as we did before and finally form the direct sum $H = \sum H^{(n)}$. The measure spaces (X_n, μ_n) may be assembled by disjoint union into a standard measure space (X, μ) and then $L^\infty(X, \mu)$, which is essentially the product of the spaces $L^\infty(X_n, \mu_n)$, acts as a von Neumann algebra on H by

$$(f \cdot \phi)_n = f|_{X_n} \cdot \phi_n,$$

where $f \in L^\infty(X, \mu)$ and $\phi = (\phi_n) \in H$. It is a standard theorem that if $\mathcal{M}$ is any abelian von Neumann algebra acting on a separable Hilbert space K, then there are (X_n, μ_n) as above and a unitary equivalence U of K with $H = \sum L^2(X_n, \mu_n, H_n)$ such that $U\mathcal{M}U^{-1} \cong L^\infty(X, \mu)$ [Dixmier 1969a, p. 117].

Thus whenever we have an abelian subalgebra $\mathcal{A}$ of $\mathcal{B}(H)$, H may be regarded by this result as a space of functions f on $X = \bigcup X_n$ with $f(x) \in H_n$ for $x \in X_n$. It is often convenient to introduce the notation $H_x = H_n$ for $x \in X_n$ so that $\{H_x\}$ may be thought of as a "field" of Hilbert spaces or a Hilbert bundle; the functions f satisfy $f(x) \in H_x$ and can be thought of as (square-integrable) sections. The notion of measurability of such a function is clear: it should be measurable on each set X_n as a function into $H_n = H_x$. What we have in fact described is the *direct integral* construction defined by the abelian subalgebra $\mathcal{A}$, and one writes

$$H = \int_X H_x \, d\mu(x)$$

as the direct integral of the spaces H_x. In the sequel we will freely think of elements f of H in this situation as vector-valued functions.

A more specific kind of example that we have in mind is described as follows: X is a connected C^∞ manifold, μ is a σ-finite measure absolutely continuous with respect to Euclidean measure on X, and $E \to X$ is a Hermitian vector bundle on X — that is, a complex vector bundle with each fibre given an Hermitian inner product which varies continuously from fibre to fibre. Denoting the fibre of E over $x \in X$ by H_x, we obtain a field of Hilbert spaces $\{H_x\}$ of constant (finite) dimension. It is easy to find a Borel trivialization of E, that is, a field of unitary isomorphisms φ_x of H_x with a fixed Hilbert space H_n so that these maps define a Borel isomorphism of the total space E of the bundle with $X \times H_n$. With H the set of square-integrable measurable sections of E, (equivalently $H = \int H_x \, d\mu(x)$ or $H = L^2(X, H_n)$), and with $\mathcal{A} = L^\infty(X, \mu)$ acting by multiplication on H, we obtain exactly the kind of abstract structure described above.

Given such a pair $H, \mathcal{A}$, we want to define what it means for an operator T on H to be locally traceable relative to $\mathcal{A}$. To motivate this, consider a one-dimensional subspace V of H and choose a unit vector φ in V. Viewing H as a direct integral of a field H_x

$$H = \int_X H_x \, d\mu(x)$$

we can think of φ as a function $\varphi(x)$ with $\varphi(x) \in H_x$ and then form $|\varphi(x)|^2$. This is an integrable function of norm one, or equivalently the measure $|\varphi(x)|^2 \, d\mu(x)$ is a probability measure which we denote $\mu_{P(V)}$. Its measure class is intrinsic to V and in particular does not depend on the choice of the measure μ used to write $\mathcal{A} = L^\infty(X, \mu)$. (Recall that μ could be replaced by any measure equivalent to μ in the sense of absolute continuity.) This measure $\mu_{P(V)}$ has μ-total mass one — the dimension of V — and can be thought of as describing how the dimension of V is "spread out over" the space X or also how the dimension of V "localizes." More generally, if V is any finite-dimensional subspace of H, let us choose an orthonormal basis $\varphi_1, \dots, \varphi_n$ for V. Then it is an elementary and well known calculation that $\sum_{i=1}^n |\varphi_i(x)|^2$ is independent of the choice of the orthonormal basis and consequently that the measure $\mu_{P(V)}$ defined by

$$d\mu_{P(V)} = \sum_{i=1}^n |\varphi_i(x)|^2 \, d\mu(x)$$

is independent of all choices. Its total mass is n, the dimension of V, and again $\mu_{P(V)}$ can be thought of as describing how the total dimension of V is distributed or localized over the space X.

In the same way we argue that if T is any finite rank operator and if $\varphi_1, \dots, \varphi_n$ is any orthonormal basis for the range of T (or for the orthogonal complement of the kernel of T), then the measure μ_T defined by

$$d\mu_T(x) = \sum_{i=1}^n ((T\varphi_i)(x), \varphi_i(x)) \, d\mu(x),$$

where the inner product is taken pointwise in H_x, is a signed measure of total mass equal to the trace of T and which again describes how this total trace is distributed over the space X. If $T = P(V)$ is the orthogonal projection onto a finite-dimensional subspace V, then this clearly coincides with the previous definition as the notation itself suggests.

With these simple examples in mind, the path of development is fairly clear and leads us to consider operators T for which a suitably defined μ_T is a σ-finite measure; or, if as in many examples X is naturally a locally compact space, then operators T for which μ_T is a Radon measure (finite on compact sets). We begin with the trace function which we view as defined on all nonnegative operators on a Hilbert space H with values in the extended positive real numbers. Denote this cone of nonnegative operators by $\mathcal{B}(H)^+$ and for $T \in \mathcal{B}(H)^+$ define $\mathrm{Tr}(T) = \sum (T\xi_i, \xi_i)$, where ξ_i is any orthonormal basis for H and where we define $\mathrm{Tr}(T)$ to be $+\infty$ if the series (of nonnegative) terms diverges. It is elementary, using the positive square root $S = T^{1/2}$ of T, to see that the sum is independent of the choice of basis. As a map from $\mathcal{B}(H)^+$ to $\bar{\mathbb{R}}^+$, Tr satisfies certain conditions (see [Dixmier 1969b, pp. 93, 81]):

(1) $\mathrm{Tr}(T_1 + T_2) = \mathrm{Tr}(T_1) + \mathrm{Tr}(T_2)$.

(2) $\mathrm{Tr}(\lambda T) = \lambda\,\mathrm{Tr}(T)$ if $\lambda \geq 0$.

(3) $\mathrm{Tr}(A^*A) = \mathrm{Tr}(AA^*)$ if $A \in \mathcal{B}(H)$.

(4) For any increasing net T_α in $\mathcal{B}(H)^+$ with $T = \mathrm{lub}\, T_\alpha$ in the sense of the order on $\mathcal{B}(H)^+$,

$$\mathrm{Tr}(T) = \mathrm{lub}\,\mathrm{Tr}(T_\alpha)$$

Such mappings defined on the positive cone in any von Neumann algebra are called *normal traces*. Condition (3) is equivalent to the condition

(3′) $\mathrm{Tr}(UTU^{-1}) = \mathrm{Tr}(T)$ for T in $\mathcal{B}(H)^+$ and U unitary.

If one drops (3) altogether such functions are called *normal weights*; in this connection see [Haagerup 1979] for a discussion of the continuity condition (4).

Suppose now that $\mathcal{A}$ is an abelian von Neumann algebra on H; then $\mathcal{A} \cong L^\infty(X, \mu)$ and for convenience we use the same symbol for a function and the corresponding operator. (We note parenthetically that for most of this $\mathcal{A}$ could be any von Neumann algebra, but as we do not have any significant applications in mind except for abelian $\mathcal{A}$ we shall not pursue this level of generality.)

Proposition 1.1. *Let $f \in \mathcal{A} \cong L^\infty(X; \mu)$ and nonnegative, and let $T \in \mathcal{B}(H)^+$. Then*

$$\mathrm{Tr}(f^{1/2}Tf^{1/2}) = \mathrm{Tr}(T^{1/2}fT^{1/2}),$$

where $f^{1/2}$ and $T^{1/2}$ are the nonnegative square roots of f and T.

Proof. Let $S = f^{1/2}T^{1/2}$; then $S^* = T^{1/2}f^{1/2}$ and the formula of the statement results immediately from the fact that $\mathrm{Tr}(AA^*) = \mathrm{Tr}(A^*A)$. □

This shows first of all that for fixed nonnegative T, the left hand side above is linear in f for f nonnegative. The continuity and additivity properties of the trace and the fact that $g \to T^{1/2}gT^{1/2}$ is order preserving and weak operator continuous show that if we define for any measurable subset E of X,

$$\mu_T(E) = \mathrm{Tr}(f_E T f_E),$$

where f_E is the characteristic function of E, then μ_T is a positive countably additive measure on X, absolutely continuous with respect to μ in that $\mu(E) = 0$ implies $\mu_T(E) = 0$. The same reasoning and an approximation argument shows that for any $f \geq 0$

$$\mathrm{Tr}(f^{1/2}Tf^{1/2}) = \int_X f \, d\mu_T.$$

The crucial problem, and this will lead us to the definition, is that μ_T may and often does fail to be σ-finite in the sense that

$$X = \bigcup_{i=1}^{\infty} X_i,$$

where the family X_i is an increasing sequence of sets of finite μ_T measure. At this point one has a choice of two closely related definitions of local traceability of T. On the one hand one could say that T is locally traceable if μ_T is σ-finite, and this is perfectly satisfactory, but for applications we want something a bit different which reflects extra structure on X. Namely suppose we are given in X an increasing family of subsets (X_i) which exhaust X. The idea is that μ_T should be not just σ-finite relative to any exhaustion of X, but that $\mu_T(X_i) < \infty$ for this particular choice of X_i. We have in mind the example of X a locally compact second countable space with X_i a countable fundamental family of compact sets. The condition above just means that μ_T is a Radon measure.

Definition 1.2. If (X_i) is an exhaustion of X by increasing Borel sets, one says that a positive operator T on H is *locally traceable* (relative to this exhaustion) if $\mu_T(X_i) < \infty$ for all i. The measure μ_T is called the *local trace* of T.

Agreeing to call a Borel subset of X *bounded* if it is contained in some X_i, we can rephrase slightly the definition of local traceability as follows: a positive operator T is locally traceable if and only if fTf is trace class for every nonnegative f in $\mathcal{A} = L^\infty(X, \mu)$ of bounded support.

It is evident from Proposition 1.1 and the continuity properties of the trace that we have the following properties for local traces which we state without proof.

Proposition 1.3. *Basic properties of the local trace*:

(1) $\mu_{T+S} = \mu_T + \mu_S$.

(2) $\mu_{\lambda T} = \lambda \mu_T$.

(3) *If* $0 \leq S \leq T$ *and* T *is locally traceable then so is* S.

(4) *If* $T(\alpha)$ *is a net converging upward to* T *then*

$$\mu_T(E) = \lim \mu_{T(\alpha)}(E)$$

for every measurable set E.

For nonpositive operators one extends the notion of local traceability using linearity.

Definition 1.4. If T is any operator on H, then T is *locally traceable* (relative to a given exhaustion of X) if we can write

$$T = \sum_{i=1}^{n} \lambda_i P_i,$$

where P_i are nonnegative locally traceable operators and λ_i are complex numbers. The *local trace* of such a T is by definition

$$\mu_T = \sum \lambda_i \mu_{P_i}.$$

This last statement requires a little explanation. First, the local trace is indeed well defined, for if T can be written in two different ways as a linear combination of positive locally traceable operators, it is easy to see using the additivity properties that μ_T comes out to be the same. Second, the measure μ_T is not quite a standard kind of object, for as a "measure" defined on all Borel subsets of X, it is all too likely to involve inadmissible expressions like $\infty - \infty$. What we have is a complex-valued measure defined on the σ-ring of all Borel sets of X which are contained in some X_i (i.e., the bounded Borel sets) for the given exhaustion and which is countably additive on the (relative) σ-field of Borel subsets of each X_i.

If an operator T is locally traceable, with local trace μ_T, then for every positive f in $\mathcal{A}$ of bounded support, $f^{1/2}Tf^{1/2}$ is a trace class operator and we have

$$\mathrm{Tr}(f^{1/2}Tf^{1/2}) = \int f \, d\mu_T,$$

where the integral on the right is well defined since f has bounded support.

We record some elementary consequences of these definitions which extend the integral formula above. For the following note that the set of complex-valued measures defined above is a (two-sided) module over $\mathcal{A} = L^\infty(X, \mu)$ by multiplication of measures by functions with the left and right actions being the same.

Proposition 1.5. *The class of locally traceable operators is closed under adjoints and is a two-sided module over $\mathscr{A}$. Moreover the local trace is a two-sided module map.*[1]

Proof. We have already seen that the locally traceable operators are closed under adjoints. To see that this class is a two-sided module over $\mathscr{A}$, it suffices, by taking linear combinations, to show that gP is locally traceable when P is nonnegative locally traceable, and $g \in \mathscr{A}$. To do this we show that the self adjoint operators $gP + Pg^*$ and $i(gP - Pg^*)$ are locally traceable. Writing $P = Q^2$ and observing that

$$R = (Q + Qg^*)^*(Q + Qg^*) = Q^2 + gQ^2 + Q^2g^* + gQ^2g^*,$$

we see that $gP + Pg^*$ is a linear combination of the positive operators P, gPg^*, and R. The first is given as locally traceable. To see that the second is also, let f be an element of bounded support in $\mathscr{A}$ and observe that $fgPg^*f = g(fPf)g^*$ is of trace class since fPf is. Hence gPg^* is locally traceable. For the third, the definition of R shows that $gP + Pg^* \leq P + gPg^*$ and hence that $R \leq 2(P + gPg^*)$. By monotonicity, R is locally traceable and it follows that $gP + Pg^*$ is locally traceable. A similar argument can be used for the imaginary part of gP, establishing that gP is locally traceable.

To see that the local trace is a bimodule map, consider an operator $S = hTk$ with T locally traceable, and h, k positive elements in $\mathscr{A}$. The local trace μ_S satisfies

$$\text{Tr}(f^{1/2}Sf^{1/2}) = \int f \, d\mu_S \tag{1.6}$$

for every positive f in $\mathscr{A}$ of bounded support, and this property characterizes μ_S since μ_S is uniquely determined by the integrals above. But now

$$\begin{aligned}\text{Tr}(f^{1/2}hTkf^{1/2}) &= \text{Tr}(h^{1/2}h^{1/2}f^{1/2}Tf^{1/2}k^{1/2}k^{1/2}) \\ &= \text{Tr}(k^{1/2}h^{1/2}f^{1/2}Tf^{1/2}k^{1/2}h^{1/2}),\end{aligned}$$

using the fact that $f^{1/2}Tf^{1/2}$ is trace class and the commutativity properties of the trace. By the definition of μ_T the last expression can be written as the integral of the nonnegative function khf, which is of bounded support, against the measure μ_T. Combining these equalities we see that

$$\text{Tr}(f^{1/2}Sf^{1/2}) = \int f \, d\mu_S = \int fhk \, d\mu_T.$$

By unicity we find

$$\mu_{hTk} = kh(\mu_T)$$

[1] In the first edition, this proposition had an additional part to it concerning the positive and negative parts of a self-adjoint operator. This second statement was false.

at least for h and k positive. By linearity this holds for all h and k and so the local trace is a bimodule map. □

We isolate as a separate statement a useful formula implicit in the preceding proof.

Corollary 1.7. *If T is locally traceable and $h, k \in \mathcal{A}$ are of bounded support, then hTk is traceable and*

$$\mathrm{Tr}(hTk) = \int hk \, d\mu_T.$$

The local trace has a further rather straightforward invariance property. Suppose that u is a unitary operator in the normalizer of the abelian algebra $\mathcal{A}$; that is, $u\mathcal{A}u^{-1} = \mathcal{A}$. Then conjugation by u defines a $*$-isomorphism of $\mathcal{A} = L^\infty(X, \mu)$ and by point realization theorems [Mackey 1962], there is a Borel automorphism θ of X such that $\theta_* \mu \sim \mu$, so that

$$ufu^{-1}(x) = f(\theta^{-1}(x)) \qquad \text{for } f \in L^\infty(X, \mu) = \mathcal{A}.$$

Recall that $\theta_* \mu(E) = \mu(\theta^{-1}(E))$ for any Borel set E. Now if (X_i) is a given exhaustion of X as introduced earlier in this section, we know what bounded sets are and we want θ to map bounded sets to bounded sets. Then the expected fact concerning this situation is true, and we omit the short proof.

Proposition 1.8. *If μ and θ are as above, and if T is a locally traceable operator with local trace μ_T, then uTu^{-1} is locally traceable with local trace $\theta_*(\mu_T)$.*

Many of the most common examples of locally traceable operators are self-adjoint projections. If $V \subset H$ is a closed subspace and $P(V)$ the orthogonal projection onto it, then we say that the subspace V is *locally finite-dimensional* if $P(V)$ is locally traceable. The local trace $\mu_{P(V)}$ is called the *local dimension* of the subspace V, and for brevity we will write it simply as μ_V.

Now let us suppose that X is a locally compact space denumerable at ∞, and let the exhaustion $\{X_i\}$ of X consist of a fundamental sequence of compact sets (every compact set K is eventually in some X_i). Further suppose that ξ is a finite dimensional Hermitian vector bundle over X and that the Hilbert space H is the space of (equivalence classes of) L^2 sections of ξ relative to some Radon measure μ on X, which without loss of generality we take to have support equal to all of X. Then it makes sense to talk about the continuous sections in H; this is the (dense) subspace C of H consisting of those equivalence classes (mod null sections) which contain a continuous section of ξ. If such a continuous section exists in a given class, it is of course unique. We make the following definition.

Definition 1.9. An operator S from H to H is *smoothing of order zero* if $S(H)$ is contained in C, the space of continuous sections.

The following result will provide large classes of interesting and important locally traceable operators — the exhaustion here is understood to be by compact subsets of X.

Theorem 1.10. *Let $S_i, i = 1, \ldots, n$ be operators on H which are smoothing of order zero. Then $T = \sum_{i=1}^{n} S_i S_i^*$ is locally traceable.*

Proof. It clearly suffices to consider one such S. If $v \in H$, then the element $S(v)$ of H lies in C and is represented by a unique continuous section $S(v)(\cdot)$. Then for fixed $x \in X$ and for a fixed vector ϕ in the dual space E_x^* of the fibre E_x of ξ at x, we can define $\phi(S(v)(x))$. By a standard argument in functional analysis using the closed graph theorem, this is a continuous linear functional $b(x, \phi)$ of v. Moreover, if $\phi(x)$ is a continuous section of the dual bundle ξ^* of ξ, it is clear that $b(x, \phi(x))$ is a continuous function of x. From all of this it follows that we can find for each $x \in X$, a measurable section $K(x, \cdot)$ of the bundle End(ξ) with $|K(x, \cdot)|$ square-integrable for each x such that

$$S(v)(x) = \int K(x, y)v(y)\, d\mu(y).$$

It is an easy matter to choose this function K to be jointly measurable in its two variables by the von Neumann selection theorem [Zimmer 1984, p. 196], and, by continuity in x, the L^2 norm of $|K(x, \cdot)|$ is bounded as x runs over compact sets. Since the Hilbert–Schmidt norm of $K(x, y)$ is at most a constant multiple of its operator norm because the fibre is finite-dimensional, the same statement holds for this norm. Thus if f is a bounded Borel function of compact support viewed both as a function and as the corresponding multiplication operator, the operator fS can be written as

$$(fS)(v)(x) = \int f(x)K(x, y)v(y)\, d\mu(y).$$

The kernel $f(x)K(x, y)$ has compact support in x and it follows from our remarks above and the Fubini theorem that the Hilbert–Schmidt norm

$$|f(x)K(x, y)|_{HS}$$

is an L^2 function on $X \times X$. This implies that fS is a Hilbert–Schmidt operator, and hence that $(fS)(fS)^* = fSS^*\bar{f}$ is a traceable operator. This means by definition that SS^* is locally traceable, and we are done. □

As an example of this theorem, consider a closed subspace V of H which consists of continuous functions. Then it follows immediately that the projection $P(V)$ onto V is locally traceable and that V is locally finite-dimensional.

By far the most important example of this for us is the following: X a C^∞ manifold which is *not* necessarily compact, ξ an Hermitian vector bundle over X, and D' a differential operator from ξ to ξ which we assume to be elliptic [Taylor 1979]. We form the space H of square-integrable sections of ξ and form the corresponding unbounded operator D on H. This is of course somewhat inexact, for one could form many such operators with different domains. The smallest such would be the closure of the operator D' acting on the space of compactly supported sections. The largest would be the Hilbert space adjoint of the formal adjoint $(D')^*$ defined on the compactly supported sections. For our purposes here D can be any closed operator between these two. (As a remark for future chapters, we note that in the specific cases to be treated later these two extreme operators defined by D' coincide—see Corollary 7.24—so there is no ambiguity about the unbounded operator D on H.) With such a D we form its kernel $V = \operatorname{Ker} D$. The elements v of V will be by definition weak solutions of the differential equation $D'v = 0$ and hence by ellipticity actually C^∞ sections. By Theorem 1.10 and the comments following it, $\operatorname{Ker} D$ is locally finite-dimensional; its local dimension, which we write μ_D, is a Radon measure on X. If D^* is the Hilbert space adjoint of D, the same considerations apply and we can form the local dimension μ_{D^*} of the kernel of D^*.

Definition 1.11. The *local index* ι_D of D is the difference

$$\iota_D = \mu_D - \mu_D^*,$$

a signed Radon measure on X.

If X is compact, then of course these are all finite measures and the total mass of ι_D, necessarily an integer, is the usual index of D. The classical Atiyah–Singer index theorem provides a formula for this in terms of topological invariants. The object of the Connes index theorem for foliations is to provide a similar formula in the following context: X a compact foliated space, D a differential operator assumed to be tangentially elliptic (see Chapter VII) so that for any leaf ℓ of the foliated space the differential operator $D|_\ell \equiv D_\ell$ will be elliptic in the usual sense and will define a local index on each leaf ℓ. The leaves ℓ are not necessarily compact and hence $\operatorname{Ker} D_\ell$ is not necessarily finite-dimensional. The theorem then provides a formula for the average of these local indices, the average being taken over all leaves. This averaging process is by no means straightforward and requires a whole subsequent chapter, Chapter IV, to explain.

The framework of locally traceable operators provides a convenient bridge to the work of Atiyah [1976] on the index theorem for covering spaces. Let X be a manifold (not necessarily compact) and let $\widetilde{X} \to X$ be a covering space with fundamental domain U and covering group Γ. Then

$$L^2(\widetilde{X}) = L^2(U) \otimes L^2(\Gamma),$$

where X is given volume measure, $\widetilde{X}$ is given the pullback measure, and Γ acts by the left regular representation. With respect to this decomposition the commutant of Γ is the von Neumann algebra

$$\widetilde{A} = \mathcal{B}(L^2(U)) \otimes \mathcal{R},$$

where $\mathcal{R}$ is the algebra corresponding to the right regular representation. There is a natural trace τ on $\widetilde{A}$ corresponding to the usual trace on $\mathcal{B}$ tensor with the canonical trace on $\mathcal{R}$. Suppose that $\widetilde{T}$ is a bounded operator on $L^2(\widetilde{X})$ which commutes with the action of Γ. Then $\widetilde{T}$ has the form

$$\widetilde{T} = \sum_{\gamma} T_\gamma \otimes R_\gamma$$

with respect to the decomposition above. Atiyah defines

$$\operatorname{ind}_\Gamma(\widetilde{T}) = \tau(f\widetilde{T}f),$$

where f is the characteristic function of U. We may simplify this to read

$$\operatorname{ind}_\Gamma(\widetilde{T}) = \text{ Trace } (fTf),$$

where $T = T_{\text{id}} \otimes I$.

Let $A = L^\infty(X)$ acting upon $L^2(\widetilde{X})$ by multiplication, and, by restriction, A acts on $L^2(U)$. Then A is isomorphic to $L^\infty_c(U)$ acting upon $L^2(U)$ by multiplication. Write $T = T_{\text{id}}$ acting upon $L^2(U)$. Then it is clear that $\operatorname{ind}_\Gamma(\widetilde{T})$ is precisely the integral of the local trace:

$$\operatorname{ind}_\Gamma(\widetilde{T}) = \int_X d\mu_T.$$

Atiyah's theorem may be understood simply as relating μ_T to the lift of μ_T to $\widetilde{X}$.

The content of Theorem 1.10 can be rephrased somewhat with no reference to topology; namely if $H = L^2(X, \mu)$ (or finite dimensional vector-valued functions) on a measure space, let T be a bounded linear transformation on H to itself such that $T(H) \subset L^\infty(X, \mu)$. That is, the image of T consists of bounded functions. Then we claim that TT^* is locally traceable and that there is a very simple formula for the local trace. Actually the same idea would work if $T(H)$ were contained in a suitably defined space of locally bounded functions too, but for simplicity let us stick to globally bounded functions.

First we observe that an application of the closed graph theorem shows that T is bounded as a map of $L^2(X)$ into $L^\infty(X)$. Further it is an easily shown fact [Dunford and Schwartz 1958, p. 499] that whenever T is a bounded linear map from a separable Banach space M into $L^\infty(X)$, there is a measurable bounded function $k(x)$ from X into the dual M^* of M such that $(\mathrm{Tm})x = k(x)(m)$ for $m \in M$. Application of this yields a bounded map $x \to k(x)$ from X to $L^2(X)$ which serves as a "kernel" for T. The following is proved in exactly the same way that Theorem 1.10 is.

Proposition 1.12. *If T maps $L^2(X,\mu)$ into $L^\infty(X,\mu)$ then TT^* is locally traceable (relative to any exhaustion by sets of finite μ-measure) and its local trace is the measure $|k(x)|^2\,d\mu(x)$, where k is as above.*

It is a standard fact that the L^2-valued measurable function can be written as $k(x)(y) = K(x,y)$ for a jointly measurable function. Then

$$(Tf)(x) = \int K(x,y)f(y)\,d\mu(y)$$

is, as we observed already, an integral kernel operator.

Because the issue will come up in the construction of operator algebras associated with groupoids and foliations, we recall briefly some sufficient conditions for a kernel $K(x,y)$ to define a bounded operator.

Definition 1.13. A kernel $K(x,y)$ on $X \times X$ is *integrable* (with respect to a measure μ on X) if

$$\operatorname*{ess\,sup}_x \int |K(x,y)|\,d\mu(y) < \infty \quad \text{and} \quad \operatorname*{ess\,sup}_y \int |K(x,y)|\,d\mu(x) < \infty.$$

One may define an operator $T = T_K$ from functions on X to functions on X formally by

$$(Tf)(x) = \int K(x,y)f(y)\,d\mu(y).$$

If $f \in L^1 \cap L^\infty$ then the integral at least makes sense and the two conditions in the definition above show immediately that $|Tf|_1$ is bounded by a constant times $|f|_1$ and that $|Tf|_\infty$ is bounded by a constant times $|f|_\infty$. It is an easy and standard interpolation result using the Riesz convexity theorem [Dunford and Schwartz 1958, p. 525] that T defines a bounded operator on each L^p to L^p for each p with a norm no worse than the larger of the two bounds in the definition.

Proposition 1.14. *If the kernel K is integrable, then $T = T_K$ defines a bounded operator on $L^2(X)$. If in addition*

$$k(x) = \left(\int |K(x,y)|^2\,dy\right)^{1/2}$$

is essentially bounded in x, then T maps $L^2(X)$ to $L^\infty(X)$ and the local trace of TT^* is $k^2(x)\,d\mu(x)$.

The ideas developed above find other interesting applications and it is our purpose in the balance of this chapter to look at some of these. Specifically, let G be a locally compact second countable abelian group. Let $H = L^2(G,\mu_G)$ with $\mathcal{A} = L^\infty(G,\mu_G)$ acting by multiplication, where μ_G is Haar measure. If E is any Borel subset of the dual group $\widehat{G}$, we construct the subspace $V(E)$ of H consisting of functions $\varphi \in H$ whose Fourier transform $\hat{\varphi}$ vanishes outside of E. We recall that if μ_G is any Haar measure on G, then there is a uniquely determined choice of Haar measure $\mu_{\widehat{G}}$ on $\widehat{G}$ with the property that the Fourier inversion formula holds exactly, not just up to a scalar, when μ_G and $\mu_{\widehat{G}}$ are used. Specifically, if

$$\hat{\varphi}(\alpha) = \int \overline{(\alpha, x)}\varphi(x)\, d\mu_G(x) \quad \text{and} \quad \hat{\psi}(x) = \int (\alpha, x)\psi(\alpha)\, d\mu_{\widehat{G}}(\alpha),$$

then $(\hat{\varphi})\hat{} = \varphi$ for suitable functions φ, where $(\cdot, \cdot)$ is the duality pairing of $\widehat{G} \times G$ to the circle group.

Let us assume that the subset E of $\widehat{G}$ has finite dual Haar measure. Then by the Fourier inversion theorem, the elements of $V(E)$ are back transforms of elements of $L^2(E) \subset L^2(\widehat{G})$. But since E has finite measure, $L^2(E) \subset L^1(E)$, and consequently the elements of $V(E)$ are back transforms of integrable functions on $\widehat{G}$. It follows that $V(E)$ consists of continuous functions and so by Theorem 1.10, $V(E)$ is locally finite-dimensional. Let μ_E be the local dimension of $V(E)$. The unitary operator u_g induced by left translation leaves $V(E)$ invariant and normalizes $\mathcal{A}$. Proposition 1.8 tells us then that μ_E is invariant under left translation by elements of G. Thus μ_E is a Haar measure; the only question is which one. This is not difficult to answer.

Proposition 1.15. *Let μ_G be a Haar measure on G, let $\mu_{\widehat{G}}$ be its dual Haar measure on $\widehat{G}$, and let E be a subset of finite measure in $\widehat{G}$. Then the local dimension of $V(E)$ is given by*

$$\mu_E = \mu_{\widehat{G}}(E)\mu_G.$$

Proof. First we observe that the answer written above does not depend on the original choice of μ_G in view of the way $\mu_{\widehat{G}}$ changes when we change μ_G. To obtain the result we note that the projection operator P_E onto $V(E)$ is given as a convolution operator with the kernel

$$K(x, y) = \int_E (xy^{-1}, \alpha)\, d\mu_{\widehat{G}}(\alpha).$$

Now for f positive, bounded and of compact support, the operator $P_E f^{1/2}$ is given by convolution with the L^2 kernel $K(x, y) f^{1/2}(y)$. Since $P_E^2 = P_E$, we have

$$f^{1/2} P_E f^{1/2} = (P_E f^{1/2})^*(P_E f^{1/2})$$

and is given as a convolution operator with kernel

$$f^{1/2}(x)K(x, y) f^{1/2}(y)$$

which is the convolution of $K(x, y) f^{1/2}(y)$ with its adjoint. Consequently we can calculate the trace of $f^{1/2} P_E f^{1/2}$ by integrating the kernel on the diagonal

$x = y$. So

$$\begin{aligned}\mathrm{Tr}(f^{1/2}P_E f^{1/2}) &= \int (f^{1/2}(x))^2 K(x,x)\, d\mu_G(x)\\ &= \int f(x) \int_E (1,\alpha)\, d\mu_{\widehat{G}}(\alpha)\, d\mu_G(x)\\ &= \int f(x)\mu_{\widehat{G}}(E)\, d\mu_G(x).\end{aligned}$$

Thus $\mu_E = \mu_{\widehat{G}}(E)\mu_G$ as desired. □

Let us continue this discussion a little further; suppose that G is a unimodular locally compact second countable group, and let π be a square-integrable irreducible representation. This means that π occurs as a summand of the left regular representation on $L^2(G)$, or that one (equivalently each) of its matrix coefficients is square-integrable. Associated to such a representation is a number d_π called the *formal degree* of π [Dixmier 1969b, 14.4], which can be defined by the equation

$$\int (\pi(g)x, y)\overline{(\pi(g)u, v)}\, d\mu_G(g) = d_\pi^{-1}(x,u)\overline{(y,v)}.$$

Of course d_π depends on the choice of Haar measure μ_G, but it is clear that the product $d_\pi \mu_G$ is intrinsic. This suggests, as we shall show in a moment, that the formal degree is not properly a number, but rather a Haar measure.

Proposition 1.16. *Let G be a unimodular group, π a square-integrable irreducible representation, and let $V(\pi)$ be any irreducible subspace of the left regular representation equivalent to π. Then $V(\pi)$ has locally finite dimension; the local dimension is a multiple of Haar measure given by*

$$\mu_\pi = d_\pi \mu_G,$$

where d_π is the usual formal degree.

Proof. It follows from the usual discussion of square-integrable representations that any subspace $V(\pi)$ can always be realized as the set of matrix coefficients $\{(\pi(g)^{-1}y, x_0)\}$, where x_0 is fixed and y varies over $H(\pi)$, the Hilbert space upon which π is realized. This demonstrates immediately that $V(\pi)$ consists of continuous functions and hence by Theorem 1.10 is locally finite-dimensional. The same argument as in the abelian case shows that the local dimension is a multiple of Haar measure. In order to compute the multiple, we realize $V(\pi)$ as the set of matrix coefficients

$$\{c_x : x \in H(\pi)\},$$

where $c_x = (\pi(g^{-1})x, x_0)$. By the orthogonality relations the square norm of c_x is $d_\pi^{-1}(x_0, x_0)(x,x)$. Normalizing x_0 by $(x_0, x_0) = d_\pi$, we see that $x \to c_x$ is an isometry. Now let $\{e_i\}$ be an orthonormal basis in $H(\pi)$ and let c_i be the corresponding vectors in $V(\pi)$. Further let V_n be the span of $(c_1, \ldots, c_n)$. By the introductory comments in the chapter, the local trace μ_n of V_n is given by

$$d\mu_n = \sum_{i=1}^{n} |c_i(g)|^2 \, d\mu_G(g).$$

As n tends to ∞, the projection onto V_n increases monotonically to the projection onto V. By (4) of Proposition 1.3, $\mu_n(E)$ increases upward to $\mu_\pi(E)$, where μ_π is the local dimension of $V(\pi)$. But $\sum_{i=1}^{n} |c_i(g)|^2$ increases monotonically to the infinite sum

$$\sum_{i=1}^{\infty} |c_i(g)|^2 = \sum_{i=1}^{\infty} |(\pi(g^{-1})e_i, x_0)|^2 = |\pi(g)x_0|^2 = d_\pi.$$

It follows that $d\mu_\pi = d_\pi \, d\mu_G$ as desired. □

If the group G is *nonunimodular* the situation becomes more complicated as one might guess from [Duflo and Moore 1976] and [Pukanszky 1971]. Suppose that π is an irreducible square-integrable representation of G. This means that π occurs as a summand of the left regular representation, but now some, but not all matrix coefficients are square-integrable. Let $P(\pi)$ be the closed linear span of all irreducible summands of $L^2(G)$ equivalent to π. Then $P(\pi)$ is also invariant under right translation and as a $G \times G$ module is isomorphic to $\pi \times \tilde{\pi}$, where $\tilde{\pi}$ is the contragredient of π [Mackey 1976]. As $\tilde{\pi}$ is also square-integrable, and as $P(\pi)$ is primary for the left and the right actions, there are, once we fix a left Haar measure on G, two canonically defined formal degree operators on $P(\pi)$, namely D_π for the left action and $\widetilde{D}_\pi$ for the right action [Mackey 1976]. Each is an unbounded positive operator affiliated to the von Neumann algebras associated to the left and right actions respectively, and semi-invariant under these actions. If we change Haar measure by a scalar factor c, then D_π and $\widetilde{D}_\pi$ change by c^{-1} so that symbolically the products $D_\pi \, d\mu_G$ and $\widetilde{D}_\pi \, d\mu_G$ are intrinsic. We recall that both the left and right von Neumann algebras are isomorphic to $\mathcal{B}(H)$, the algebra of all bounded operators, and so have canonically defined traces.

Now suppose that $V \subset P(\pi)$ is a subspace of $P(\pi)$ invariant under the right action. We would like to know when V is locally finite-dimensional and in those cases we want a formula. As before, the local dimension, if it exists, is a multiple of left Haar measure. The subspace V, being left invariant, defines a projection P_V in the right von Neumann algebra on $P(\pi)$ as these two algebras are commutants of each other. We now try to make sense out of the expression

$$(\widetilde{D}_\pi)^{1/2} P_V (\widetilde{D}_\pi)^{1/2}$$

as a bounded positive operator. In fact it will be a well-defined bounded operator precisely when the range of P_V is included in the domain of $(\tilde{D}_\pi)^{1/2}$. When this happens and when in addition this bounded positive operator has a trace, we see that P_V or V itself is *finite* relative to $\tilde{D}_\pi$. Another way to say this very much in the spirit of [Pedersen and Takesaki 1973] is to observe that $\tilde{D}_\pi$ defines a weight ψ on the von Neumann algebra of the right action given by

$$T \to \mathrm{Tr}(D_\pi^{1/2} T D_\pi^{1/2})$$

(see [Moore 1977]) and the condition on P_V is that ψ is finite on this element. Our result is the following.

Proposition 1.17. *The subspace V of $P(\pi)$ has locally finite dimension if and only if P_V is finite relative to $\tilde{D}_\pi$. The local dimension is then*

$$\mu_V = \mathrm{Tr}(\tilde{D}_\pi^{1/2} P_V \tilde{D}_\pi^{1/2}) \mu_G.$$

We omit the proof of this fact and simply remark that if G is unimodular, then D_π and $\tilde{D}_\pi$ become scalar multiples of the identity, namely $d_\pi \cdot 1$, where d_π is the usual (scalar) formal degree. Then the statement above is exactly the same as in the unimodular case. It is interesting that, contrary to the unimodular case, not all irreducible summands of $P(\pi)$ have finite local dimension, and moreover that there are irreducible subspaces of $P(\pi)$ with arbitrarily small local dimension.

These special cases suggest the form of the general result which is as follows: Let μ_G be left Haar measure on G. Then there are semifinite normal weights semi-invariant for the modular functions ψ on $\mathcal{L}$, the von Neumann algebra of the left regular representation, and $\tilde{\psi}$ and $\mathcal{R}$, the von Neumann algebra of the right regular representation. Normalize these so that Fourier transform becomes an isometry. Then if V is an invariant subspace for the left regular representation, then the projection P_V onto V is in the algebra $\mathcal{R}$ of the right regular representation.

Proposition 1.18. *The local dimension of the subspace V is finite if and only if $\tilde{\psi}(P_V) < \infty$; in this case it is given by*

$$\mu_V = \tilde{\psi}(P_V) \mu_G.$$

We again omit the proof of this result.

□ □□□□□ □□□□

Locally traceable operators have been used by John Roe [1993] as part of his work on coarse cohomology $HX^*(M)$ for open manifolds. Briefly, let H denote the Hilbert space of L^2-sections of a vector bundle over a complete Riemannian manifold M. Let A_H denote the algebra of all bounded operators with finite propagation speed (see Section VII-B), and let B_H denote the ideal of those which are locally traceable. Suppose that H is graded, $F \in A_H$ is odd with respect to the grading, and $F^2 - 1 \in B_H$. Then F is a generalized Fredholm operator and so has an index $\mathrm{Ind}(F) \in K_0(B_H)$ (as defined in Section VII-A). A generalized Dirac operator D gives rise to such an operator and we let $\mathrm{Ind}(D) = \mathrm{Ind}(F)$. For any class $\phi \in HX^{2q}(M)$, Roe uses cyclic cohomology to construct an associated complex-valued index $\mathrm{Ind}_\phi(D)$. He then establishes an index theorem of the form

$$\mathrm{Ind}_\phi(D) = \frac{q!}{(2q)!(2\pi i)^q} \langle I_D \cup c(\phi), [M] \rangle,$$

where $I_D \in H^*(M)$ is the usual index class and $c : HX^*(M) \to H_c^*(M)$ is a character map. (This is the form for M even-dimensional; there is also a theorem for odd-dimensional M.) Roe has applied this theorem in several contexts, one of which bears on the nonexistence of manifolds of positive scalar curvature.

CHAPTER II

Foliated Spaces

In this chapter we introduce the basic definitions and elementary properties of foliated spaces.

The local picture of a foliated space is a topological space of the form $L \times N$, where L is a copy of $\mathbb{R}^p$ and N is a separable metric space, not necessarily a manifold. A *tangentially smooth* function

$$f : L \times N \to \mathbb{R}$$

is a continuous function with the following properties:

(1) For each $n \in N$, the function $f(\cdot, n) : L \to \mathbb{R}$ is smooth.

(2) All partial derivatives of f in the L directions are continuous on $L \times N$.

We denote the tangentially smooth functions as $C_\tau^\infty(L \times N)$. A function

$$f : L \times N \to \mathbb{R}^k$$

is *tangentially smooth* if each of the composites $\pi_i f$ are tangentially smooth, where the π_i are the coordinate projections. Finally, if

$$U \subset L \times N \quad \text{and} \quad U' \subset L' \times N'$$

are open sets, a function $f : U \to U'$ is *tangentially smooth* if locally it has the form

$$f(t, n) = \big(f_1(t, n),\ f_2(n) \big),$$

with $f_2 : N \to N'$ continuous and $f_1 : L \times N \to L'$ tangentially smooth.

Let X be a separable metrizable space. A *foliated chart* (U, φ) is an open set $U \subseteq X$ and a homeomorphism

$$\varphi : U \longrightarrow \varphi(U) \subseteq L \times N.$$

with $\varphi(U)$ open in $L \times N$. We define $C_\tau^\infty(U)$ as the set of all functions $f : U \to \mathbb{R}$ such that $\varphi^{-1} f \in C_\tau^\infty(L \times N)$. A *plaque* P of X is a set of the form $\varphi^{-1}(L \times \{n\})$. It is evident that U is the union of its plaques and that each plaque has a natural structure as a smooth manifold of dimension p. So U is foliated by its plaques.

Two foliated charts (U, φ) and (V, ψ) of X are *coherently foliated* if for every choice of plaques $P \subset U$ and $Q \subset V$, the set $P \cap Q$ is open both in P and in

Q. A *foliated atlas* is a collection $\mathcal{U} = \{(U_\alpha, \varphi_\alpha)\}$ of mutually coherent foliated charts of X of the same dimension p such that $\{U_\alpha\}$ is an open cover of X.

Two foliated atlases are equivalent if their union is a foliated atlas. Each equivalence class of foliated atlases of X determines a foliated space structure on X as follows. Using [Candel and Conlon 2000, Lemma 11.2.9], we may assume without loss of generality that our atlas $\mathcal{U}$ is *regular*; that is:

(1) Given a foliated chart $(U, \varphi) \in \mathcal{U}$, there exists a foliated chart $(V, \psi) \in \mathcal{U}$ with $U \subseteq \overline{T} \subseteq V$, $\overline{T}$ compact in V, and $\psi|_U = \varphi$. (Thus we can take the closure of a plaque and stay within some other overlapping plaque.)

(2) The open cover $\{U_\alpha\}$ is locally finite.

(3) Given foliated charts (U, φ) and (V, ψ) and plaque $P \subset U$, then P meets at most one plaque in $\overline{V}$.

Fix a regular foliated atlas. A *plaque path* $P_1, \ldots P_k$ is a collection of plaques of X such that $P_i \cap P_{i+1} \neq \varnothing$ for all i. Now fix one plaque P and take the union of all of the plaques that can be reached from P by plaque paths. This will be a topological manifold ℓ of dimension p called a *leaf*. It is clear that X is foliated by leaves. This is not enough, however. We want our leaves to be smooth manifolds. Here is how to do it.

Definition 2.1. A *foliated space* X of dimension p is a separable metrizable space equipped with a regular foliated atlas $\mathcal{U} = \{(U_\alpha, \varphi_\alpha)\}$ such that whenever $U_\alpha \cap U_\beta \neq \varnothing$ then the composition

$$\varphi_\alpha(U_\alpha \cap U_\beta) \xrightarrow{\varphi_\alpha^{-1}} U_\alpha \cap U_\beta \xrightarrow{\varphi_\beta} \varphi_\beta(U_\alpha \cap U_\beta)$$

is tangentially smooth. A *tangentially smooth* function $f : X_1 \to X_2$ of foliated spaces is a continuous function such that if $U_i \subset X_i$ are foliated charts with associated maps

$$\varphi_i : U_i \longrightarrow L_i \times N_i,$$

then the composition

$$\varphi_1(U_1 \cap f^{-1}(U_2)) \xrightarrow{\varphi_1^{-1}} U_1 \cap f^{-1}(U_2) \xrightarrow{f} f(U_1) \cap U_2 \xrightarrow{\varphi_2} L_2 \times N_2$$

is tangentially smooth. We let $C_\tau^\infty(X_1, X_2)$ denote the space of tangentially smooth maps $X_1 \to X_2$.

If X_2 is a smooth manifold foliated as one leaf, then the condition reduces to showing that for any foliated chart

$$\varphi : U \longrightarrow L \times N,$$

the composite $f\varphi^{-1}$ is tangentially smooth. In particular, we may take $X_2 = \mathbb{R}$ or $\mathbb{C}$ and let $C_\tau^\infty(X)$ to denote the set of tangentially smooth (real or complex-valued) functions on the foliated space X. Note that $C_\tau^\infty(X)$ is a commutative algebra, unital if X is compact, and normed by the sup norm. It is almost never complete in that norm. If X is a smooth manifold regarded as a foliation with one leaf, then

$$C_\tau^\infty(X) \cong C^\infty(X).$$

Since coordinate changes smoothly transform the level surface $n =$ constant to $n' =$ constant, the level surfaces coalesce to form maximal connected sets called *leaves*, and the space X is foliated by these leaves. Each leaf ℓ is a smooth manifold of dimension p.

The main examples of foliated spaces are, of course, foliated manifolds [Lawson 1977; Candel and Conlon 2000] of class C^∞ or of class $C^{\infty,0}$ as in [Connes 1979]. We pause to exhibit some standard examples of foliated manifolds. Our reference is [Lawson 1977], upon whom we have relied heavily.[1] We encourage the reader interested in a deeper and elegant treatment of foliations themselves to read these books.

The simplest example of a foliated manifold is just $M = L^p \times B^q$, where L and B are smooth manifolds and M is foliated with leaves of the form $L \times \{b\}$. The projection map $f : M \to B$ is a *submersion* (i.e., $df_x : TM_x \to TB_x$ is surjective for all x).

More generally, if $f : M^{p+q} \to B^q$ is any submersion then M has a p-dimensional foliation with leaves corresponding to connected components of some $f^{-1}(b)$. If

$$F^p \to M^{p+q} \to B^q$$

is a fibre bundle in the category of smooth manifolds with F and B connected then M^{p+q} is foliated by the inverse images $F_b \equiv f^{-1}(b) \cong F$. For instance, the Hopf fibration

$$S^1 \to S^3 \to S^2$$

and a closed connected subgroup H of a Lie group G

$$H \to G \to G/H$$

yield foliations of S^3 and of G respectively.

A different sort of example arises by taking a connected Lie group G acting smoothly on a manifold M. Assume that the isotropy group at x, $\{g \in G \mid gx = x\}$, has dimension independent of x. Then M is foliated by the orbits of G. (If

[1] In the first edition we relied upon [Lawson 1977] as a basic reference for foliations, and this is still a valuable source. The more recent books [Candel and Conlon 2000; 2003] give an extensive and thorough treatment of the geometric and topological structure of foliated manifolds and foliated spaces. The books and their authors have been very helpful to us in the preparation of the second edition. There is a symbiotic aspect to this, as our introduction of the concept of foliated space in the first edition had some impact on the direction of some of the research there.

H acts on G for H a closed connected subgroup then this coincides with the previous example.)

Foliations may also be described in terms of the foliation bundle FM. Let $M = T^2 = \mathbb{R}^2/\mathbb{Z}^2$ and fix a smooth one-form

$$\omega = a_1 dx_1 + a_2 dx_2$$

with $a_1 a_2 \neq 0$. It is evident that $d\omega = 0$. Let

$$FM = \{v \in TM \mid \omega(v) = 0\}.$$

This is an involutive subbundle and hence foliates the torus. If $a_1/a_2 \in \mathbb{Q}$ then each leaf is a circle. If $a_1/a_2 \notin \mathbb{Q}$ then each leaf is dense, in fact a copy of $\mathbb{R}$ sitting densely in the torus, which corresponds to an irrational flow on the torus.

Next we construct bundles with discrete structural group. Let F be a space, let B^p be a manifold (connected for simplicity), and let $\widetilde{B} \to B$ denote the universal cover. Suppose given a homomorphism $\varphi : \pi_1(B) \to \text{Homeo}(F)$. Form the space

(2.2) $$M = \widetilde{B} \times_{\pi_1(B)} F$$

as a quotient of $\widetilde{B} \times F$ by the action of $\pi_1(B)$ determined by deck transformations on $\widetilde{B}$ and by φ on F. The action on $\widetilde{B} \times F$ is free and properly discontinuous, hence M is a foliated space. It is foliated by leaves ℓ_x which are the images of $\widetilde{B} \times \{x\}$ as $x \in F$. There is a natural map $M \to B$ and the composite $\ell_x \to M \to B$ is a covering space. If F is a manifold and φ takes values in $\text{Diff}(F)$ then M is a smooth manifold.

A very special case of the above construction is of considerable importance. Suppose given a single homeomorphism $\theta \in \text{Homeo}(F)$. Then $\pi_1(S^1) = \mathbb{Z}$ acts on Homeo (F) via θ and there results a bundle

(2.3) $$M = \mathbb{R} \times_{\mathbb{Z}} F \to S^1$$

called the *suspension* of the homeomorphism θ. For instance, if $\theta \in \text{Diff}(\mathbb{R})$ is the map $\theta(y) = -y$ then $\mathbb{R} \times \mathbb{R}$ has a $\mathbb{Z}$-action given by $(x, y) \mapsto (x+1, -y)$ and $M = \mathbb{R} \times_{\mathbb{Z}} \mathbb{R}$ is the Möbius strip.

(2.4)

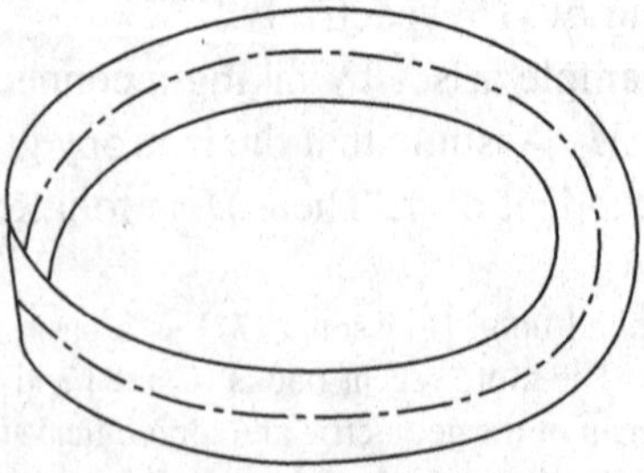

Each leaf ℓ_y is a circle wrapping around twice except for the core circle ℓ_0 (corresponding to $\mathbb{R} \times \{0\}$) which wraps once.

Finally we describe the Reeb foliation of S^3. This is constructed in stages. First foliate the open strip $\mathbb{R} \times [-1, 1]$ as shown:

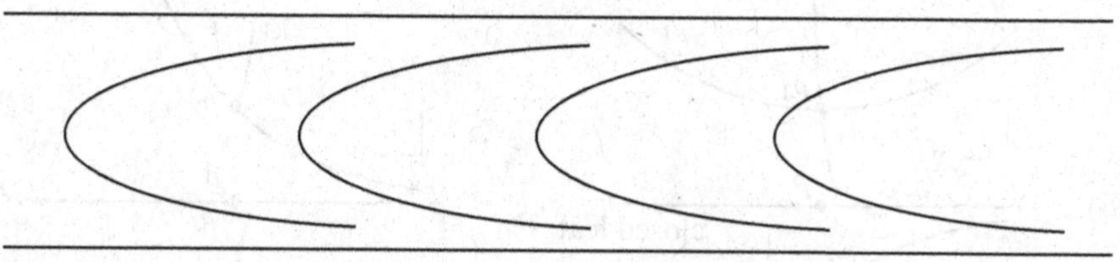

Then spin the strip about the x-axis to obtain a solid infinite cylinder (thought of as a collection of snakes, each eating the tail of the next):

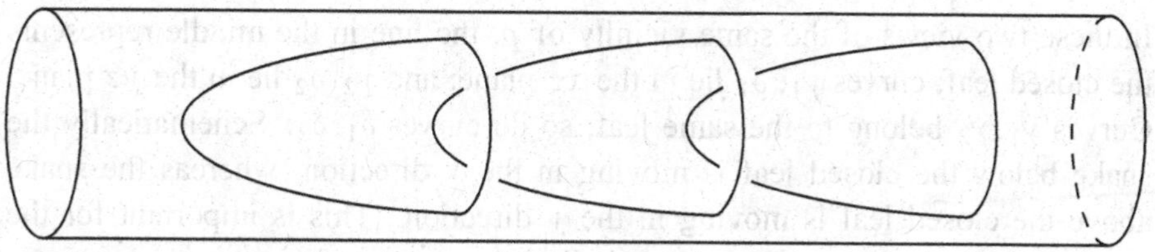

Next identify (x, y, z) with $(x+1, y, z)$ to obtain a solid torus foliated by copies of $\mathbb{R}^2$ and the boundary leaf, which is of course the torus.

(2.5)

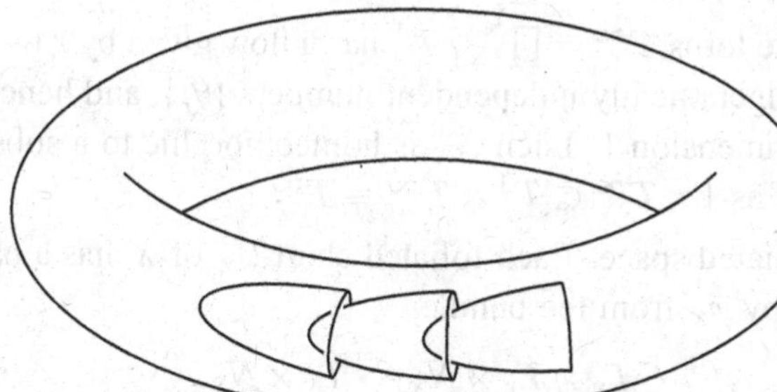

(This is to be thought of as a collection of snakes, each eating its own tail.) Finally, S^3 may be obtained by gluing two copies of a solid torus along the boundary torus. Taking two copies of the solid torus above, one obtains S^3 foliated by leaves of dimension two. Along the boundary of the two solid tori there is a closed leaf diffeomorphic to T^2. All other leaves are copies of $\mathbb{R}^2$. No leaf is dense: the closure of a typical copy of $\mathbb{R}^2$ is $\mathbb{R}^2$ together with the closed leaf T^2. Note that each point p on the closed leaf is a sort of saddle point in the sense that curves in leaves nearby (above and below) have the property illustrated schematically here:

(2.6)

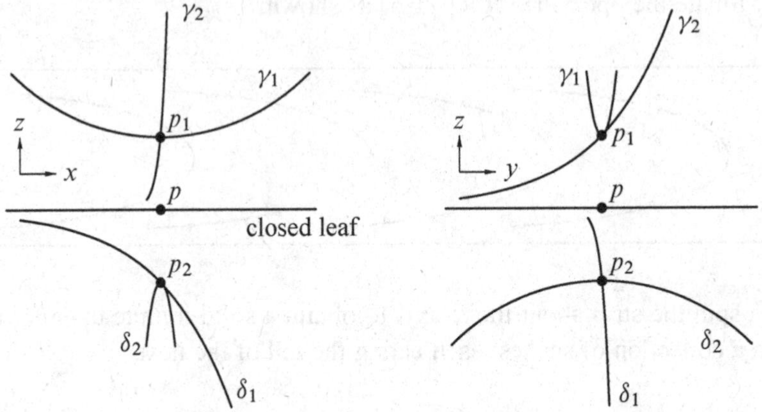

In these two views of the same vicinity of p, the line in the middle represents the closed leaf; curves γ_1, δ_1 lie in the xz plane; and γ_2, δ_2 lie in the yz plane. Curves γ_1, γ_2 belong to the same leaf; so do curves δ_1, δ_2. Schematically the snake below the closed leaf is moving in the x direction, whereas the snake above the closed leaf is moving in the y direction. This is important for the resulting holonomy property, as we shall see.

The notion of foliated space is strictly more general than that of a foliated manifold. Here are two examples:

(1) A solenoid is a foliated space ($p = 1$) with each N_x homeomorphic to a subspace of a Cantor set.

(2) The infinite torus $T^\infty = \prod_{j=1}^\infty T^1$ has a flow given by $r \mapsto \lambda_0 + \prod e^{ir\theta_j}$ for fixed algebraically independent numbers $\{\theta_j\}$, and hence is a foliated space of dimension 1. Each N_x is homeomorphic to a subspace of T^∞, thought of as $1 \times T^\infty \subset T^1 \times T^\infty \equiv T^\infty$.

Let X be a foliated space. Each foliated chart U_x of X has a natural tangent bundle, induced by φ_x from the bundle

$$T_x \times T_x \times N_x \to T_x \times N_x.$$

The transition functions $\{\varphi_x\}$ preserve smoothness in the leaf direction and hence these coalesce to form a p-plane bundle over X, called the *tangent bundle* or foliation bundle of the foliated space and denoted $p : FX \to X$. We frequently write $F = FX$ and also write $FX_x \equiv F_x = p^{-1}(x)$ for the fibre over $x \in X$.

Proposition 2.7. (a) *A tangentially smooth map $f : X \to Y$ induces a bundle map $df : FX \to FY$ which over leaves corresponds to the usual differential.*

(b) *Let X^δ denote the disjoint union of the leaves of X (each leaf having its smooth manifold topology). Then X^δ is a (usually nonseparable) smooth* *manifold of dimension p, the identity map* $i : X^\delta \to X$ *is tangentially smooth, and* $i^* FX = T(X^\delta)$, *the tangent bundle of* X^δ.

A vector bundle $\pi : E \to X$ of (real) dimension k over a foliated space X of dimension p is *tangentially smooth* if E has the structure of a foliated space of dimension $p+k$ which is compatible with the local product structure of the bundle and if the map $\pi : E \to X$ is tangentially smooth. The tangent bundle is tangentially smooth. We let $\Gamma_\tau(E)$ or $\Gamma_\tau(X, E)$ denote the $C_\tau^\infty(X)$-module of tangentially smooth sections of the bundle $E \to X$.

The following series of properties (2.8–2.15) serves to let us assume freely that all bundles which arise in our study are tangentially smooth. Tranverse continuity is essential here; Proposition 2.8 is false if one assumes only transverse measurability.

Proposition 2.8. *Every open cover of a foliated space X has a subordinate tangentially smooth partition of unity.*

Proof. (Compare [Hirsch 1976, 2.2.1].) Let $\mathcal{U} = \{U_i\}_{i \in I}$ be an open cover of X. There is a locally finite atlas on X, say $\mathcal{V} = \{\varphi_\alpha, V_\alpha\}$, such that $\{\overline{V}_\alpha\}$ refines $\mathcal{U}$; and we may assume that each image

$$\varphi_\alpha(V_\alpha) \subset T_\alpha \times N_\alpha \subset \mathbb{R}^p \times N_\alpha$$

is bounded and each $\overline{V}_\alpha \subset \overline{X}$ is compact. There is a shrinking $\{W_\alpha\}_{\alpha \in J}$ of $\mathcal{V}$, and each $\overline{W}_\alpha \subset V_\alpha$ is compact. It suffices to find a tangentially smooth partition of unity subordinate to $\mathcal{V}$.

For each α, cover the compact set $\varphi_\alpha(\overline{W}_\alpha) \subset \mathbb{R}^p \times N_\alpha$ by a finite number of closed balls

$$B(\alpha, 1), \ldots, B(\alpha, k(\alpha))$$

contained in $\varphi_\alpha(V_\alpha)$. Choose tangentially smooth maps

$$h_{\alpha,j} \in C_\tau^\infty(\mathbb{R}^p \times N_\alpha)$$

with $0 \le h_{\alpha,j}(x,n) \le 1$ and such that

$$h_{\alpha,j}(x) > 0 \quad \text{if and only if} \quad x \in \operatorname{Int} B(\alpha, j).$$

Let

$$h_\alpha = \sum_{j=1}^{k(a)} h_{\alpha,j} : \mathbb{R}^p \times N_\alpha \to [0, \infty).$$

Then

$$\begin{aligned} h_\alpha(x) > 0 &\quad \text{if } x \in \varphi_\alpha(\overline{W}_\alpha), \\ h_\alpha(x) = 0 &\quad \text{if } x \in \mathbb{R}^p \times N_\alpha - \textstyle\bigcup_j B(\alpha, j). \end{aligned}$$

Let $m_\alpha : M \to [0,\infty)$ be defined by

$$m_\alpha(x) = \begin{cases} h_\alpha \varphi_\alpha(x) & \text{if } x \in V_\alpha, \\ 0 & \text{if } x \in X - V_\alpha. \end{cases}$$

Then m_α is tangentially smooth, $m_\alpha > 0$ on $\overline{W}_\alpha$, and $\operatorname{supp} m_\alpha \subset V_\alpha$. Define $r_\alpha = m_\alpha / \sum_\alpha m_\alpha$. Then the $\{r_\alpha\}$ form a tangentially smooth partition of unity subordinate to $\mathcal{V}$. □

For foliated spaces X and Y, let $C^0_\ell(X,Y)$ denote the continuous functions from X to Y taking leaves to leaves and let $C^\infty_\tau(X,Y)$ denote the subset of tangentially smooth maps. We topologize $C^0_\ell(X,Y)$ by the strong topology as follows. Let $\Phi = \{\varphi_i, U_i\}_{i\in\Lambda}$ and $\Psi = \{\psi_i, V_i\}_{i\in I}$ be locally finite sets of charts on X and Y respectively. Let $\mathcal{K} = \{K_i\}_{i\in I}$ be a family of compact subsets of X, with $K_i \subset U_i$, let $\mathcal{E} = \{\epsilon_i\}_{i\in I}$ a family of positive numbers, and let $f \in C^0_\ell(X,Y)$ with $f(K_i) \subset V_i$. A *strong basic neighborhood* $N^0(f;\Phi,\Psi,\mathcal{K},\mathcal{E})$ is the set of maps $g \in C^0_\ell(X,Y)$ such that $g(K_i) \subset V_i$ for all $i \in I$ and

$$\left\| (\psi_i f \varphi_i^{-1})(x) - (\psi_i g \varphi_i^{-1})(x) \right\| < \epsilon_i \qquad \text{for all } x \in \varphi_i(K_i).$$

The strong topology has all possible sets of this form for a base. If X is compact then this topology coincides with the weak (= compact-open) topology on $C^0_\ell(X,Y)$. We refer the reader to [Hirsch 1976], from which we have freely borrowed.

Proposition 2.9. *Let $X = T \times N$ and $X' = T' \times N'$ be trivial foliated spaces (with $T \subset R^p$, $T' \subset R^{p'}$). Then $C^\infty_\tau(X,X')$ is dense in $C^0_\ell(X,X')$.*

Proof. Since all functions preserve leaves we may assume that $X' = T' = \mathbb{R}^n$, regarded as a foliated space with one leaf. We must show that $C^\infty_\tau(X,\mathbb{R}^n)$ is dense in $C^0(X,\mathbb{R}^n)$ in the strong topology.

Let $\{V_\alpha\}$ be a locally finite open cover of X and for each α let $\epsilon_\alpha > 0$. Let $f : X \to \mathbb{R}^n$ be continuous, and suppose we want a C^∞_τ map g to satisfy $|f - g| < \epsilon_\alpha$ on V_α for all α. For each $x \in X$, let $W_x \subset X$ be a neighborhood of x meeting only finitely many V_α. Set

$$\delta_x = \min\{\epsilon_\alpha : x \in V_\alpha\} > 0.$$

Let $U_x \subset W_x$ be an open neighborhood of x so small that

$$|f(y) - f(x)| < \delta_x \qquad \text{for all } y \in U_x.$$

Define constant maps $g_x : U_x \to \mathbb{R}^n$ by $g_x(y) = f(x)$. Relabeling the cover $\{U_x\}$ and the maps $\{g_x\}$, we have shown that there is an open cover $\{U_i\}_{i\in I} = \mathcal{U}$ of X and C^∞_τ maps $g_i : X \to \mathbb{R}^n$ such that

$$|g_i(y) - f(y)| < \epsilon_\alpha \qquad \text{whenever } y \in U_i \cap V_\alpha.$$

Let $\{r_i\}_{i\in I}$ be a C^∞_τ partition of unity subordinate to $\mathcal{U}$. Define $g : X \to \mathbb{R}^n$ by

$$g(y) = \sum_i r_i(y) g_i(y).$$

Then $g \in C^\infty_\tau(X, \mathbb{R}^n)$, and

$$|g(y) - f(y)| = \left|\sum r_i(y)g_i(y) - \sum r_i(y) f(y)\right| \leq \sum r_i(y)\,|g_i(y) - f(y)|.$$

Hence $y \in V_\alpha$ implies $|g(y) - f(y)| < \sum r_i(y)\epsilon_\alpha = \epsilon_\alpha$. □

The following relative approximation lemma allows us to globalize the preceeding proposition.

Lemma 2.10. *Let $U = L \times N \subset \mathbb{R}^p \times N$ and $V = L' \times N' \subset \mathbb{R}^{p'} \times N'$ be open sets, $K \subset U$ a closed set, $W \subset U$ an open set, and let $f \in C^0_\ell(U, V)$ be tangentially smooth on a neighborhood of $K - W$. Then every neighborhood N of f in $C^0_\ell(U, V)$ contains a map $h : U \to V$ which is tangentially smooth on a neighborhood of K and agrees with f on $U - W$.*

Proof. Since all maps send leaves to leaves and since $C^0(U, L')$ is open in $C^0(U, \mathbb{R}^p)$ we may assume that $V = L' = \mathbb{R}^n$. Let $A \subset U$ be an open set containing the set $K - W$ such that $f|A$ is C^∞_τ. Let $W_0 \subset U$ be open with

$$K - A \subset W_0 \subset \overline{W}_0 \subset W.$$

Let $\{r_0, r_1\}$ be a C^∞_τ partition of unity for the open cover $\{W, U - \overline{W}_0\}$ of U. Define

$$G : C^0(U, \mathbb{R}^n) \to C^0(U, \mathbb{R}^n)$$

by

$$G(g)(x) = r_0(x)g(x) + r_1(x) f(x).$$

Then

$$G(g)|_{W_0} = g|_{W_0}$$

and

$$G(g)|_{U-W} = f|_{U-W}.$$

Further, $G(g)$ is C^∞_τ on every open set on which both f and g are C^∞_τ, and G is clearly continuous.

Since $G(f) = f$, there is an open set $N_0 \subset C^0(U, \mathbb{R}^n)$ containing f such that $G(N_0) \subset N$. By Proposition 2.9 there is a C^∞_τ map $g \in N_0$ (since $C^\infty_\tau(U, \mathbb{R}^n)$ is dense in $C^0(U, \mathbb{R}^n)$). Then $h = G(g)$ has the required properties. □

We now prove the basic approximation theorem.

Theorem 2.11. *Let X and Y be foliated spaces. Then $C^\infty_\tau(X, Y)$ is dense in $C^0_\ell(X, Y)$ with the strong topology.*

Corollary 2.12. *Let X be a foliated space and M a C^∞ manifold, regarded as a foliated space with one leaf. Then $C^\infty_\tau(X, M)$ is dense in $C^0(X, M)$.*

Proof. Let $f : X \to Y$ be in C^0_ℓ. Let $\Phi = \{\varphi_i, U_i\}_{i \in I}$ be a locally finite atlas for X and let $\Psi = \{\psi_i, V_i\}_{i \in I}$ be a family of charts for Y such that for all $i \in I$, $f(U_i) \subset V_i$. Let $\mathscr{C} = \{C_i\}_{i \in I}$ be a closed cover of X, $C_i \subset U_i$. Let $\mathscr{E} = \{\mathscr{E}_i\}$ be a family of positive numbers and put $N = N(f; \Phi, \psi, \mathscr{C}, \mathscr{E}) \subset C^0_\ell(X, Y)$. We look for a $g \in N$ which is C^∞_τ. The set I is countable; we therefore assume that $I = \{1, 2, 3, \dots\}$ or, if X is compact, $I = \{1, 2, \dots, s\}$.

Let $\{W_i\}_{i \in I}$ be a family of open sets in X such that

$$C_i \subset W_i \subset \overline{W}_i \subset U_i.$$

We shall define by induction a family of C^∞_τ maps $g_k \in N$ having the following properties: $g_0 = f$ and, for $k \geq 1$, the maps g_k and g_{k-1} coincide on $X - W_k$ and g_k is C^∞_τ on a neighborhood of $\bigcup_{0 \leq j \leq k} C_j$.

Assuming for the moment that the g_k exist, define $g : X \to Y$ by $g(x) = g_{\kappa(x)}(x)$, where $\kappa(x) = \max\{k \mid x \in \overline{T}_k\}$. Each x has a neighborhood on which $g = g_{\kappa(x)}$. This shows that $g \in C^\infty_\tau$ and $g \in N$, and the theorem is proved.

It remains to construct the g_k. Put $g_0 = f$; then the hypotheses are true vacuously. Suppose that $0 < m$ and we have maps $g_k \in N, 0 \leq k < m$, satisfying the inductive hypothesis. Define a space of maps

$$\mathscr{G} = \{h \in C^0_\ell(U_m, V_m) \mid h = g_{m-1} \text{ on } U_m - W_m\}.$$

Define $T : \mathscr{G} \to C^0_\ell(X, Y)$ by

$$T(h) = \begin{cases} h & \text{on } U_m, \\ g_{m-1} & \text{on } X - U_m. \end{cases}$$

It is evident that T is continuous, $T(g_{m-1}|_{U_m}) = g_{m-1}$, and hence $T^{-1}(N)$ is nonempty.

Form the closed subset $K = \bigcup_{k \leq m} C_k \cap U_m$ of U_m. Then $g_{m-1} : U_m \to V_m$ is C^∞_τ on a neighborhood of $K - W_m$. Since U_m and V_m are trivially foliated spaces we can apply the previous proposition to $C^0_\ell(U_m, V_m)$. We conclude that the maps in $\mathscr{G}$ which are C^∞_τ in a neighborhood of K are dense in $\mathscr{G}$. Therefore $T^{-1}(N)$ contains such a map h. Define $g_m = T(h)$; then $g_m \in N$ satisfies the inductive hypothesis at stage m, completing the proof. □

Theorem 2.13 (Relative Approximation Theorem). *Let $f \in C^0_\ell(X, Y)$ and suppose f is tangentially smooth on some neighborhood of a (possibly empty) closed set $A \subset X$. Then every neighborhood N of f in $C^0_\ell(X, Y)$ contains a map $h \in C^\infty_\tau(X, Y)$ with $h = f$ on some neighborhood of A.*

Proof. If X and Y are product foliations this follows from the relative approximation Lemma 2.10. The local-global process is much the same as in the proof of Theorem 2.11, where we show that $C^\infty_\tau(X, Y)$ is dense in $C^0_\ell(X, Y)$. In the construction of the maps $\{g_k\}$, add the additional condition that $g_k = f$ on A. In the induction assume that every map in $\mathscr{G}$ agrees with f on some neighborhood of A. The relative approximation Lemma 2.10 allows the same argument to proceed. □

Lemma 2.14. *Let $f \in C_\ell^0(X, \mathbb{R}^p \times N)$, let A be a closed subset of X, and suppose that f is tangentially smooth on some neighborhood of A. Then there is a homotopy $H \in C_\ell^0(X \times \mathbb{R}, \mathbb{R}^p \times N)$ with the following properties:*

(1)
$$H(x,t) = \begin{cases} f(x) & \text{for } t \le 0, \\ H(x,1) & \text{for } t > 1, \\ f(x) & \text{for } x \in A. \end{cases}$$

(2) $H(x,1) \in C_\tau^\infty(X, \mathbb{R}^p \times N)$.

(3) *For each t, $H(\cdot\,, t)$ is arbitrarily close to f on compact subsets.*

Proof. Write $f(x) = (f_1(x), f_2(x))$. By the preceding theorem, there exists a map $g \in C_\tau^\infty(X, \mathbb{R}^p \times N)$ with $g = f$ on some neighborhood of A and g arbitrarily close to f. We may assume that $g = (g_1, f_2)$. Let $\delta \in C^\infty(\mathbb{R}, \mathbb{R})$ be a monotone function with $\delta(t) = 0$ for $t \le 0$ and $\delta(t) = 1$ for $t \ge 1$. Define $H : X \times \mathbb{R} \to \mathbb{R}^p \times N$ by

$$H(x,t) = \big(f_1(x)(1 - \delta(t)) + g(x)\delta(t), f_2(x)\big).$$

Then H has the required properties. □

Theorem 2.15. *Let $f \in C_\ell^0(X, Y)$ and suppose that f is tangentially smooth on some neighborhood of a closed subset A. Then there is a homotopy $H \in C_\ell^0(X \times \mathbb{R}, Y)$ satisfying the following properties:*

(1)
$$H(x,t) = \begin{cases} f(x) & \text{for } t \le 0, \\ H(x,1) & \text{for } t \ge 1, \\ f(x) & \text{for } x \in A. \end{cases}$$

(2) $g = H(x,1) \in C_\tau^\infty(X, Y)$.

(3) *$H(\cdot\,, t)$ is arbitrarily close to f on compact subsets.*

The function $g \in C_\tau^\infty(X, Y)$ is unique up to tangentially smooth homotopy ($rel\, A$) and hence defines a unique map $f^* : H_\tau^*(Y) \to H_\tau^*(X)$. (Here H_τ^* is tangential cohomology, which will be formally introduced in Chapter III.)

Proof. Let $\Psi = \{V_i\}$ be a family of coordinate patches for Y and let $\Phi = \{U_i\}$ be a family of coordinate patches for X with $f^{-1}(V_i) \subset U_i$. Let $\mathscr{C} = \{C_i\}$ be a closed cover of X with $C_i \subset U_i$. Let $\mathscr{E} = \{\mathscr{E}_i\}$ be a family of positive numbers, and let

$$N = (f\pi, \Psi \times \mathbb{R}, \Psi \times \mathbb{R}, \mathscr{C}, \mathscr{E}) \subset C_\ell^0(X \times \mathbb{R}, Y),$$

where $\pi : X \times \mathbb{R} \to X$ is the projection and $\Phi \times \mathbb{R}$ is the pullback along π of Φ. Choose open sets W_i with $C_i \subset W_i \subset \overline{W}_i \subset U_i$.

We shall define a family of maps $g_k \in C^0_\ell(X \times \mathbb{R}, Y)$ with the following properties:

(1) $$g_k(x,t) = \begin{cases} f(x) & \text{for } t \leq 0, \\ g_k(x,1) & \text{for } t \geq 1, \\ f(x) & \text{for } x \in A. \end{cases}$$

(2) $g_k(x,1)$ is tangentially smooth on a neighborhood of

$$(L_1 \cup \cdots \cup L_k) \times [1, \infty).$$

(3) $g_k(\cdot, t)$ is close to f on compact subsets.

(4) $g_0(x,t) = f(x)$.

(5) $g_k = g_{k-1}$ on $(X \times \mathbb{R}) - (W_k \times \mathbb{R})$.

Suppose for the moment that the g_k exist. Define $H : X \times \mathbb{R} \to Y$ by

$$H(x,t) = g_{\kappa(x)}(x,t),$$

where $\kappa(x) = \max\{k \mid x \in \overline{T}_k\}$. Each point (x,t) has a neighborhood on which $H(x,t) = g_{\kappa(x)}(x,t)$. Thus $H(x,1) \in C^\infty_\tau(X, Y)$. The other conditions on H are evident, so H has been constructed as required.

Here is the construction of the g_k, by induction. Set $g_0(x,t) = f(x)$. Suppose that $m > 0$ and we have maps $g_k \in N$ with $0 \leq k < m$ satisfying the inductive hypotheses. Define a space of maps $\mathcal{G}$ by

$$\mathcal{G} = \{h \in C^0_\ell(U_m \times \mathbb{R}, V_m) \mid h = g_{m-1} \text{ on } (U_m - W_m) \times \mathbb{R} \text{ and } h = f \text{ on a neighborhood of } (U_m \cap A) \times \mathbb{R}\}.$$

Define $T : \mathcal{G} \to C^0_\ell(X \times \mathbb{R}, Y)$ by

$$T(h) = \begin{cases} h & \text{on } U_m \times \mathbb{R}, \\ g_{m-1} & \text{on } (X - U_m) \times \mathbb{R}. \end{cases}$$

Clearly T is continuous and $T(g_{m-1}|U_m) = g_{m-1}$, so $T^{-1}(N)$ is nonempty.

Let $K = \bigcup_{k \leq m}(C_k \cap U_m) \times \mathbb{R}$. Then K is a closed subset of $U_m \times \mathbb{R}$ and $g_{m-1} \in C^0_\ell(U_m \times \mathbb{R}, V_m)$ is tangentially smooth on a neighborhood of $K \times (W_m \times \mathbb{R})$. Since $U_m \times \mathbb{R}$ and V_m are product foliated spaces, we may apply the previous proposition to $C^0_\ell(U_m \times \mathbb{R}, V_m)$. We conclude that the maps in $\mathcal{G}$ which are tangentially smooth on some neighborhood of K are dense in $\mathcal{G}$. Therefore $T^{-1}(N)$ contains such a map h. Define $g_m = T(h)$. Then $g_m \in N$ satisfies the inductive hypotheses at stage m. This completes the proof of the existence of the homotopy H.

It remains to demonstrate that $g = H(\cdot, 1)$ is unique up to tangentially smooth homotopy which fixes A. Suppose that g and $\bar{g}$ are both constructed by the above procedure with $g = H(\cdot,1)$ and $\bar{g} = \overline{H}(\cdot,1)$ and $g = \bar{g}$ on A. An obvious construction yields a homotopy $M \in C^0_\ell(X \times \mathbb{R}, Y)$ with

$$M(x,t) = \begin{cases} g(x) & \text{for } t \le 0, \\ \bar{g}(x) & \text{for } t \ge 1, \\ g(x) & \text{for } x \in A \end{cases}$$

and M is close to g as usual. Let

$$\widetilde{A} = X \times [(-\infty,0] \cup [1,\infty)] \cup (A \times \mathbb{R}).$$

Apply the first part of the theorem with X replaced by $X \times \mathbb{R}$, f replaced by M, and A replaced by $\widetilde{A}$. We obtain a function $\widetilde{M} \in C^\infty_\tau(X \times \mathbb{R}, Y)$ with

$$\widetilde{M}(x,t) = \begin{cases} g(x) & \text{for } t \le 0, \\ \bar{g}(x) & \text{for } t \ge 1, \\ g(x) & \text{for } x \in A \end{cases}$$

and $\widetilde{M}$ is close to g as usual. Thus g is homotopic to $\bar{g}$ via a tangentially smooth homotopy fixing A. □

We consider next the consequences of Theorem 2.15 for vector bundles.

Proposition 2.16. *Every continuous (real or complex) vector bundle E over a compact foliated space X has a compatible tangentially smooth bundle structure; and such a structure is unique up to C^∞_τ isomorphism.*

Proof. Let $g : X \to G_n$ be a classifying map for $E \to X$, where $G_n = G_n(\mathbb{R}^{n+k})$ or $G_n(\mathbb{C}^{n+k})$ denotes a suitable compact Grassmann manifold with canonical smooth bundle $E^n \to G_n$. Then g can be approximated by, and so is homotopic to, a C^∞_τ map h by Theorem 2.15. Then E is equivalent to h^*E^n, and h^*E^n is a C^∞_τ-bundle, since E^n is a smooth bundle and h is of class C^∞_τ.

If E_0 and E_1 are C^∞_τ bundles that are isomorphic as C^0-bundles, there is a continuous map $H : X \times I \to G_n$ such that $H^*_0(E^n) = E_0$ and $H^*_1(E^n) = E_1$. Approximate H by a map $\hat{H}$ in C^∞_τ fixing H_0 and H_1; then $\hat{H}^*_\tau(E^n)$ is a C^∞_τ equivalence between E_0 and E_1. □

The proposition implies that tangentially smooth K-theory (i.e., K-theory defined via tangentially smooth bundles) on locally compact foliated spaces coincides with the usual K-theory. In the next chapter we shall introduce tangential de Rham cohomology. This does *not* agree with ordinary de Rham cohomology, as will become evident.

Let X be a foliated space of dimension p. The next order of business is the construction of the holonomy groupoid or graph of X, denoted G or $G(X)$. Our construction follows that of [Winkelnkemper 1983] as closely as possible.

Recall that a *plaque* is a component of $U \cap \ell$, where ℓ is some leaf and U is some coordinate patch. Every point of X has a neighborhood which consists of a union of plaques with respect to some U and, with respect to the same U, two different plaques $\mathfrak{p}$, $\mathfrak{p}'$, can be on the same leaf. A *regular covering* is a covering of X by open coordinate patches U_i such that each plaque in U_i meets at most one plaque in U_j. We henceforth assume (without any loss of generality) that our covers are always regular.

We recall the definition and elementary properties of the concept of *holonomy*. Let ℓ be a leaf of X and α an arc in ℓ starting at a and ending at b. Subdivide the arc α into small enough subarcs by means of points $a = a_0, a_1, \ldots, a_k = b$ so that each point a_i has a neighborhood U_i consisting entirely of plaques, so that if we choose a plaque $\mathfrak{p}_0$ of U_0, there is a unique plaque $\mathfrak{p}_1 \subset U_1$ which intersects $\mathfrak{p}_0$, a unique plaque $\mathfrak{p}_2 \subset U_2$ which intersects $\mathfrak{p}_1$, etc., and finally a unique plaque $\mathfrak{p}_k \subset U_k$.

Let N_a and N_b be transversals through a and b respectively. For points $n \in N_a$ which are sufficiently close to a, we define $H^\alpha_{ab}(n) \in N_b$ by the above procedure. That is, find the unique plaque $\mathfrak{p}_0 \subset U_0$ which contains n, follow the plaque to plaque $\mathfrak{p}_k \subset U_k$, and define $H^\alpha_{ab}(n)$ to be the unique element in $\mathfrak{p}_k \cap N_b$. Then H^α_{ab} is a homeomorphism from a neighborhood of a in N_a to a neighborhood of b in N_b, and $H^\alpha_{ab}(n)$ lies on the same leaf as n. Choosing the partition $\{a_i\}$ and the neighborhoods $\{U_i\}$ differently changes H^α_{ab}, but the new and old maps will coincide on some smaller neighborhood. Thus the germ of H^α_{ab} does not depend on these choices. Altering α by a homotopy in ℓ which fixes endpoints preserves the germ of H^α_{ab}.

If $a = b$ and $N_a = N_b$, composing the germs is a well-defined operation under which the holonomy germs form a group G^a_a. The natural map $\pi_1(\ell, a) \to G^a_a$ given by $\alpha \mapsto H^\alpha_{aa}$ is a surjective homomorphism, so if ℓ is simply connected then $G^a_a = \{0\}$ for each $a \in \ell$. The group G^a_a is the *holonomy group* of the leaf ℓ at the point a. (The notation comes from groupoids and will become apparent.) The set $\{x \in X \mid G^x_x = 0\}$ is a dense G_δ, by Epstein, Millet, and Tischler [Epstein et al. 1977] and independently by Hector, so that in that sense at least trivial holonomy is generic.

The set $\{x \in G \mid G^x_x \neq 0\}$ may have positive measure. For example, let K be a Cantor subset of the unit circle of positive measure. Choose a homeomorphism of the circle which has K as its fixed point set. The associated foliation of the torus has closed leaves corresponding to each point of K and each of these leaves has nontrivial holonomy.

For example, if we foliate the annulus as shown at the top of the next page, then $G^a_a = \mathbb{Z}$ for each $a \in \ell$, since with respect to the arc α which traverses the leaf once clockwise the holonomy map $H : I \to I$ is monotone decreasing and hence of infinite order in G^a_a. Similarly, the other closed leaf has nontrivial holonomy. Each of the remaining leaves is homeomorphic to $\mathbb{R}$ (and thus simply connected) and hence has trivial holonomy.

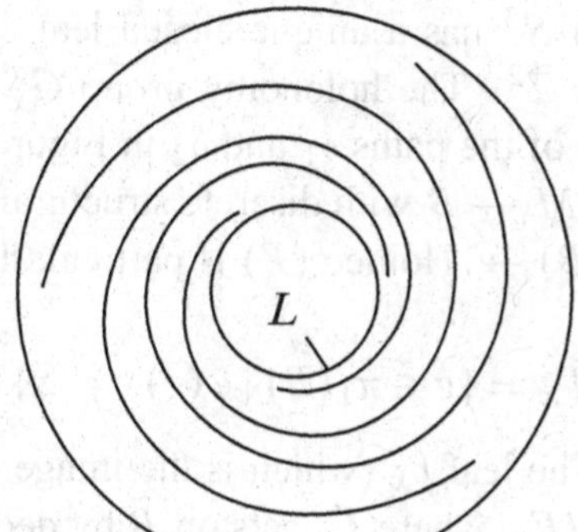

Let $\widetilde{X}$ be the foliated space shown:

(2.17)

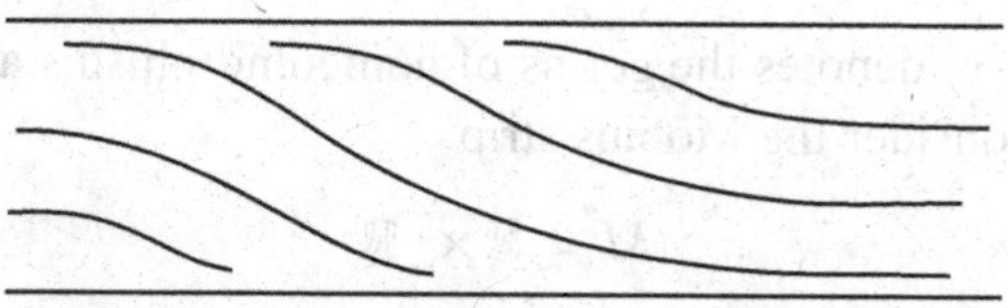

This is noncompact, of course. Every leaf is simply connected, so all of the holonomy groups are trivial. The exponential map yields a tangentially smooth map $\widetilde{X} \to X$, and this is a covering space.

Here are some more examples to illustrate the concept.

Consider the torus, foliated as indicated below. There are closed leaves through A, B, C, and a family of closed leaves intercepting the line segment DA (with ℓ_E as a typical closed leaf in this family). Each closed leaf ℓ is a circle, with $\pi_1(\ell) = \mathbb{Z}$. The leaf ℓ_E has trivial holonomy, since a small transverse disk meets only the adjacent family of closed leaves which are plaque paths. The leaves ℓ_A, ℓ_B, ℓ_C, and ℓ_D each have holonomy group $\mathbb{Z}$. Note that for the leaf ℓ_D a disk placed between D and E is acted upon trivially; the disk must overlap the $C - D$ area to see the holonomy.

(2.18)

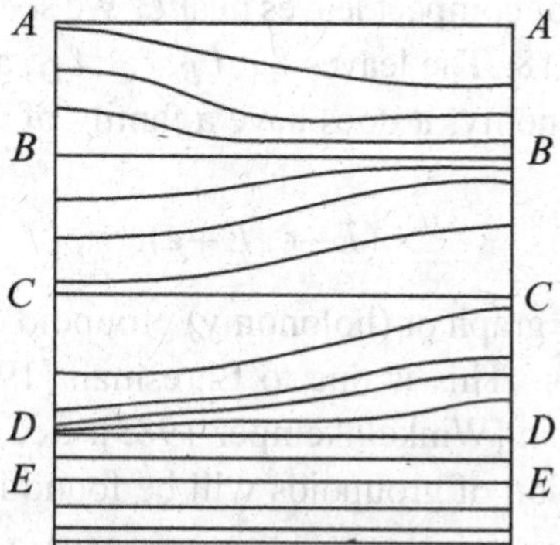

The Reeb foliation of S^3 has a unique closed leaf ℓ_0 diffeomorphic to the torus T^2 with $\pi_1(\ell_0) = \mathbb{Z}^2$. The holonomy group G_x^x for $x \in \ell_0$ is also $\mathbb{Z}^2$, generated by the images of the paths δ_1 and δ_2 in Figure 2.6.

The case of a bundle $M \to B$ with discrete structural group (2.2) given by a homomorphism $\varphi : \pi_1(B) \to$ Homeo (F) is particularly pleasing. For $x \in F$, let

$$\Gamma_x = \{g \in \pi_1(B) \mid \varphi(g)x = x\}$$

be the isotropy group. The leaf ℓ_x (which is the image of $\widetilde{B} \times \{x\}$ in M) may be expressed as $\ell_x = \widetilde{B}/\Gamma_x$, where Γ_x acts on $\widetilde{B}$ by deck transformations. The holonomy group G_x^x is the image of the homomorphism

$$\pi_1(\ell_x) \cong \Gamma_x \to \mathrm{Homeo}(F, x),$$

where Homeo(F, x) denotes the germs of homeomorphisms at x which fix x.

For instance, consider the Möbius strip

$$M = \mathbb{R} \times_{\mathbb{Z}} \mathbb{R}$$

foliated by circles corresponding to the images of $\mathbb{R} \times \{y\}$ for various values of $y \in \mathbb{R}$ (see Figure 2.4). If $y \neq 0$ then $\pi_1(\ell_y) = \mathbb{Z}$ acts trivially upon Diff$(\mathbb{R}, y)$, and hence $G_y^y = 0$. However, the holonomy group G_0^0 of the core circle is the group $\mathbb{Z}/2$, since the diffeomorphism $\theta(y) = -y$ which creates M does lie in Diff$(\mathbb{R}, 0)$, and $\theta^2 = 1$.

Holonomy is a critically important internal property of foliations. As evidence we cite a special case of the Reeb stability theorem and refer the reader to [Lawson 1977] for more information.

Theorem 2.19 (Reeb). *Let M^{p+q} be a smooth foliated manifold with a compact leaf ℓ with trivial holonomy. Then there exists a neighborhood U of ℓ in M such that U is a union of leaves and a diffeomorphism $f : \ell \times D^q \to U$ which preserves leaves.*

Thus M has a family of compact leaves near ℓ. We see this theorem at work in the example of Figure 2.18. The leaves $\ell_A, \ell_B, \ell_C, \ell_D$, and ℓ_E are all compact. Only ℓ_E has trivial holonomy; it does have a family of closed leaves near it, of the form

$$\ell \times (E - \epsilon, E + \epsilon).$$

We next introduce the graph or (holonomy) groupoid of a foliation and verify its elementary properties. This is due to Ehresman [1963], Thom [1964] and Reeb, and is expounded in [Winkelnkemper 1983]. See also [Phillips 1987]. A more systematic discussion of groupoids will be found in Chapter IV.

Definition 2.20. The *holonomy graph* or *groupoid* $G(X)$ of the foliated space X is defined to be the collection of all triples $(x, y, [\alpha])$, where x and y lie on the same leaf ℓ, α is a continuous path from x to y in ℓ, and $[\alpha]$ is the holonomy equivalence class of α: α is equivalent to β if $\alpha\beta^{-1} = 1$, the identity in G_y^y.

There are canonical maps as follows:

(1) $\Delta : X \to G(X)$ by

$$\Delta(x) = (x, x, [0]),$$

where 0 denotes the constant path at x.

(2) An involution $i : G(X) \to G(X)$ given by

$$i(x, y, [\alpha]) = (y, x, [\alpha^{-1}]).$$

(3) projections $p_1, p_2 : G(X) \to X$ defined by

$$p_1(x, y, [\alpha]) = x, \qquad p_2(x, y, [\alpha]) = y.$$

Frequently p_1 is written as r (= range) and p_2 is written as s (= source). Note that if ℓ_x is the leaf through x in X, then $p_1^{-1}(x)$ will turn out to be $\tilde{\ell}_x$, the covering space of ℓ_x corresponding to the holonomy kernel and $\tilde{\ell}_x / G_x^x = \ell_x$. Thus the construction "'unwraps' all leaves of X simultaneously with respect to their correct topology as well as their holonomy" [Winkelnkemper 1983, 0.3].

(4) Let

$$G(X) \oplus G(X) = \{(u, v) \in G(X) \times G(X) \mid p_1(u) = p_1(v)\}.$$

Then we have $m : G \oplus G \to G$ defined by

$$m((x, y, [\alpha]), (x, z[\beta])) = (y, z, [\beta\alpha^{-1}])$$

with $m \circ \text{diag} = \Delta p_2$, $m(u, v) = i \circ m(v, u)$, and

$$m(u, \Delta \circ p_1(u)) = i(u).$$

The p-dimensional foliation on X induces a $2p$-dimensional foliation on $G(X)$: the leaf in $G(X)$ through the point $(x_0, y_0[\alpha_0])$ does not depend on $[\alpha_0]$ and consists of all triples $(x, y, [\alpha])$ with $x, y \in \ell_{x_0} = \ell_{y_0}$ with $[\alpha]$ arbitrary. With the leaf topology it is diffeomorphic to $p_1^{-1}(x) \times p_2^{-1}(y) \cong \tilde{\ell}_x \times \tilde{\ell}_y$.

Next we define the topology on $G(X)$. Let $z = (a, b, [\alpha])$ be a point in $G(X)$. Choose a path α which represents $[\alpha]$, a family $\mathcal{U} = \{U_1, \ldots, U_k\}$ of coordinate patches which implements the holonomy map H_{ab}^{α} and an open tranversal N upon which H_{ab}^{α} is defined. We may assume that the projection $n : U_1 \to N$ is surjective. Suppose that x is an element of U_1. There is a path s_x in the plaque of x (unique to holonomy) from x to $n(x)$. By the setup above, there is a canonical (up to holonomy) path α_x from $n(x)$ to $H_{ab}^{\alpha}(n(x))$. Let $q(x)$ be the unique plaque in U_k which contains H_{ab}^{α}. Then for $y \in q(x)$ there is a path t_{yx}

in $q(x)$ (unique up to holonomy) from $H^{\alpha}_{ab}(n(x))$ to y. As a subbase for the topology of $G(X)$ we take the subsets

$$V_{z,\alpha,\mathfrak{U},N} = \{(x, y, [t_{yx}\alpha_x s_x]) : x \in U_1, y \in q(x)\}.$$

Since each leaf, being a smooth p-manifold, has a countably generated fundamental group, it follows that this topology has a countable base.

Proposition 2.21. *With the above topology $G(X)$ is Hausdorff if and only if for all x and y, the holonomy maps along two arbitrary arcs α and β from x to y and with respect to the same transversals N_x, N_y are already the same if they coincide on an open subset of their domain whose closure contains x.*

Proof. Since X is Hausdorff, it is enough to separate points $z = (x, y, [\alpha])$ and $z' = (x, y, [\alpha'])$ in order to show that $G(X)$ is Hausdorff.

Suppose any two neighborhoods of z and z' had a point $z'' = (x'', b'', [\alpha''])$ in common. Then z'' lies in

$$V_{z,\alpha} \cap V_{z',\alpha'} = \{(\tilde{x}, \tilde{y}, \beta_n) \in G(X) \mid \tilde{x} \in \mathfrak{p}_x(n), \tilde{y} \in H^{\alpha}_{xy}(\mathfrak{p}_x(n)) \cap H^{\alpha'}_{xy}(\mathfrak{p}_x(n))\},$$

where $\beta_n = s_{\tilde{x}} \cup \alpha_n \cup s_{\tilde{y}} \cong s'_{\tilde{x}} \cup \alpha'_n \cup s_{\tilde{y}}$. Since the short arcs $s_{\tilde{x}}, s_{\tilde{y}}$ do not affect holonomy, the holonomy along both α and α' would have to coincide with the holonomy defined by α'' on its domain. The domain of the holonomy of α'' contains x in its closure.

Conversely, if the holonomy along α and α' coincided on an open set, containing x in its closure, then from the definition of the sets $V_{z\alpha}$ above any neighborhood of z will intersect any neighborhood of z'. □

Corollary 2.22. *If $G^x_x = 0$ for all $x \in X$ then $G(X)$ is Hausdorff.*

This is the case, for instance, if each leaf is simply-connected.

Consider the graph of Example 2.18. Is it Hausdorff? Following Proposition 2.21, it suffices to examine the foliation at leaves with nontrivial holonomy, in this case leaves ℓ_A, ℓ_B, ℓ_C, and ℓ_D. Intuitively the question is whether the holonomy is one-sided. Leaves ℓ_B and ℓ_C cause no difficulty. However, leaves ℓ_A and ℓ_D do indeed cause difficulty. Take ℓ_D, for example. Here is the picture:

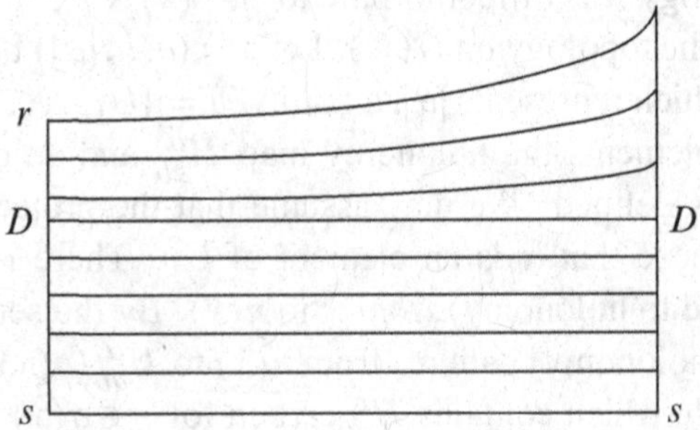

Let α be the horizontal circle through D and let β be the constant path at D. Let N be the transversal (r, s) and let N' be the tranversal (D, s). We have already determined that $G_D^D = \mathbb{Z}$ generated by $[\alpha]$, and thus

$$(D, D, [\alpha]) \neq (D, D, [\beta])$$

in the graph. However the transversal N' (which contains D in its closure) does not detect the presence of holonomy. Proposition 2.21 implies that the points $(D, D, [\alpha])$ and $(D, D, [\beta])$ cannot be separated by disjoint open sets, so the graph is not Hausdorff.

The graph of the Reeb foliation of S^3 is also not Hausdorff, though this is for more subtle reasons. The point is that the holonomy corresponding to the spreading out in the γ_2 direction is seen by a closed path in the leaf parallel to δ_1, so that if one cuts the foliation then a cross-section appears just as Figure 2.6 and the same nonseparation problem occurs.

Definition. A topological space is said to be *locally Hausdorff* if every point has an open neighborhood which is Hausdorff.

Proposition 2.23. *Each point of $G(X)$ has a neighborhood which is tangentially diffeomorphic to an open neighborhood of $\mathbb{R}^{2p} \times N_a$. Hence $G(X)$ is locally Hausdorff.*

Proof. Pick $(a, b, [\alpha]) \in G(X)$ and a path α representing $[\alpha]$. Choose neighborhoods $U_1, \ldots, U_k$ and tangential coordinate patches $(t_i, n_i) : U_i \to \mathbb{R}^p \times N$ corresponding to α.

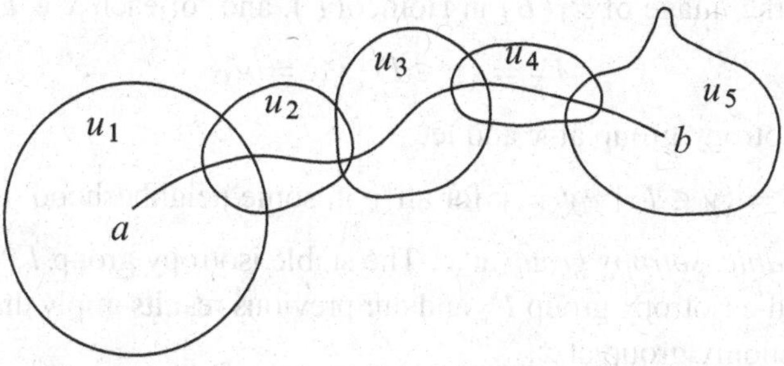

Let $N_a = n_1(U_1)$ and $N_b = n_k(U_k)$. After a possible shrinking of U_1 and U_k there results the holonomy map $H_{ab}^{\alpha} : N_a \to N_b$.

Given $x \in U_1$, there is a unique plaque relating $n_1 x$ with $H_{ab}^{\alpha}(n_1 x)$. If $y \in U_k$ with $n_k y = H_{ab}^{\alpha}(n_1 x)$, the unique plaque path determines a path β from x to y in $\bigcup_i U_i$. Now β is not unique, but $[\beta]$ is unique, and of course $H_{xy}^{\beta}(n_1 x) = n_k y$. Let $W \subset G(X)$ be the set of all points $(x, y, [\beta])$ such that:

(1) $x \in U_1, \quad y \in U_k$;

(2) $n_k y = H_{ab}^{\alpha}(n_1 x)$;

(3) β is determined as above.

Note that if $(x, y, [\beta]) = (x, y, [\beta'])$ in W then $[\beta] = [\beta']$. Further, define $\Phi : W \to \mathbb{R}^p \times \mathbb{R}^p \times N$ by

$$\Phi(x, y, [\beta]) = (t_1 x, t_k y, n_1 x).$$

We claim that Φ is a bijection. It is clear that Φ must be injective by our restriction on β. Suppose that $(r_1, r_2, r_3) \in \mathbb{R}^p \times \mathbb{R}^p \times N$, (or an open subset if the t_i and n_i are not surjective). Choose $x \in U_1$ with $t_1 x = r_1$ and $n_1 x = r_3$. Choose $y \in U_k$ with $t_k y = r_2$ and $n_k y = H^{\alpha}_{ab}(r_3)$. Since $n_k y = H^{\alpha}_{ab}(n_1 x)$, there is a leaf path β in $\bigcup U_i$ from x to y. Then $\Phi(x, y, [\beta]) = (r_1, r_2, r_3)$, so Φ is surjective. It is clear that Φ is tangentially smooth. □

Our final topic in this chapter is a close examination of the equivalence relation and (in anticipation of the Chapter IV discussion) the topological structure of the groupoid of a foliated space in the case of a foliated bundle with discrete structural group and the case of the Reeb foliation.

Recall from the beginning of this chapter that the initial data for a foliated bundle are a manifold B^p with universal cover $\widetilde{B}$, a space F and a homomorphism $\varphi : \pi_1(B) \to \mathrm{Homeo}(F)$. The resulting space (2.2),

$$M = \widetilde{B} \times_{\pi_1(B)} F,$$

is a foliated space of dimension p, and the natural map $\pi : M \to B$ restricts to a covering space

$$\widetilde{B} \times \{x\} \to \ell \xrightarrow{\pi} B.$$

Let Γ be the image of $\pi_1(B)$ in $\mathrm{Homeo}(F)$, and for each $x \in F$ let

$$\Gamma_x = \{\gamma \in \Gamma \mid \gamma x = x\}$$

denote the isotropy group at x and let

(2.24) $\quad \Gamma^x = \{\gamma \in \Gamma \mid \gamma y = y \text{ for all } y \text{ in some neighborhood of } x \text{ in } F\}$

denote the *stable isotropy group* at x. The stable isotropy group Γ^x is a normal subgroup of the isotropy group Γ_x and our previous results imply that $\Gamma_x / \Gamma^x \cong G^x_x$, the holonomy group at x.

Let $b \in B$ be a basepoint, let $\tilde{b} \in \widetilde{B}$ be some preimage of b, and let N be the image of $\tilde{b} \times F$ in M. The map $\tilde{b} \times F \to N$ is a homeomorphism since $\pi_1(B)$ acts freely on $\widetilde{B}$, so N is a copy of F sitting as a complete transversal to the foliated space.

Let G^N_N be the subgroupoid $\bigcup_{m,n \in N} G^n_m$, so that the elements of G^N_N are triples $(n, m, [\alpha])$ with $n, m \in N$ and $[\alpha]$ some holonomy class of a path in the leaf ℓ_n of M from n to m. If we regard G as a category, G^N_N is the full subcategory with objects N. Results from [Hilsum and Skandalis 1983] (see Theorem 6.14 on page 139 below) imply that the C^*-algebra of the foliation of M is determined by the C^*-algebra of the groupoid G^N_N. (In fact G^N_N is Morita equivalent to $G(X)$; see [Ramsay 1982]). As G_N^N is much simpler to understand than the full groupoid of the foliation, we explore its structure.

Theorem 2.25. *If $M = \widetilde{B} \times_{\pi_1(B)} F$ is a foliated bundle as above with complete transversal $N \cong F$, there is natural homeomorphism of topological groupoids*

$$G_N^N \cong (G \times \Gamma)/\approx,$$

where $(x, \gamma) \approx (y, \delta)$ if and only if $x = y$, and $\delta^{-1}\gamma$ lies in the stable isotropy group Γ^x. Thus G_N^N is completely determined by the action of

$$\Gamma = \mathrm{Im}(\pi_1(B) \to \mathrm{Homeo}(F))$$

on F.

We note some consequences of the result.

Corollary 2.26. *With the notation of Theorem 2.25, if the holonomy groups G_x^x are trivial for all $x \in F$ then*

$$G_N^N \cong (F \times \Gamma)/\sim,$$

where $(x, \gamma) \sim (y, \delta)$ if and only if $x = y$ and $\delta^{-1}\gamma$ lies in the isotropy group Γ_x (i.e., if and only if $x = y$ and $\gamma x = \delta x$).

The corollary is immediate from the identification $G_x^x \cong \Gamma_x/\Gamma^x$.

Note that the stable isotopy groups Γ^x vanish for all x if and only if for each $\gamma \in \Gamma$ the fixed point set of γ has no interior. This condition is quite frequently satisfied in practice. For instance, if F is a Riemannian manifold F^q, Γ acts as isometries and each nonzero element γ moves some element of F, then the fixed point set of each $\gamma \in \Gamma$ is a manifold of dimension at most $(q-1)$ and hence has no interior. Indeed any real analytic action satisfies this condition. For an example where the condition is violated, see Figure 2.28 below.

Corollary 2.27. *With the notation of Theorem 2.25, if for each $\gamma \in \Gamma$ the fixed point set of γ has no interior then there is a natural isomorphism of topological groupoids*

$$G_N^N \cong F \times \Gamma.$$

Proof. Each stable isotropy group Γ^x vanishes and so the result follows from Theorem 2.25. □

Proof of Theorem 2.25. We shall show that $G_N^N \cong (N \times \Gamma)/\approx$, which suffices. Define a map

$$\sigma : (N \times \Gamma)/\approx \to G_N^N$$

as follows. Let $(n, \gamma) \in N \times \Gamma$. Represent γ by some based loop α in B. Lift α to a path $\hat{\alpha}$ in the leaf ℓ_n of $n \in M$ with $\hat{\alpha}(0) = n$. Then $\hat{\alpha}(1) \in N \cap \ell_n$ and $(n, \hat{\alpha}(1), [\hat{\alpha}])$ represents an element $\sigma(n, \gamma) \in G_N^N$. We argue that σ is well-defined as follows. Independence of choice of lifts $\hat{\alpha}$ of α is clear. Suppose that $(n, \gamma) \approx (n, \delta)$, so that $\delta^{-1}\gamma \in \Gamma^n$. Represent γ and δ by loops α and β

respectively, and lift these loops to paths $\hat{\alpha}$ and $\hat{\beta}$ in ℓ_n with $\hat{\alpha}(0) = \hat{\beta}(0) = n$. Then $\hat{\beta}^{-1} \circ \hat{\alpha}$ is a loop in ℓ_n whose holonomy class is trivial, since $\delta^{-1}\gamma \in \Gamma^n$. Thus $\sigma(n, \gamma) = \sigma(n, \delta)$ and σ is well-defined.

The map σ is obviously continuous. If $\sigma(n, \gamma) = \sigma(n, \delta)$ then $\delta^{-1}\gamma$ must lift to a loop $\hat{\beta}^{-1}\hat{\alpha}$ with trivial holonomy in G_n^n. This implies that $\delta^{-1}\gamma \in \Gamma^n$ and hence σ is a monomorphism. If $(n, m, [\alpha]) \in G_N^N$ then the composite

$$[0,1] \xrightarrow{\alpha} M \xrightarrow{\pi} B$$

is a loop (since $\pi n = \pi m$) and $\sigma(n, \pi\alpha) = (n, m, [\alpha])$. Thus σ is a homeomorphism.

The groupoid structure on $(N \times \Gamma)/\approx$ is obtained as follows. The unit space is N, of course, and $s(n, \gamma) = n$. The range map r is given by $r(n, \gamma) = \hat{\alpha}(1)$, where $\hat{\alpha}$ is a lift of a realization of the loop γ as earlier in this proof. Thus (n, γ) and (m, δ) may be multiplied when $\hat{\alpha}$ lifts γ and $\hat{\alpha}(1) = m$, and then

$$(n, \gamma) \cdot (m, \delta) = (n, \delta\gamma).$$

With this structure, σ is clearly a homeomorphism of topological groupoids. □

In practice Theorem 2.25 is rather easy to use. For instance, consider the Möbius strip $M = \mathbb{R} \times_{\mathbb{Z}} \mathbb{R}$ of Figure 2.4. The equivalence relation is simply the union of the $y = x$ and $y = -x$ lines in the plane, a figure X. The group Γ is $\mathbb{Z}/2$ acting nonfreely since Γ fixes $0 \in \mathbb{R}$. This is an isolated fixed point and certainly has no interior; thus $G_N^N \cong \mathbb{R} \times \mathbb{Z}/2$ with the obvious structure of a (Hausdorff) smooth manifold by Corollary 2.27. The map $G_N^N \to \{(x, y) \mid y = \pm x\}$ is a homeomorphism except at the origin, where it is two-to-one in the obvious way, corresponding to the fact that $G_0^0 \cong \mathbb{Z}/2$, $G_n^n = 0$ for $n \neq 0$.

Next we consider the manifold M constructed as the suspension of the action of $\mathbb{Z}$ on $\mathbb{R}$ given by θ, where

$$\theta(n)(t) = \begin{cases} 2^n t & \text{for } t > 0, \\ t & \text{for } t \leq 0. \end{cases}$$

The element $\theta(1)$ fixes $(-\infty, 0]$ and hence the condition of Corollary 2.27 is violated. The equivalence relation for G_N^N has the following form:

(2.28) 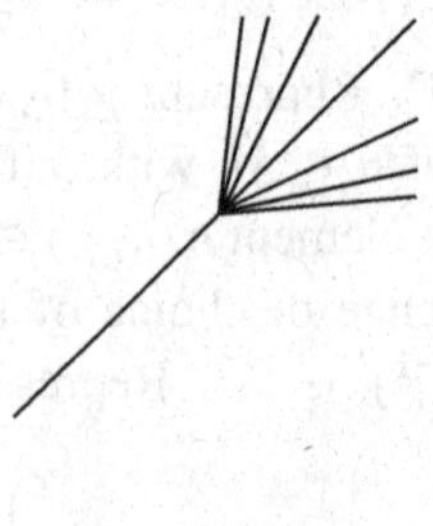

The groups Γ_t are given by $\Gamma_t = \mathbb{Z}$ for $t \leq 0$ and $\Gamma_t = 0$ for $t > 0$, and using Theorem 2.25 we have

$$G_N^N = (\mathbb{R} \times \mathbb{Z})/\approx,$$

where

$$(t,n) \approx (t,m) \quad \text{if and only if} \quad m = n \text{ or } t < 0,$$

and hence G_N^N is the (path-connected) non-Hausdorff one-manifold

(2.29)

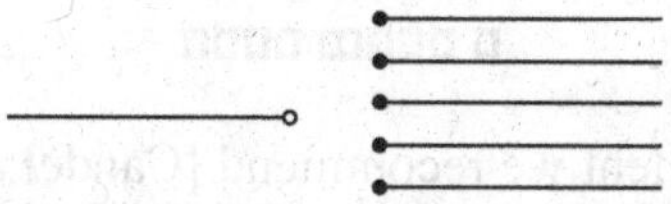

Finally we move away from foliated bundles and consider the Reeb foliation of S^3 [Candel and Conlon 2000; Lawson 1977]. Take a transversal $N = (-1, 1)$ which starts near the closed leaf, tunnels through the solid snake in time $(-1, 0)$, passes through the closed leaf at time 0, and tunnels through the other solid snake in $(0, 1)$, stopping near (but not at) the closed leaf. Then N is a complete transversal. The corresponding equivalence relation for G_N^N is the following subset of the plane with the relative topology:

(2.30)

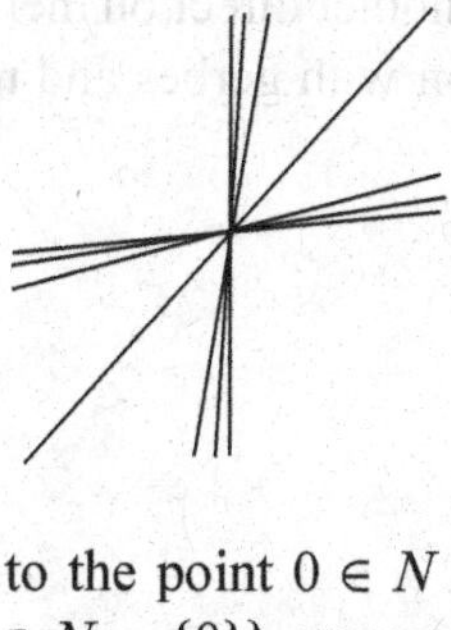

The point $(0, 0)$ corresponds to the point $0 \in N$ which lies on the closed leaf ℓ_0. A sequence $\{(t, 2^n t) : t \in N - \{0\}\}$ corresponds to choosing a point $t \in N - \{0\}$, going around a corresponding holonomy path of degree n and returning to $\ell_t \cap [-1, 1]$.

The map from G_N^N to the equivalence relation is a bijection except that $(0, 0)$ has preimage $\mathbb{Z}^2$, corresponding to the fact that the closed leaf ℓ_0 has holonomy group $\mathbb{Z}^2$. So as a set fibred over the transversal N, G_N^N has structure

(2.31)

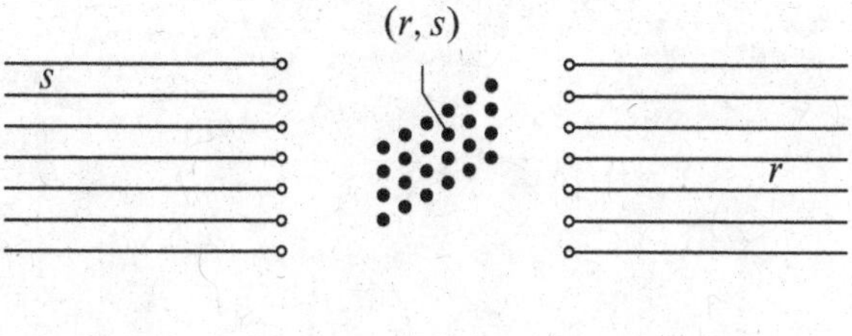

Write the lines for $t < 0$ as $(0, s, [-1, 0))$ and the lines for $t > 0$ as $(r, 0, (0, 1])$. Then the set

$$(0, s, [-1, 0)) \cup \{(r, s)\} \cup (r, 0, (0, 1])$$

is diffeomorphic to $[-1, 1]$ in the topology of G_N^N. These sets serve as coordinate patches which exhibit G_N^N as a (non-Hausdorff) smooth topological groupoid. As an exercise, the reader is invited to show that the fundamental group $\pi_1(G_N^N)$ is the free group on two generators.

[illegible]

For general enlightenment we recommend [Candel and Conlon 2000; 2003], as well as the new text [Moerdijk and Mrčun 2003]. There has been an explosion in the study of foliated spaces (or *laminations*, as they are more commonly called these days) in low-dimensional topology, and we refer to [Gabai and Oertel 1989; Gabai 2001; Calegari 2003] as representative of this development. We would also include [Bedford and Smillie 1999], which studies the dynamics of polynomial automorphisms of $\mathbb{C}^2$ on their Julia set. In another direction, there is a whole industry at work on symplectic, Poisson, and related groupoids. We refer to the fine book [Cannas da Silva and Weinstein 1999] as a general reference for this area. In yet another direction there is a lot of work on groupoids with structure and their relation with gerbes and related matters; see [Moerdijk 2003].

CHAPTER III

Tangential Cohomology

In this chapter we discuss certain cohomology groups associated with a foliated space, which we shall call tangential cohomology groups. It will be in these groups that invariants connected with the index theorem will live. Similar groups have been considered, for instance, in [Kamber and Tondeur 1975; Molino 1973; Vaisman 1973; Sarkaria 1978; Heitsch 1975; El Kacimi-Alaoui 1983; Haefliger 1980] (we discuss Haefliger's work at the end of chapter IV). The similarities and differences between the three situations are easy to describe; all involve differential forms which are smooth in the tangential direction of the foliation. The difference comes in the assumptions on the transverse behavior: for foliated manifolds (Kamber, Tondeur, and others), forms are C^∞ in the transverse direction; for foliated spaces (the present treatment), the forms are to be continuous in the transverse directions, since that is all that makes sense; and finally for foliated measure spaces, the forms are to be measurable in the transverse direction, for again that is all that makes sense.

Thus, we let X be a metrizable foliated space with foliation tangent bundle $FX \to X$, as defined in Chapter II. The quickest and simplest way to introduce the tangential cohomology is via sheaf theory and sheaf cohomology, but for those readers who are not familiar with such notions we show how to define the groups via a de Rham complex and also show in an appendix how to give a completely algebraic definition. For details concerning sheaves and their cohomology, consult [Godement 1973] and [Wells 1973].

We consider the sheaf $\mathcal{R}_\tau$ on X of germs of continuous real-valued tangentially locally constant functions. Specifically, this sheaf assigns to each open set U of X the set of continuous real-valued functions on U that are locally constant in the tangential direction on the foliated space U (given the induced foliation from X). This is obviously a presheaf and it is immediate that the additional conditions defining a sheaf [Godement 1973, p. 109] are satisfied.

Definition 3.1. The *tangential cohomology* groups of the foliated space X are the cohomology groups of the sheaf $\mathcal{R}_\tau$, $H^*(X, \mathcal{R}_\tau)$, which we normally write as $H_\tau^*(X, \mathbb{R})$ or simply $H_\tau^*(X)$.

These cohomology groups can be defined by construction of resolutions (see [Godement 1973, p. 173]) or perhaps more simply by the Čech method using cocycles defined on open covers of X [Godement 1973, p. 203], but for us the most useful and transparent way of dealing with them is via a de Rham complex.

Definition 3.2. A *tangential differential* k*-form* at $x \in X$ is an alternating k-form on the tangent space FX_x at x, i.e., an element of $\Lambda^k(F^*X_x)$. These fit together to yield a vector bundle denoted $\Lambda^k(F^*)$ on X which is just the k-th exterior power of the cotangent bundle, and it is quite evidently tangentially smooth in the sense of the previous chapter.

We assign to each open set U the tangentially smooth sections $\Gamma_\tau(\underline{\Lambda}^k(F^*))$ (defined on U). Just as before, this gives a sheaf which we denote by $\underline{\Lambda}^k(F^*)$ — the *sheaf of germs of tangentially smooth* k*-forms*.

There is an obvious differential

$$d : \Gamma_\tau(\underline{\Lambda}^k(F^*)) \longrightarrow \Gamma_\tau(\underline{\Lambda}^{k+1}(F^*))$$

which can be defined in an elementary way in terms of local coordinates. If $U \cong L^p \times N$ is a local coordinate patch with $x_1, \dots, x_p$ coordinates on the open ball L^p in $\mathbb{R}^p$ and $n \in N$, then a tangential differential k-form is an object that can be written locally as

$$\omega = \sum_{(i_\ell)} a(x_1, \dots x_p, n)\, dx_{i_1} \wedge \cdots \wedge dx_{i_k} \tag{3.3}$$

with a and all of its derivatives with respect to the x_i continuous in all variables. Then $d\omega$ is defined just as one does classically for a k-form with n playing the role of a parameter:

$$d\omega = \sum_{(i_\ell), j} \frac{\partial a}{\partial x_j}(x_1, \dots, x_p, n) dx_j \wedge dx_{i_1} \wedge \cdots \wedge dx_{i_k}. \tag{3.4}$$

We evidently have $d^2 = 0$ and so we have a sequence of sheaves with maps

$$0 \to \mathcal{R}_\tau \to \underline{\Lambda}^0(F^*) \xrightarrow{d} \underline{\Lambda}^1(F^*) \to \cdots \to \underline{\Lambda}^p(F^*) \to 0, \tag{3.5}$$

where the first map is the natural inclusion of tangentially locally constant functions into tangentially smooth functions. The Poincaré Lemma obviously holds in this context:

Proposition 3.6 (Poincaré Lemma). *The sequence* (3.5) *above is an exact sequence of sheaves; that is, for sufficiently small open sets* U*, the kernel of each map on sections over* U *is the range of the map in one lower degree.*

Proof. On an open set of the form $L \times N$, where L is a ball in $\mathbb{R}^p$, a k-form in the kernel of d is an expression $\omega(x, n)$, where for fixed n this is an ordinary closed k form with respect to the variable $x \in L$. (The variable n plays the role of a parameter with respect to which everything varies continuously.) By the usual Poincaré Lemma, one finds a $k-1$ form φ_n, one for each n, so that

$d\varphi_n = \omega(\cdot, n)$ and what is at issue is that we can choose φ_n to be continuous as n varies over N so that φ_n defines a section of $\Lambda^{k-1}(F^*)$ over U. This is a routine exercise the details of which we omit. □

Moreover, just as in the usual case, one sees that the sheaves $\underline{\Lambda}^k(F^*)$ are fine [Godement 1973, p. 157] and consequently by the general machinery of sheaf theory one can calculate the cohomology of the sheaf $\mathcal{R}_\tau$ from this resolution — a de Rham type theorem. Let

$$\Omega_\tau^k \equiv \Omega_\tau^k(X) = \Gamma_\tau(\underline{\Lambda}^k(F^*)) = \Gamma_\tau(\underline{\Lambda}^k(F^*))$$

denote the global tangentially smooth sections of the sheaf $\underline{\Lambda}^k(F^*)$.

Proposition 3.7. *There are isomorphisms*

$$H_\tau^k(X;\mathbb{R}) = H^k(X,\mathcal{R}_\tau) \cong \frac{\operatorname{Ker}(\Omega_\tau^k \to \Omega_\tau^{k+1})}{\operatorname{Im}(\Omega_\tau^{k-1} \to \Omega_\tau^k)}.$$

In particular, if $X = M$ foliated as one leaf then this is the usual identification of the de Rham cohomology groups $H^*(M;\mathbb{R})$. The analogous result (and indeed the entire chapter) holds with $\mathbb{R}$ replaced by $\mathbb{C}$ throughout.

From this proposition it is evident that $H_\tau^k(X,\mathbb{R}) = 0$ for $k > p$, where p is the leaf dimension of the foliated space. However, the individual cohomology groups are in general going to be infinite-dimensional, in contrast to the case of a compact manifold (with a foliation consisting of one leaf). Further, these groups, which are vector spaces, also inherit via the de Rham isomorphism the structure of (generally non-Hausdorff) topological vector spaces.

We topologize $\Omega_\tau^k(X)$ by demanding that in all local coordinate patches we have uniform convergence of the functions $a(x_1,\dots,x_p)$ of (3.3) together with all their derivatives in the tangential direction on compact subsets of the coordinate patch. The differentials are clearly continuous with respect to these topologies and so $H_\tau^n(X,\mathbb{R})$ is a topological vector space.

In general the image of d will fail to be closed and so $H_\tau^n(X,\mathbb{R})$ will not be Hausdorff in these cases. It will be useful occasionally to replace the image of d by its closure, or equivalently replace $H_\tau^n(X,\mathbb{R})$ by its quotient obtained from dividing by the closure of the identity; this is the largest Hausdorff quotient. We will denote this maximal Hausdorff quotient of $H_\tau^k(X,\mathbb{R})$ by

$$\overline{H}_\tau^k(X,\mathbb{R}) = H_\tau^k(X,\mathbb{R})/\overline{\{0\}}.$$

The point of this is twofold: first, we shall usually only care about the image of a cohomology class $[\omega]$ of $H_\tau^k(X,\mathbb{R})$ in this Hausdorff quotient, rather than the class itself, since $\int \omega\, d\nu$ depends only on the class of ω in $\overline{H}_\tau^p$; second, one at least has a chance of computing the groups $\overline{H}_\tau^*$ in certain cases. There is, however, a significant drawback. The functors $\overline{H}_\tau^*(\cdot, \mathbb{R})$ do not form a cohomology theory, since exactness is not preserved in general under the operation $H_\tau^* \mapsto \overline{H}_\tau^*$.[1]

The tangential cohomology groups are related via natural maps to the usual cohomology groups of the compact metrizable space. Since Čech cohomology and sheaf cohomology agree for such spaces [Godement 1973, p. 228], we shall simply write $H^*(X, A)$ for this cohomology for coefficients in an abelian group A. Specifically, the sheaf cohomology is defined to be the cohomology of the sheaf $\mathcal{R}$ of germs of locally constant real-valued functions. As a sheaf $\mathcal{R}$ assigns to each open set U the locally constant real-valued functions on U. The cohomology groups $H^*(X, \mathcal{R})$ are written as we indicated above as $H^*(X, \mathbb{R})$. But now there is a natural inclusion map of the sheaf $\mathcal{R}$ into the sheaf $\mathcal{R}_\tau$ of tangentially locally constant functions and we can complete this to a short exact sequence

$$0 \to \mathcal{R} \xrightarrow{r} \mathcal{R}_\tau \to \mathcal{R}_\nu \to 0, \tag{3.8}$$

where $\mathcal{R}_\nu$ is defined as the quotient sheaf of $\mathcal{R}_\tau$ by $\mathcal{R}$ [Godement 1973, p. 117]. We obtain in particular an induced homorphism

$$r_* : H^*(X, \mathbb{R}) = H^*(X, \mathcal{R}) \to H^*(X, \mathcal{R}_\tau) = H_\tau^*(X, \mathbb{R}), \tag{3.9}$$

a sort of "restriction" map from ordinary cohomology to tangential cohomology. Of course we also have a long exact sequence of cohomology corresponding to the short exact sequence of sheaves above, but we will not explore that further, and the sheaf $\mathcal{R}_\nu$ will not play any further role.

We should comment that the only reason for introducing sheaves was to obtain a natural definition of r_*. For we could have defined $H^*(X, \mathbb{R})$ as either Čech cohomology or equivalently Alexander–Spanier cohomology and we could have directly defined $H_\tau^*(X, \mathbb{R})$ as the cohomology of the tangential de Rham complex with no mention of sheaves. But then it is not at all apparent that there is a map r_* from the cohomology of X to the tangential cohomology of X. Actually, as we have suggested before, it is usually the composed map $\bar{r}_*$ from $H^*(X, \mathbb{R})$ to $\overline{H}_\tau^*(X, \mathbb{R})$ that is of more significance than r_*.

It might be helpful to look at an example and the simplest one is that of the Kronecker foliation of a two-torus T^2 by parallel lines of a fixed irrational slope λ relative to given coordinate axes. The leaves are given in parametric form as $\{(e^{it}, e^{i\lambda t}c) \mid t \in \mathbb{R}\}$ for some fixed $c \in T$. Tangential zero-forms are simply real-valued functions which are tangentially smooth. Clearly the tangent

[1] This is a familiar problem. For example, Steenrod noted that Čech homology theory did not satisfy an exactness axiom and he invented [1940] a homology theory, now called *Steenrod homology*, that does satisfy the exactness axiom [Eilenberg and Steenrod 1952]. Its maximal Hausdorff quotient is Čech homology.

bundle is a trivial bundle and in fact we can find an essentially unique tangential one-form ω which is invariant under group translation on T^2. Then the most general tangential one-form is easily seen to be of the type $f\omega$, where f is any tangentially smooth function. If θ is a group-invariant vector field on T^2 pointing in the tangential direction, then the differential

$$d : \Omega_\tau^0(F^*) \to \Omega_\tau^1(F^*)$$

is given by

$$d(g) = \theta(g)\omega$$

for a suitable normalization of θ.

To investigate this more closely we expand g in double Fourier series,

$$g(\xi_1, \xi_2) = \sum_{n,m} g_{n,m}\xi_1^n \xi_2^m,$$

and denote the Fourier coefficients of a second function f by $f_{n,m}$. The condition for g to be tangentially smooth is easily seen to be that $g_{n,m}(n+\lambda m)^k$ should be the Fourier coefficients of a continuous function, for each $k = 0, 1, \ldots$. The relation between f and g expressed by $d(g) = f\omega$ is simply that

$$f_{n,m} = (n + \lambda m)g_{n,m}. \tag{3.10}$$

Quite clearly the kernel of d consists of constants so $H_\tau^0(X, \mathbb{R}) \cong \mathbb{R}$. On the other hand if we are given $f\omega$ with f tangentially smooth, we have to find out when we can solve (3.10). An evident necessary condition is that $f_{0,0} = 0$ and indeed if $f_{0,0} = 0$ and if f is a trigonometric polynomial, we can find a trigonometric polynomial g solving the equation, as λ is irrational and $n + \lambda m$ is not zero unless $n = m = 0$. Since one easily sees that the set

$$\{f\omega \mid f_{0,0} = 0, f \text{ a trigonometric polynomial}\}$$

is dense in all $f\omega$ with $f_{0,0} = 0$ in the topology described above, one can conclude immediately that

$$\overline{H}_\tau^1(X, \mathbb{R}) \cong \mathbb{R}.$$

It is interesting to note that the closed tangential cohomology $\overline{H}_\tau^*(X, \mathbb{R})$ in this case is the cohomology over $\mathbb{R}$ of a circle. However

$$H_\tau^1(X, \mathbb{R}) \neq \overline{H}_\tau^1(X, \mathbb{R})$$

and the former is in fact infinite-dimensional, for (3.10) results in a classic "small denominator problem." Indeed, choose a sequence $(n(k), m(k))$ with

$$n(k) + \lambda m(k) = \xi(k)$$

a summable sequence, and define $f_{n,m} = 0$ unless $(n, m) = (n(k), m(k))$ and $f_{n(k),m(k)}$ any sequence in k asymptotic to $\xi(k)^{-1}$. Then

$$f_{n,m}(n + \lambda m)^k,$$

where $f_{n,m} \neq 0$, is the Fourier series of a continuous function for each k, since this holds for $k = 0$ and since $(n + \lambda m)$ is bounded (in fact tends to zero). But quite evidently

$$f_{n,m}(n + \lambda m)^{-1} = g_{n,m}$$

is not the Fourier series of a continuous function as $g_{n,m}$ does not tend to zero. This shows that $H^1_\tau(X, \mathbb{R})$ is infinite-dimensional and of course non-Hausdorff since $\overline{H}^1_\tau(X, \mathbb{R})$ is one-dimensional.

We remark that if one uses differential forms which also are required to be C^∞ in the transverse direction then the result is quite different. Haefliger [1980] has shown that for such forms the associated first cohomology groups of the Kronecker flow on the torus has either infinite dimension or dimension one, depending upon whether the irrational slope is Liouville or diophantine.

Let

$$L \to X \to B$$

be a fibre bundle with X compact and with leaves L_b corresponding to preimages of points $b \in B$ assumed to be smooth. Then the tangential cohomology of X has a simple description. Form a vector bundle E over B with

$$E_b \cong H^*(L_b).$$

(It is locally trivial.) Then $H^*_\tau(X)$ is isomorphic to the continuous cross-sections of E. (This suggests that for more general fibrations

$$F \to X \to B$$

of foliated spaces there should be a Serre spectral sequence of the type

$$H^*_\tau(B; H^*_\tau(F)) \Rightarrow H^*_\tau(X);$$

we do not pursue this direction here.)

The next order of business is a more thorough study of $H^*_\tau(X)$. Let $\mathcal{F}$ denote the category of metrizable (hence paracompact) foliated spaces and tangentially smooth leaf-preserving maps. We assume that $\mathbb{K} = \mathbb{R}$ or $\mathbb{C}$, and note once and for all that our results hold in both cases and that $\mathbb{R} \hookrightarrow \mathbb{C}$ induces an isomorphism $H^k_\tau(X; \mathbb{R}) \otimes_{\mathbb{R}} \mathbb{C} \cong H^k_\tau(X; \mathbb{C})$. Let $H^*_\tau(X) = H^*_\tau(X; \mathbb{K})$.

Proposition 3.11. *H^*_τ is a contravariant functor from $\mathcal{F}$ to the category of $\mathbb{Z}$-graded associative, graded-commutative topological $\mathbb{K}$-algebras and continuous homomorphisms, and $H^k_\tau(X) = 0$ for $k < 0$ or $k > p$, where p is the leaf dimension of X.*

Proof. The wedge product of forms yields a natural continuous map

$$\Omega_\tau^i(X) \otimes \Omega_\tau^j(X) \to \Omega_\tau^{i+j}(X),$$

which supplies the product structure in the usual way. As $\Omega_\tau^k(X) = 0$ for $k < 0$ or $k > p = \dim X$, the cohomology groups also vanish. If $f : X \to Y$ we may assume by Theorem 2.15 that f is tangentially smooth. Thus the induced map $\Omega_\tau^*(X) \to \Omega_\tau^*(X)$ is continuous and $f^* : H_\tau^*(Y) \to H_\tau^*(X)$ is continuous. □

Proposition 3.12. *If X is the topological sum of $\{X_j\}$ in $\mathcal{F}$, then*

$$H_\tau^k(X) \cong \prod_j H_\tau^k(X_j).$$ □

Proposition 3.13.

$$H_\tau^0(X) = \{f \in C_\tau^\infty(X) \mid f|_\ell \text{ is a constant for any leaf } \ell\}.$$

In particular, if X has a dense leaf then $H_\tau^0(X) \cong \mathbb{K}$. □

Definition 3.14. Let $f, g : X \to Y$ be continuous and leaf preserving functions. An $\mathcal{F}$-homotopy h between f and g is a leaf-preserving map

$$h : X \times \mathbb{R} \to Y,$$

where $X \times \mathbb{R}$ is foliated as

$$(\text{leaf of } X \times \mathbb{R}) = (\text{leaf of } X) \times \mathbb{R}$$

such that

$$h(x,t) = \begin{cases} f(x) & \text{for } t \leq 0, \\ g(x) & \text{for } t \geq 1. \end{cases}$$

Homotopy in $\mathcal{F}$ is obviously an equivalence relation. The following technical proposition leads to homotopy-invariance of H_τ^*.

Proposition 3.15. *Let $J_t : X \to X \times \mathbb{R}$ by $J_t(x) = (x,t)$. There is a $\mathbb{K}$-linear map*

$$L : \Omega_\tau^*(X \times \mathbb{R}) \to \Omega_\tau^*(X)$$

such that

(1) $L(\Omega_\tau^k(X \times \mathbb{R})) \subset \Omega_\tau^{k-1}(X)$ *and*

(2) $dL + Ld = J_1^* - J_0^*$.

That is, L is a chain-homotopy from J_0 to J_1.

Proof. By a tangentially smooth partition of unity argument, we may assume that $X = \mathbb{R}^p \times N$. Then any k-form in $\Omega_\tau^k(X \times \mathbb{R})$ with $k \geq 1$ may be written uniquely as a sum of monomials of the form

$$\alpha = a\, dx_I$$

or

$$\beta = b\, dx_I \wedge dt.$$

Define $L \mid \Omega^0_\tau(X \times \mathbb{R}) \equiv 0$, $L(\alpha) = 0$, and

$$L\beta = \left(\int_0^1 b\, dt \right) dx_I.$$

Then $L(\Omega^k_\tau(X \times \mathbb{R})) \subset \Omega^{k-1}_\tau(X)$. If $f \in \Omega^0_\tau(X \times \mathbb{R})$ then

$$(dL + Ld)f = L\left(\frac{\partial f}{\partial t}\, dt\right) + L\left(\sum_i \frac{\partial f}{\partial x_i} dx_i\right) = \int_0^1 \frac{\partial f}{\partial t}\, dt = (J_1^* - J_0^*)f.$$

On forms of type α,

$$(dL + Ld)\alpha = Ld\alpha = \left(\int_0^1 \frac{\partial a}{\partial t}\, dt \right) dx_I = \left(J_1^* - J_0^*\right)\alpha.$$

On forms of type β we have $J_I^*\beta = J_0^*\beta = 0$ and so

$$dL\beta = -Ld\beta = \sum_{i=1}^{p} \left(\frac{\partial b}{\partial x_i}\, dt \right) dx_i \wedge dx_I.$$

This shows that $dL + Ld = J_1^* - J_0^*$ on monomials and hence in general. □

Theorem 3.16. *If $f, g : X \to Y$ are $\mathcal{F}$-homotopic, then*

$$f^* = g^* : H^*_\tau(Y) \to H^*_\tau(X).$$

Proof. This is immediate from Proposition (3.15). □

Corollary 3.17. *If $f : X \to Y$ is a continuous leaf-preserving map, f induces a unique continuous map $f^* : H^*_\tau(Y) \to H^*_\tau(X)$.*

Proof. Say $f \simeq g$ and $f \simeq g'$, where $g, g' \in C^\infty_\tau$. Then $g^* = g'^*$ by Theorem 3.16, so declare $f^* = g^*$. □

Corollary 3.18. *Suppose that X and Y are foliated spaces and $f : X \to Y$ is a leaf-preserving homeomorphism. Then*

$$f^* : H^*_\tau(Y) \longrightarrow H^*_\tau(X)$$

is an isomorphism. Thus H^*_τ is a leaf-preserving topological invariant.

Proof. The map f^{-1} is also leaf-preserving. By Corollary 3.17 the maps f, f^{-1} induce f^*, $(f^{-1})^*$, and clearly $(f^{-1})^* = (f^*)^{-1}$. □

Corollary 3.19 (Homotopy-type invariance). *Two foliated spaces that have the same "leaf-preserving homotopy type" have isomorphic tangential cohomology.*

Proof. Let $f : X \to Y$ be a leaf-preserving homotopy equivalence with leaf-preserving homotopy inverse g, so $fg \simeq 1_Y$ and $gf \simeq 1_X$ via $\mathcal{F}$-homotopies. By Corollary 3.17, f^* and g^* exist, and then $f^* = (g^*)^{-1}$. □

Next we introduce cohomology with compact supports. The *support* of a form $\omega \in \Omega_\tau^k(X)$ is the closure of $\{x \in X \mid \omega(x) \neq 0\}$. Let $\Omega_{\tau c}^k(X) \subset \Omega_\tau^k(X)$ denote the forms of compact support. The groups $\Omega_{\tau c}^k(X)$ form a complex, as $d : \Omega_\tau^k(X) \to \Omega_\tau^{k+1}(X)$ decreases supports. Define *tangential cohomology with compact support* by

$$H_{\tau c}^k(X) = H^k(\Omega_{\tau c}^*(X)). \tag{3.20}$$

The inclusion $\Omega_{\tau c}^*(X) \hookrightarrow \Omega_\tau^*(X)$ is the inclusion of a differential subalgebra, thus inducing a map of $\mathbb{Z}$-graded $\mathbb{K}$-algebras

$$H_{\tau c}^k(X) \to H_\tau^k(X), \tag{3.21}$$

which is an isomorphism if X is compact. The following proposition summarizes the elementary properties of $H_{\tau c}^*$.

Proposition 3.22. (1) *$H_{\tau c}^*$ is a contravariant functor from $\mathcal{F}$ and proper $\mathcal{F}$-maps to $\mathbb{Z}$-graded associative, graded commutative topological $\mathbb{K}$-algebras and continuous homomorphisms.*

(2) *If X is the topological sum of $\{X_j\}$ in $\mathcal{F}$, then there is a natural isomorphism*

$$H_{\tau c}^k(X) \cong \textstyle\bigoplus_j H_{\tau c}^k(X_j).$$

(3) *$H_{\tau c}^*(X)$ is a unital algebra if and only if X is compact, in which case $H_{\tau c}^*(X) \cong H_\tau^*(X)$ naturally.*

(4) *$H_{\tau c}^*(X)$ is a covariant functor with respect to inclusions of open sets $U \subset X$.*

An $\mathcal{F}$-homotopy $h : X \times \mathbb{R} \to Y$ is *proper* if $h|_{X \times I}$ is proper.

Proposition 3.23. *Let X be a foliated space. There is a chain equivalence*

$$L : \Omega_{\tau c}^*(X \times \mathbb{R}) \xrightarrow{\simeq} \Omega_{\tau c}^{*-1}(X),$$

and hence an isomorphism

$$H_{\tau c}^*(X \times \mathbb{R}) \cong H_{\tau c}^{*-1}(X).$$

Proof. We borrow the proof from [Bott and Tu 1982, pp. 37–39]. By using tangentially smooth partitions of unity, we may assume that $X = \mathbb{R}^p \times N$, as usual. Let $\pi : X \times \mathbb{R} \to X$ be the projection. We will define the maps L above and also a chain map

$$e_* : \Omega_{\tau c}^*(X) \longrightarrow \Omega_{\tau c}^{*+1}(X \times \mathbb{R})$$

and a linear map

$$K : \Omega_{\tau c}^*(X \times \mathbb{R}) \longrightarrow \Omega_{\tau c}^{*-1}(X \times \mathbb{R})$$

with the property that

$$1 - e_* L = (-1)^q (dK - Kd) \qquad \text{and} \qquad Le_* = 1$$

on $\Omega^q_{\tau c}(X \times \mathbb{R})$, which implies the result.

The map L is defined as follows. Every tangentially smooth compactly supported form on $X \times R$ is a linear combination of forms of the following two types:

$$\text{(I)} \quad \pi^* \varphi \cdot f(x,t), \qquad\qquad \text{(II)} \quad \pi^* \varphi \cdot f(x,t)\, dt,$$

where φ is a tangentially smooth form on X, not necessarily with compact support, and $f(x,t)$ is a function of compact support. Define L by

$$\text{(I)} \quad L\big(\pi^* \varphi \cdot f(x,t)\big) = 0,$$

$$\text{(II)} \quad L\big(\pi^* \varphi \cdot f(x,t)\, dt\big) = \varphi \int_{-\infty}^{\infty} f(x,t)\, dt.$$

One verifes directly that $dL = Ld$; L is a chain map.

To define the map e_* we first choose $e = e(t)\, dt$ to be any compactly supported 1-form on $\mathbb{R}$ with total integral 1, and define

$$e_* : \Omega^*_{\tau c}(X) \longrightarrow \Omega^{*+1}_{\tau c}(X \times \mathbb{R})$$

by

$$e_*(\varphi) = (\pi^* \varphi) \wedge e.$$

(Some construction of this sort is necessary since π^* takes forms to forms that almost never have compact support. The fact that e has compact support on $\mathbb{R}$ implies that $e_*(\varphi)$ has compact support on the space $X \times \mathbb{R}$.) The map

$$K : \Omega^*_{\tau c}(X \times \mathbb{R}) \longrightarrow \Omega^{*-1}_{\tau c}(X \times \mathbb{R})$$

is defined by

$$\text{(I)} \quad K\big(\pi^* \varphi \cdot f(x,t)\big) = 0,$$

$$\text{(II)} \quad LK\big(\pi^* \varphi \cdot f(x,t)\, dt\big) = \varphi \int_{-\infty}^{t} f(x,t)\, dt - \varphi\, A(t) \int_{-\infty}^{\infty} f(x,t),$$

where

$$A(t) = \int_{-\infty}^{t} e.$$

One checks directly that

$$1 - e_* L = (-1)^q (dK - Kd) \qquad \text{and} \qquad Le_* = 1. \qquad \square$$

Theorem 3.24. *If f, g are proper $\mathcal{F}$-homotopic continuous maps then $f^* = g^*$ on $H^*_{\tau c}$.*

Proof. The homotopy may be regarded as a function $X \times \mathbb{R} \to X$ and then Proposition 3.23 implies the result. □

Corollary 3.25. *Let $h : X \to Y$ be a leaf-preserving homeomorphism. Then h induces an isomorphism*

$$h^* : H^*_{\tau c}(Y) \xrightarrow{\cong} H^*_{\tau c}(X). \qquad \square$$

Note that $H^*_{\tau c}$ is *not* an invariant of homotopy type: two spaces (even smooth manifolds foliated so as to have exactly one leaf) can be homotopy equivalent and yet have different compactly supported cohomology. The simplest example is Euclidean space, for every $\mathbb{R}^n$ is homotopy equivalent to a point, and hence to one another, but $H^*_{\tau c}(\mathbb{R}^n)$ depends upon n.

In preparation for the Thom isomorphism theorem, we introduce a third sort of cohomology which best suits the total space of vector bundles. (The book [Bott and Tu 1982] is an excellent general reference.) Suppose that $\pi : E \to X$ is a tangentially smooth real vector bundle over X with E foliated by leaves which locally are of the form

$$(\text{leaf of } X) \times E_x,$$

where $E_x = \pi^{-1}(x) \cong \mathbb{R}^n$. Let $\Omega^k_{\tau v}(E)$ be the space of those forms $\omega \in \Omega^k_\tau(E)$ which are compactly supported on each fibre E_x. Then $\Omega^*_{\tau v}(E)$ is a subcomplex; let $H^*_{\tau v}(E)$ be the associated cohomology groups. We shall refer to them as *tangential compact vertical* or more simply as *tangential vertical* cohomology groups. If X is compact then $\Omega^*_{\tau v}(E) = \Omega^*_{\tau c}(E)$ and so $H^*_{\tau v}(E) = H^*_{\tau c}(E)$; in general these groups differ.

Theorem 3.26 (Mayer–Vietoris). *Let U, V be open subspaces of the foliated space X. The Mayer–Vietoris sequence (with usual maps)*

$$0 \to \Omega^*_\tau(U \cup V) \to \Omega^*_\tau(U) \oplus \Omega^*_\tau(V) \to \Omega^*_\tau(U \cap V) \to 0$$

is exact. Hence there is a long exact sequence

$$(3.26) \qquad \cdots \to H^k_\tau(U \cup V) \to H^k_\tau(U) \oplus H^k_\tau(V) \to$$
$$\to H^k_\tau(U \cap V) \to H^{k+1}_\tau(U \cup V) \to \cdots$$

Similarly, if $\pi : E \to X$ is a tangentially smooth bundle over X, X_1 and X_2 are open sets in X and

$$X_1 \cup X_2 = X, \qquad U = \pi^{-1}(X_1) \qquad V = \pi^{-1}(X_2),$$

then the sequence

$$0 \to \Omega^k_{\tau v}(E) \to \Omega^k_{\tau v}(U) \oplus \Omega^k_{\tau v} V \to \Omega^k_{\tau v}(U \cap V) \to 0$$

is exact and so there is a long exact sequence

$$\cdots \to H^k_{\tau v}(E) \to H^k_{\tau v}(U) \oplus H^k_{\tau v}(V) \to H^k_{\tau v}(U \cap V) \to H^{k+1}_{\tau v}(E) \to \cdots$$

Proof. Let $\omega_U \in \Omega^k_\tau(U)$, $\omega_V \in \Omega^k_\tau(V)$, and suppose that

$$\omega_U|_{U\cap V} = \omega_V|_{U\cap V}.$$

Define $\omega \in \Omega^k_\tau(U \cup V)$ by

$$\omega(x) = \begin{cases} \omega_U(x) & \text{if } x \in U, \\ \omega_V(x) & \text{if } x \in V. \end{cases}$$

Then ω maps to (ω_U, ω_V). This shows exactness of the first sequence. The other verifications are as trivial. □

Proposition 3.27. *There is a natural associative continuous external product pairing*

$$\alpha : H^i_\tau(X) \otimes H^j_\tau(Y) \to H^{i+j}_\tau(X \times Y)$$

and similarly

$$\alpha_c : H^i_{\tau c}(X) \otimes H^j_{\tau c}(Y) \to H^{i+j}_{\tau c}(X \times Y)$$

respecting $H^*_{\tau c} \to H^*_\tau$.

Proof. Let

$$X \xleftarrow{\pi_x} X \times Y \xrightarrow{\pi_y} Y$$

be the projections. Define the first pairing by

$$H^i_\tau(X) \otimes H^j_\tau(Y) \xrightarrow{\pi_x^* \otimes \pi_y^*} H^i_\tau(X \times Y) \otimes H^j_\tau(X \times Y) \xrightarrow{\text{multiply}} H^{i+j}_\tau(X \times Y)$$

and similarly for $H^*_{\tau c}$. □

Proposition 3.28. *Let X be a foliated space and let M be a smooth connected manifold. Foliate $X \times M$ as (leaf of X) $\times M$. Then α induces natural continuous isomorphisms*

$$H^*_\tau(X) \otimes H^*(M) \to H^*_\tau(X \times M)$$

and

$$H^*_{\tau v}(X) \otimes H^*_c(\mathbb{R}^n) \to H^*_{\tau v}(X \times \mathbb{R}^n).$$

Proof. There is a natural isomorphism of sheaves

$$\mathcal{R}_\tau(X) \otimes \mathcal{R}_\tau(M) \cong \mathcal{R}_\tau(X \times M)$$

corresponding to the pairing α. This is clear since (on a local patch and hence globally) a function on $X \times M$ which is constant on leaves corresponds uniquely to a function on X which is constant on leaves and a constant function on M. This proves the first isomorphism. For the second we regard $X \times \mathbb{R}^n$ as a trivial bundle over X. The homotopy inverse to the Künneth pairing above is given by integration along the fibre

$$H^k_{\tau v}(X \otimes \mathbb{R}^n) \to H^{k-n}_\tau(X) \cong H^{k-n}_\tau(X) \otimes H^n_c(\mathbb{R}^n)$$

as in [Bott and Tu 1982, p. 61]. □

We fix once and for all an orientation for $\mathbb{R}^n$ and let

$$u_n \in H_c^n(\mathbb{R}^n) \cong H^n(S^n) \cong \mathbb{R}$$

be the corresponding generator. Note that there are exactly two choices for an orientation, and switching orientations corresponds with replacing u_n by $-u_n$.

Theorem 3.29. *Let X be a foliated space. Define*

$$u_n^X = \alpha(1^X \otimes u_n) \in H_{\tau v}^n(X \times \mathbb{R}^n).$$

(1) *$H_{\tau v}^*(X \times \mathbb{R}^n)$ is a free $H_\tau^*(X)$-module on u_n^X.*

(2) *If $f : X \to Y$ in $\mathcal{F}$ then $(f \times 1)^* u_n^Y = u_n^X$.*

(3) *$\bar{\alpha}(u_n^X \otimes u_m^Y) = u_{n+m}^{X \times Y}$ (explained below).*

The class u_n^X is called the *Thom class* of the trivial oriented bundle

$$X \times \mathbb{R}^n \to X.$$

The map $\bar{\alpha}$ is the composition

$$\begin{array}{ccc} H_{\tau v}^n(X \times \mathbb{R}^n) \otimes H_{\tau v}^m(X \times \mathbb{R}^m) & \xrightarrow{\alpha} & H_{\tau v}^{n+m}(X \times \mathbb{R}^n \times Y \times \mathbb{R}^m) \\ & {\scriptstyle \bar{\alpha}} \searrow & \downarrow \cong \ (\tilde{t} \text{ defined below}) \\ & & H_{\tau v}^{n+m}(X \times Y \times \mathbb{R}^{n+m}) \end{array}$$

Proof. Apply Proposition 3.28 to $X \times \mathbb{R}^n$. Then

$$H_{\tau v}^{k+n}(X \times \mathbb{R}^n) \cong \bigoplus_j H_\tau^j(X) \otimes H_c^{k+n-j}(\mathbb{R}^n) \cong H_\tau^k(X) \otimes H_c^n(\mathbb{R}^n).$$

Since $H_c^n(\mathbb{R}^n) \cong \mathbb{R}$ on u_n, the class

$$u_n^X = 1^X \otimes u_n$$

generates $H_{\tau v}^{k+n}(X \times \mathbb{R}^n)$ as an $H_\tau^k(X)$-module. This proves (1).

For (2), we compute

$$(f \times 1)^* u_n^Y = (f \times 1)^*(1^Y \otimes u_n) = f^*(1^Y) \otimes u_n = 1^X \otimes u_n = u_n^X,$$

as required.

For (3), consider the following graded commutative diagram, where t generically denotes twist maps:

$$\begin{array}{ccc}
H^0_\tau(X)\otimes H^n_c(\mathbb{R}^n)\otimes H^0_\tau(Y)\otimes H^m_c(\mathbb{R}^m) & \xrightarrow{1\otimes t\otimes 1} & H^0_\tau(X)\otimes H^0_\tau(Y)\otimes H^n_c(\mathbb{R}^n)\otimes H^m_c(\mathbb{R}^m) \\
\downarrow{\scriptstyle \alpha\otimes\alpha} & & \downarrow{\scriptstyle \alpha\otimes\alpha} \\
H^n_{\tau v}(X\times\mathbb{R}^n)\otimes H^m_{\tau v}(Y\times\mathbb{R}^m) & & H^0_\tau(X\times Y)\otimes H^{n+m}_c(\mathbb{R}^{n+m}) \\
\downarrow{\scriptstyle \alpha} & & \downarrow{\scriptstyle \alpha} \\
H^{n+m}_{\tau v}(X\times\mathbb{R}^n\times Y\times\mathbb{R}^m) & \xrightarrow{\tilde{t}} & H^{n+m}_{\tau v}(X\times Y\times\mathbb{R}^{n+m})
\end{array}$$

Then

$$\begin{aligned}
\bar{\alpha}(u^X_n\otimes u^Y_m) &= \tilde{t}\alpha(u^X_n\otimes u^Y_m) \\
&= \tilde{t}\alpha(\alpha\otimes\alpha)(1^X\otimes u_n\otimes 1^Y\otimes u_m) \\
&= \alpha(\alpha\otimes\alpha)(1\otimes t\otimes 1)(1^X\otimes u_n\otimes 1^Y\otimes u_m) \\
&= \alpha(\alpha\otimes\alpha)(1^X\otimes 1^Y\otimes u_n\otimes u_m) \\
&= \alpha(1^{X\times Y}\otimes u_{n+m}) \qquad\qquad (\text{since } \alpha(u_n\otimes u_m)=u_{n+m}) \\
&= u^{X\times Y}_{n+m}.
\end{aligned}$$

□

Theorem 3.30 (Thom Isomorphism Theorem). *For any compact foliated space X and for any tangentially smooth real oriented n-plane bundle $p: E\to X$ there is a unique Thom class $u_E\in H^n_{\tau c}(E)$ with the following properties:*

(1) *If $f: X\to X'$ in $\mathcal{F}$ and E' is a real oriented bundle over X', then*

$$f^*u_{E'} = u_E.$$

(2) *Let $x\in X$ and let E_x denote the fibre over X in E. Then the inclusion $E_x\subset E$ induces a map*

$$H^n_{\tau c}(E)\to H^n_c(E_x)\cong H^n_c(\mathbb{R}^n)$$

under which u_E is sent to u_n.

The $\mathbb{K}$-algebra $H^*_{\tau c}(E)$ is a free $H^*_\tau(X)$-module on the Thom class u_E; precisely, there is a continuous Thom isomorphism

(3.31)
$$\Phi_\tau : H^k_\tau(X) \xrightarrow{\cong} H^{n+k}_{\tau c}(E)$$

given by

(3.32)
$$\Phi_\tau(\omega) = u_E\omega.$$

If E and E' are bundles over X as above then

$$u_{E\oplus E'} = u_E u_{E'}.$$

If E' denotes the bundle E with its orientation reversed then $u_{E'} = -u_E$.

Proof. We shall establish the Thom theorem in somewhat greater generality than stated above. Let us say that a bundle E over X is *r-trivial* if there exist a finite open cover $X_1, \ldots, X_r$ of X such that the bundle E is trivial when restricted to any X_i. We shall prove that the Thom theorem in the form

$$\Phi_\tau : H^k_\tau(K) \xrightarrow{\cong} H^{n+k}_{\tau v}(E)$$

holds for X a foliated space (compact or not) and $E \to X$ any oriented r-trivial bundle. This implies Theorem 3.30 since if X is compact then every vector bundle over X is r-trivial for some r and also

$$H^*_{\tau v}(E) \cong H^*_{\tau c}(E).$$

We proceed by induction on r. If $r = 1$ then E is a trivial bundle. Theorem 3.29 establishes the existence and uniqueness of the classes $u^X_n \equiv u_E$ with the properties (1) and (2) compatible with orientation. Suppose inductively that for all bundles E' which are k-trivial for some $k < r$ we have shown uniqueness of the Thom class $u_{E'}$ compatible with orientations. Let $\pi : E \to Y$ be an oriented bundle which is oriented r-trivial, via open sets $X_1, \ldots, X_r$. Let $U = \pi^{-1}(X_1 \cup \cdots \cup X_{r-1})$ and $V = \pi^{-1}(X_r)$. Then U and V are open sets in E with $E = U \cup V$. The Mayer–Vietoris sequence of Theorem 3.26 yields the long exact sequence

$$\cdots \to H^{n-1}_{\tau v}(U \cap V) \to H^n_{\tau v}(E) \to H^n_{\tau v}(U) \oplus H^n_{\tau v}(V) \to H^n_{\tau v}(U \cap V) \to \cdots.$$

Since $U \cap V \subset \pi^{-1}(X_r)$ we have

$$U \cap V \cong \big((X_1 \cup \cdots \cup X_{r-1}) \cap X_r\big) \times \mathbb{R}^n.$$

Thus $H^{n-1}_{\tau v}(U \cap V) = 0$ by Corollary 3.25. By induction, the classes

$$u^U_n \in H^n_{\tau v}(U) \qquad \text{and} \qquad u^V_n \in H^n_{\tau v}(V)$$

exist and are unique, and they each restrict to the class

$$u^{U\cap V}_n \in H^n_{\tau v}(U \cap V),$$

by uniqueness and orientability. Exactness of the Mayer–Vietoris sequence implies that there is a unique class $u_E \in H^n_{\tau v}(E)$ which maps to (u^U_n, u^V_n). This establishes the existence and uniqueness of the Thom classes u_E for all r-trivial bundles E. Define

$$\Phi_\tau : H^k_\tau(X) \to H^{n+k}_{\tau v}(E)$$

by $\Phi_\tau(\omega) = u_E\omega$. This is a continuous isomorphism on trivial bundles, by Corollary 3.29. A Mayer–Vietoris argument which we omit (see [Bott and Tu 1982, p. 64]) implies that Φ_τ is an isomorphism for all r-trivial bundles. □

Remark. Let $E \to X$ be a tangentially smooth real oriented n-plane bundle over the space X. Let $z : X \to E$ be the zero-section. Define

$$\tilde{e}_\tau(E) \in H^n_\tau(X)$$

by

$$\tilde{e}_\tau(E) = z^* u_E.$$

The class $\tilde{e}_\tau$ is called the *tangential Euler class* of the bundle. Similarly we may construct tangential Chern classes and the tangential Chern character in this manner. Since u_E lies in cohomology with real or complex (but not integer) coefficients, characteristic classes constructed in this manner are not visibly integral classes. We shall pursue this theme in Chapter V.

Our final topic in this chapter is the introduction of tangential homology. Recall that the tangential forms $\Omega^k_\tau(X)$ and $\Omega^k_{\tau c}(X)$ have been topologized by demanding that in all coordinate patches we have uniform convergence of the functions $a(x_1, \ldots, x_p, n)$ together with all their derivatives in the tangential direction on compact subsets of the coordinate patch. The differential d is continuous. Define

$$\Omega^\tau_k(X) = \mathrm{Hom}_{\mathrm{cont}}(\Omega^k_{\tau c}(X), \mathbb{R}), \tag{3.33}$$

where $\mathrm{Hom}_{\mathrm{cont}}$ denotes *continuous* homomorphisms. Elements $c \in \Omega^\tau_k$ are called *tangential currents*. The natural differential

$$d_* : \Omega^\tau_k \to \Omega^\tau_{k-1}$$

is given by

$$\langle \omega, d_* c \rangle = (-1)^{k-1} \langle d\omega, c \rangle,$$

where $c \in \Omega^\tau_k$, $\omega \in \Omega^{k-1}_\tau$, and $\langle \cdot, \cdot \rangle$ denotes the evaluation of a current $c \in \Omega^\tau_*$ on a form ω. (Our sign convention dictates that forms are placed on the left, currents on the right, in $\langle \omega, c \rangle$.) It is immediate that $d_*^2 = 0$. Let $\Omega^{\tau c}_k \subset \Omega^\tau_k$ be those currents which have compact support in the obvious sense. This is a differential submodule. Define *tangential homology* by

$$H^\tau_k(X; \mathbb{R}) = \frac{\mathrm{Ker}\, d_* : \Omega^\tau_k \to \Omega^\tau_{k-1}}{\mathrm{Im}\, d_* : \Omega^\tau_{k+1} \to \Omega^\tau_k}, \tag{3.34}$$

and similarly for $H^{\tau c}_*(X; \mathbb{R})$.

Proposition 3.35. (1) *Each H^τ_k is a covariant functor from foliated spaces and tangentially smooth maps to real (or complex) vector spaces and continuous homomorphisms.*

(2) *If f and g are tangentially homotopic maps $X \to Y$ then*

$$f_* = g_* : H^\tau_*(X; \mathbb{R}) \to H^\tau_*(Y; \mathbb{R}).$$

(3) *The pairings*

$$\langle\cdot,\cdot\rangle : \Omega^*_\tau \otimes \Omega^{\tau c}_* \to \mathbb{R} \qquad \textit{and} \qquad \langle\cdot,\cdot\rangle : \Omega^*_{\tau c} \otimes \Omega^{\tau}_* \to \mathbb{R}$$

induce continuous pairings

$$\langle\cdot,\cdot\rangle : H^*_\tau(X;\mathbb{R}) \otimes H^{\tau c}_*(X:\mathbb{R}) \to \mathbb{R},$$
$$\langle\cdot,\cdot\rangle : H^*_{\tau c}(X:\mathbb{R}) \otimes H^{\tau}_*(X,\mathbb{R}) \to \mathbb{R}$$

and an isomorphism

$$H^\tau_k(X) \cong \mathrm{Hom}_{\mathrm{cont}}(H^k_{\tau c}(X), \mathbb{R}).$$

(4) *If $X = M$ foliated as one leaf then*

$$H^\tau_*(X;\mathbb{R}) \cong H_*(X;\mathbb{R}).$$

All of these results continue to hold if $\mathbb{R}$ is replaced by $\mathbb{C}$.

Proof. Only (3) requires comment. Compactness (on one side or the other) guarantees that the pairings exist at the chain level. There is a natural continuous pairing

$$(\text{cocycles}) \otimes (\text{cycles}) \to \mathbb{R}$$

given by evaluation. If $\omega = d\omega'$ then

$$\langle\omega, c\rangle = \langle d\omega', c\rangle = \pm\langle\omega', d_*c\rangle$$

But $d_*c = 0$ since c is a cycle; thus $\langle\omega, c\rangle$ vanishes. Similarly, if c is a boundary we have

$$\langle\omega, c\rangle = \langle\omega, d_*c'\rangle = \pm\langle d\omega, c'\rangle = 0.$$

since $d\omega = 0$. Thus there are pairings as indicated. The isomorphism comes on purely algebraic grounds from the fact that $\mathrm{Hom}_{\mathrm{cont}}(\cdot, \mathbb{R})$ is an exact functor. □

□ □□□□□□

Here we rephrase the construction of the tangential de Rham complex so as to make the algebraic essentials of the construction clear and to show the essential unity of this construction with ordinary Lie algebra cohomology. In this we will be following what is folklore. We start with a pair consisting of a commutative associative algebra A over a field k and a Lie algebra L also over k. We assume that we have a representation of L as a Lie algebra of derivations of A, and we write the action of $\Theta \in L$ on an element $a \in A$ as just $\Theta(a)$. We further assume that L as a linear space is a module over A, but not that L is a Lie algebra over A. Rather one assumes

$$[\Theta, b\psi] = b[\Theta, \psi] + \Theta(b)\psi, \tag{3.36}$$

where $a\psi$ is left multiplication of $a \in A$ on $\psi \in L$. We call (A, L) a *Lie-assocative pair*. Note that if $\Theta(b) = 0$ for all Θ and b and then L is a Lie algebra over A. A *module* M for the pair (A, L), called an (A, L)*-module*, is simply a vector space over k with a module structure for A and with a representation of L on M (as vector space) satisfying

$$\begin{aligned} \Theta(am) &= a \cdot \Theta(m) + \Theta(a) \cdot m, \\ (a\Theta)(m) &= a(\Theta(m)) \quad \text{for } a \in A, \Theta \in L, m \in M, \end{aligned} \tag{3.37}$$

where $\Theta(m)$ is the Lie algebra action and $b \cdot m$ is the left module action.

Proposition 3.38. *The algebra A itself, given the structure of A module by left multiplication, and the defining representation of L as derivations of A, is an* (A, L) *module.*

Proof. That the key identities (3.37) are satisfied in the first case is just the fact that L is given to act as derivations of A. □

As noted previously this structure already contains ordinary Lie algebras by taking for instance $A = k$ in which case modules as defined above are ordinary L modules. However, the motivating example for this is given by a C^∞ manifold X, with $A = C^\infty(X)$ and L the C^∞ vector fields. More generally X could be a foliated space with A the tangentially smooth functions $C_\tau^\infty(X)$ and L the tangentially smooth sections of the tangent bundle $\Gamma_\tau(FX)$. That L is a Lie algebra under commutator brackets is immediate.

The immediate point here is to define cohomology groups $H^*(M)$ for any (A, L) module M so that in the first example above ($A = k$) one obtains usual Lie algebra cohomology while in the second example, one obtains the usual de Rham cohomology of X and in the third example one obtains the tangential cohomology. The construction is patterned exactly on the classical Koszul complex [Mac Lane 1963] and the construction of differential forms. If M is an (A, L) module we let $C_A^p(L, M)$ or for short $C^p(M)$ denote the space of all alternating p-linear, *A-linear* maps from L to M. A differential $C^p(M) \to C^{p+1}(M)$ is defined as usual by

$$\begin{aligned} D\phi(\Theta_0, \ldots, \Theta_p) &= \sum_{i=0}^{p} (-1)^i \Theta_i(\phi(\Theta_1, \ldots, \hat{\Theta}_i, \ldots, \Theta_p)) \\ &\quad + \sum_{i<j} (-1)^{i+j} \phi([\Theta_i, \Theta_j], \Theta_1, \ldots, \hat{\Theta}_i, \ldots, \hat{\Theta}_j, \ldots, \Theta_p). \end{aligned} \tag{3.38}$$

What requires checking is that $d\phi$ is actually A linear since none of the individual terms on the right are A linear. Use of the basic identities (3.37) for A, L, and M produces the necessary cancellations. We omit the details. It is also evident that $d^2 = 0$ and so one as usual defines cohomology groups $H_A^p(L, M)$

or for short $H^p(M) = Z^p(M)/B^p(M)$, where $Z^p(M)$ is the kernel of d in $C^p(M)$ and $B^p(M)$ is the image of d from $C^{p-1}(M)$.

It is an easy matter to check that in the case $A = k$, this yields the usual Lie algebra cohomology of the module M as the formulas (3.38) are the standard ones [Mac Lane 1963]. It is equally easy to see that if $A = C^\infty(X)$, and L the C^∞ vector fields on X, then the cohomology $H_A^*(L, A) = H^*(A)$ is the usual de Rham cohomology of X because $C^*(A)$ is visibly the de Rham complex of differential forms with its usual differential. In the same way, when $A = C_\tau^\infty(X)$ is the tangentially smooth functions on a foliated space and L is the C^∞ tangentially smooth tangential vector fields, then $H^*(A)$ is also visibly the tangential cohomology as defined in Chapter III.

□ □□□□□ □□□□

There has been a steady use of tangential cohomology — both in the sense of this chapter and in the more traditional sense — since the first edition of this book. What is much more interesting, though, is the idea of obtaining information directly from the holonomy groupoid of the foliated space using other functors. This work is represented by two papers. In the first, [Moerdijk 1997], the author shows that the classifying space of an étale groupoid G (such as the holonomy groupoid of a complete transversal of a foliated space) is weakly equivalent to a small (discrete) category. He then shows that for any system L of coefficients on the classifying space BG of the groupoid, there is a natural isomorphism

$$H^n(BG; L) \cong H^n(G^0; \hat{L}),$$

where $\hat{L}$ is the associated sheaf on the unit space G^0 and the right-hand side denotes an appropriate sheaf cohomology theory. In [Crainic and Moerdijk 2000], the authors introduce an associated sheaf homology theory for étale groupoids. Quoting from their abstract: "We prove its invariance under Morita equivalence, as well as Verdier duality between Haefliger cohomology and this homology. We also discuss the relation to the cyclic and Hochschild homology of Connes' convolution algebra of the groupoid, and derive some spectral sequences which serve as a tool for the computation of these homologies."

In a different direction, Heitsch and Hurder [2001] take Roe's coarse cohomology theory [Higson et al. 1997; Roe 1996] and generalize it to the foliation setting.

CHAPTER IV

Transverse Measures

In this chapter we concentrate upon the measure theoretic aspects of foliated spaces, including especially the notion of transverse measures.

We begin with a general study of groupoids, first in the measurable and later in the topological context. Our examples come from the holonomy groupoid of a foliated space (2.20) and a discrete version corresponding to a complete transversal. We introduce transverse measures ν with a given modulus and discuss when these are invariant.

Next we look in the tangential direction, defining a tangential measure λ to be a collection of measures $\lambda = \{\lambda^x\}$ (one for each leaf in the case of a foliated space) which satisfies certain invariance and smoothness conditions. For instance, a tangential, tangentially elliptic operator D yields a tangential measure ι_D as follows. Restrict D to a leaf ℓ. It follows from Chapter I that Ker D_ℓ and Ker D_ℓ^* are locally finite-dimensional and hence the local index

$$\iota_{D_\ell} = \mu_{D_\ell} - \mu_{D_\ell^*}$$

is defined as a signed Radon measure on ℓ. (A priori it would seem that ι_D depends on the domains Dom D_ℓ but in Chapter VII we shall demonstrate that ι_D is well-defined.) Then $\iota_D = \{\iota_{D_\ell}\}$ is a tangential measure. Tangential measures, suitably bounded, correspond to integrands: if λ is a tangential measure and ν is an invariant transverse measure then $\lambda\, d\nu$ is a measure on X and $\int \lambda\, d\nu \in \mathbb{R}$ is defined.

Next we specialize to topological groupoids and continuous Radon tangential measures. In the case of a foliated space we recount the Ruelle–Sullivan construction of a current associated to a transverse measure and we show that the current is a cycle if and only if the transverse measure is invariant.

Finally we prove a Riesz representation theorem for (signed) invariant transverse measures on a foliated space X; they correspond precisely to elements of the topological vector space $(\overline{H}_\tau^p(X))^*$.

A groupoid, whose main feature is a partially defined associative multiplication, is best understood by two extreme special cases — a group on the one hand, and an equivalence relation on the other. We need say no more about groups, but if $\mathcal{R}$ is an equivalence relation on a set X so that $\mathcal{R}$ is a subset of $X \times X$, one can construct a partially defined associative multiplication on $\mathcal{R}$ so that it becomes a groupoid. Specifically if $u = (x, y)$ and $v = (w, z)$ are two elements of $\mathcal{R}$, the product uv is defined exactly when $y = w$, and then $uv = (x, z)$. It is suggestive to define the range of an element $u = (x, y)$, denoted $r(u)$, to be the first coordinate x and the source of u, denoted $s(u)$ to be the second coordinate y. Then uv is defined precisely when $r(v) = s(u)$. Intuitively one might think of the pair (x, y) as something starting at y and going to x so that multiplication is in some way a kind of composition.

If X is a foliated space, there is an obvious equivalence relation on X defined by the leaves, but as we saw in Chapter II a foliated space has associated to it something more, namely its graph $G(X)$ or as it is also called, the holonomy groupoid of X. This is but one example where a Borel or topological groupoid presents itself naturally—another is when one has a topological group acting on a space where the action is not necessarily free. Thus we are led to the notion of a groupoid:

Definition 4.1. A *groupoid* G with unit space X consists of the sets G and X together with several maps:

(1) $\Delta : X \to G$ (the diagonal or identity map);

(2) an involution $i : G \to G$, called inversion and written $i(u) = u^{-1}$;

(3) range and source maps $r : G \to X$ and $s : G \to X$;

(4) an associative multiplication m defined on the set G' of pairs $(u, v) \in G \times G$ such that $r(v) = s(u)$; one writes $m(u, v) = u \cdot v$ or just uv.

These maps must satisfy the obvious conditions

$$r(\Delta(x)) = x = s(\Delta(x)),$$
$$u \cdot \Delta(s(u)) = u = \Delta(r(u)) \cdot u,$$
$$r(u^{-1}) = s(u), \qquad m(u, u^{-1}) = \Delta(r(u)).$$

Alternatively, one could define a groupoid as a small category where every map has an inverse. At all events, if X is reduced to a single point, G is simply a group with identity element $\Delta(x)$, $X = \{x\}$. In general the maps r and s together yield a map $\Phi : u \to (r(u), s(u))$ of G into $X \times X$. The image of this map is an equivalence relation on X in view of the axioms above. If this map is injective, then G as a groupoid is (isomorphic to) this equivalence relation; G is called *principal* if this happens. In any case this shows that associated to any groupoid there is always a principal groupoid (i.e., an equivalence relation). A general groupoid can be viewed as a mixture or combination of this equivalence relation $\mathcal{R}$ and the other extreme case of a groupoid, namely a group.

Define

$$\begin{aligned} G_x &= \{u : s(u) = x\}, \\ G^y &= \{u : r(u) = y\}, \\ G_x^y &= G_x \cap G^y, \\ G_Y^Z &= \{u \mid r(u) \in Z, s(u) \in Y\}. \end{aligned}$$

Then G_x^x is immediately seen to be a group with identity element $\Delta(x)$. The sets G_y^x for $(x, y) \in \mathcal{R}$ are principal homogeneous spaces for G_x^x and G_y^y with G_x^x acting on the left and G_y^y acting on the right. In particular for $(x, y) \in \mathcal{R}$, G_x^x and G_y^y are isomorphic. Thus the groupoid G appears as a kind of fibre space over the equivalence relation $\mathcal{R}$ as base and with the group-like objects G_x^y as fibres. This is exactly the geometric structure that the holonomy groupoid of Chapter II displayed. Indeed we will often refer to the groups G_x^x as holonomy groups. They can also be thought of as "isotropy groups" because of another important example of groupoids coming from group actions. If a group H acts as a group of transformations on a space X, the set $G = H \times X$ becomes a groupoid, as George Mackey has emphasized in his seminal papers [1963; 1966]. The unit space is X; $\Delta(x) = x$; the range and source maps are $s(h, x) = x$, $r(h, x) = h \cdot x$, where $h \cdot x$ is the result of the group element h acting on the point x. The inverse of (h, x) is the $(h^{-1}, h \cdot x)$. Two points (g, y) and (h, x) are multipliable when $y = h \cdot x$ and then $(g, y) \cdot (h, x) = (gh, x)$. Finally the holonomy group G_x^x is visibly just the isotropy group $\{h : h \cdot x = x\}$ of the action at x.

Now that the purely algebraic structure of groupoids has been described, we impose the extra conditions appropriate for the analytic and geometrical applications.

Definition 4.2. A (standard) *Borel groupoid* (see [Mackey 1966] or [Ramsay 1971]) is a groupoid G such that G and its unit space are Borel spaces—that is, come equipped with a σ-field of sets—so that the defining maps Δ, r, s, i and m are Borel.

The set X becomes, via the diagonal map Δ, a subset of G, and it will have the relative Borel structure because Δ and r are Borel maps. (In principle it would not be necessary to separately assume that X was a Borel space.) The subset G' of $G \times G$, where m is defined, is given the product Borel structure. We will assume throughout that the Borel space G is a standard Borel space. This means that G with its Borel σ-field is isomorphic to a Borel subset of a complete and separable metric space given its Borel σ-field. The reader is referred to [Mackey 1966; Arveson 1976; Bourbaki 1958] for futher discussion of this important and pervasive regularity condition for Borel spaces. It is a condition that can be easily checked in the examples to be treated.

Proposition 4.3. *The graph $G(X)$ of a foliated space* (Definition 2.20 on p. 46) *with the σ-field generated by the open sets is a standard Borel groupoid.*

Proof. In case the graph $G(X)$ is Hausdorff, this is obvious for it is a locally compact Hausdorff second countable space and can be given a separable complete metric. In general $G(X)$ may be covered by a countable numer of open sets U_i each of which is locally compact, Hausdorff and second countable. It is easy to see that a subset E of $G(X)$ is Borel if and only if $E \cap U_i$ is Borel for all i. Since each U_i is standard as a Borel space, it follows easily that $G(X)$ is standard. □

We will impose two further conditions on our standard Borel groupoid G, both of which are very natural and immediate in the context of foliated spaces. First we shall assume that *each holonomy group G_x^x is countable.* The second condition revolves around the notion of a transversal.

Definition 4.4. If G is a standard Borel groupoid with unit space X and associated equivalence relation $\mathcal{R}$, a Borel subset S of X is called a *transversal* if S intersects each equivalence class of $\mathcal{R}$ in a countable set. (For us countable shall mean finite or countably infinite.) A transversal is *complete* if it meets every equivalence class.

If $\mathcal{R}$ is a countable standard Borel equivalence relation in the sense of [Feldman and Moore 1977] (that is, the equivalence classes are countable), then of course any Borel subset is a transversal. As we shall see, the existence of a complete Borel transversal for a general G ensures that it can be built up in a simple way from a countable standard equivalence relation.

We shall forthwith assume that $\mathcal{R}$ *always has a complete* (*Borel*) *transversal.* Note that for foliated spaces the existence of such sets is an immediate consequence of the definitions. In dealing analytically with transversals, we will have need of a very helpful result about Borel spaces that is not too well known.

Theorem 4.5. *Let X and Y be standard Borel spaces and let f be a Borel map from X into Y with property that $f^{-1}(y)$ is countable for each y. Then X can be written as the disjoint union of Borel subsets U_i so that f is injective on each U_i. Moreover $f(X)$ is a Borel subset of Y.*

We shall not include a proof. The reader is referred to the discussion in [Kuratowski 1966, Section 35, VII]. A proof may be found in [Hahn 1932, p. 381]. See also [Purves 1966].

We list some consequences of this result that will be relevant for us.

Proposition 4.6. *Let G be a standard Borel groupoid with countable holonomy groups.*

(1) *The equivalence relation $\mathcal{R}$ is a Borel subset of $X \times X$, hence a standard space.*

(2) *If S is a Borel transversal, the saturation $\mathcal{R}(S)$ of S with respect to the equivalence relation $\mathcal{R}$ is a Borel subset of X.*

(3) *If S is as in* (2), *there is a Borel map f from $\mathcal{R}(S)$ to S with $f(x) \sim x$.*

Proof. (1) The map $G \to X \times X$ given by $u \to (r(u), s(u))$ is Borel and countable to one, that is, the inverse image of any point in $X \times X$ is at most countable. Hence its image $\mathcal{R}$ is Borel.

(2) Recall that the saturation of a set S is the set of all points equivalent to a member of S. Let W be the subset of $X \times X$ given by $(S \times X) \cap \mathcal{R}$. By (1) W is a Borel set. Now let p be the projection map to the second factor. The image of W under p is nothing else but $\mathcal{R}(S)$, and since S is a transversal p on W is countable to one. Hence $p(W)$ is Borel by Theorem 4.5.

(3) By the first part of the theorem, we may with a little cutting and pasting construct a subset U of W above so that p is injective on U and $p(U) = p(W) = \mathcal{R}(S)$. Then define a map f of $\mathcal{R}(S)$ into S by the condition that $f(x)$ is the unique point so that $(f(x), x) \in U$. The graph of f is a Borel function, and it follows that f itself is Borel [Auslander and Moore 1966, Chapter I]. This is the desired function. □

The existence of a complete Borel transversal in a standard Borel groupoid G guarantees by part (3) of the proposition that the equivalence relation $\mathcal{R}$ of G is built up in a very simple way from a countable standard equivalence relation. To see this, note that a complete Borel transversal S in X defines a countable standard equivalence $\mathcal{R}_S$ on S itself:

$$\mathcal{R}_S = (S \times S) \cap \mathcal{R}.$$

The map f guaranteed by Proposition 4.6(3) from X to S with $f(x) \sim x$ displays X as a fibre space over S so that $\mathcal{R}$ is also fibred over $\mathcal{R}_S$ in the sense that two points of X are $\mathcal{R}$-equivalent if and only if their images under f are $\mathcal{R}_S$-equivalent. We shall exploit this structural representation heavily in our discussion of transverse measures.

We observe that not every standard Borel groupoid $\mathcal{R}$ satisfies our condition on the existence of a complete Borel transversal. The turbulent equivalence relations [Hjorth 2000] provide examples.

Mackey [1966], followed by many others (see [Ramsay 1971]), introduced and studied the notion of measured groupoids; these are by definition standard Borel groupoids with one more additional datum, namely a Borel measure or better an equivalence class of Borel measures on the groupoid. This class of measures has to satisfy an invariance property that reduces in the case of a principal groupoid (an equivalence relation) to the condition that $\theta_* \mu$ be equivalent to μ, where μ is any measure in the class, and θ is the flip $\theta(x, y) = (y, x)$ on the equivalence relation and $\theta_* \mu$ is the image of the measure μ under the map θ. The condition in general is somewhat more complicated but basically the same.

Definition 4.7. A measure μ on a standard Borel groupoid G is *quasi-invariant* if $\phi_*\mu$ is quasi-invariant on $\mathcal{R}$, where $\mathcal{R}$ is the principal groupoid associated to G and ϕ is the projection map $G \to \mathcal{R}$ and if, when μ is disintegrated over $\phi_*(\mu)$ into measures μ_x^y on the fibres G_x^y of the maps ϕ, then for almost all pairs (x, y) in $\mathcal{R}$, each μ_x^y is quasi-invariant under the action of the groups G_x^x and G_y^y.

In the present case when the holonomy groups G_x^x are countable this last condition can be rephrased more simply as the condition that for almost all (x, y) μ_x^y gives positive mass to each point in the countable set G_x^y. Note that $r_*(\mu)$ is equivalent to $s_*(\mu)$ and defines an equivalence class of measures on the unit space of X.

Although we have seen that a standard Borel groupoid may fail to have a complete transversal, an important result of Ramsay [1982] shows that a standard measured Borel groupoid does have such a transversal up to null sets.

Theorem 4.8. *Let G be a standard measured Borel groupoid with unit space X. Then there is a Borel subset Y of X conull for the natural measure (class) on X defined by the measure μ on G and a subset T of Y which is a complete Borel transversal for the groupoid*

$$G_Y = r^{-1}(Y) \cap s^{-1}(Y).$$

That is, T is a transversal for the original equivalence relation on X and meets every equivalence class of that relation which has a nonempty intersection with the conull subset Y.

Thus while the results to follow concerning transverse measures which all assume the existence of a complete transversal on the groupoid do not strictly apply to a measured groupoid, they will apply after one deletes an inessential null set from the unit space. Our point of view in that discussion is that *all* the points count and that one cannot delete or ignore null sets, especially when one is dealing, as we shall later, with locally compact groupoids.

The discussion to follow concerning tranvservse and tangential measures can be interpreted as an analysis of a measure on a groupoid into a product (in a Fubini type sense) of a part tangential to the orbits of the groupoid times a part transverse to the orbits. The transverse part is thus in some vague sense a measure on the space of orbits of the groupoid.

Let us now turn to the crucial topic of transverse measures. If G is a standard Borel groupoid (or more particularly an equivalence relation $\mathcal{R}$ on X) a transverse measure provides, at least intuitively, a method of integrating some kind of object over the set of equivalence classes of the principal groupoid $\mathcal{R}$

associated to G — that is over the quotient space $X/\mathcal{R}$. This quotient space is in general a very pathological space from the point of view of measure theory, containing subsets like $\mathbb{R}/\mathbb{Q}$, the real numbers modulo the rational numbers. If the quotient space $X/\mathcal{R}$ with its quotient Borel structure were a standard or even analytic Borel space (e.g., if G were to come from a foliation given by the fibres of a fibre bundle) then transverse measures would be really just ordinary measures on $X/\mathcal{R}$. For general foliations, transverse measures suitably defined have played an important role for years. In addition, as pointed out in [Connes 1979], one has to rethink one's concept of what sort of functions are suitable integrands for integrating against a transverse measure.

We will treat something a bit more general than what traditionally in the theory of foliations is called a transverse measure; transverse measures here will involve a modular function analogous to the modular function on a locally compact group. When this modular function is identically one, as is traditional in foliation theory, the transverse measure will be called invariant. Hence what in foliations is called a transverse measure, we shall call an *invariant transverse measure*.

The modular function above is simply a homomorphism from the groupoid to the group of positive real numbers $\mathbb{R}^+$ under multiplication. A homomorphism of a groupoid G to a group H (or indeed to another groupoid) is a map ϕ from G to H so that when uv is defined $\phi(u)\phi(v)$ is defined and is equal to $\phi(uv)$. When G and H are standard Borel groupoids, one insists naturally that ϕ be a Borel map. For the purposes at hand we fix a Borel homomorphism, denoted by Δ, of G into the group $\mathbb{R}^+$. We further assume that Δ is holonomy invariant in that $\Delta(u)$ depends only on $r(u)$ and $s(u)$. Put another way, there is a homomorphism Δ' of the principal groupoid (equivalence relation) $\mathcal{R}$ associated to G so that

$$\Delta(u) = \Delta'(p(u)),$$

where

$$p(u) = (r(u), s(u))$$

is the projection of G onto the equivalence relation $\mathcal{R}$.

We now consider the case when G (or $\mathcal{R}$) has countable equivalence classes. In view of our standing hypothesis that all holonomy groups are countable, the range and source maps r and s are countable to one. In [Mackey 1966], the notion of a quasi-invariant measure on X with given Radon–Nikodým derivative (or modulus) Δ is discussed, at least in the case of trivial holonomy groups; see also [Feldman and Moore 1977]. The discussion extends without change; namely we start with a measure ν on X quasi-invariant under $\mathcal{R}$ in the sense that a subset E of x is ν-null if and only if its $\mathcal{R}$ saturation — again a Borel set by Proposition 4.6 — is also ν-null. As r is countable to one, there is a unique measure ν_r on $\mathcal{R}$ which is the integral of the counting measures on the fibres of the map r over the base X. Specifically if $|C|$ is the cardinality of C, then

$$\nu_r(S) = \int_X |S \cap r^{-1}(x)|\, d\nu(x).$$

There is a similar measure ν_s defined using the source map s instead of r. As in [Feldman and Moore 1977], these measures are mutually absolutely continuous and the Radon–Nikodým derivative

$$\Delta = \frac{d\nu_r}{d\nu_s}$$

is called the *modulus* of ν. This function on G is readily seen to depend only on the projection of G onto $\mathcal{R}$. As a function on G or $\mathcal{R}$ the modulus Δ is a homomorphism up to null sets in that

$$\Delta(uv) = \Delta(u)\Delta(v)$$

for almost all u and v in the obvious sense.

We return to the case of a general standard Borel groupoid with countable holonomy groups and a complete Borel transversal. We observe that the set of all Borel transversals $\mathcal{S}$ is indeed a σ-ring, but not in general a σ-field, of subsets of X. A transverse measure will be simply a measure on this σ-ring. For each $S \in \mathcal{S}$ we can form the restriction of G to S,

$$G_S^S = \{u \in G \mid r(u), s(u) \in S\}.$$

This is a groupoid which has countable orbits and countable holonomy groups of the kind discussed a moment ago.

There is a subtle point here about whether or not Δ is constant on the holonomy groups G_x^x. There will be instances later on when we specifically will want to allow Δ to be nonconstant on some holonomy groups G_x^x; the point is that this cannot happen for too many x's, because Δ is equal almost everywhere to the Radon–Nikodým derivative of $\nu|_S$ on G_S^S, and this implies, after some null set manipulations, that Δ is constant on G_x^x for $\nu|_S$-almost all $x \in S$.

Definition 4.9. By a *transverse measure* with modulus Δ on a standard Borel groupoid we understand a measure ν on the σ-ring of Borel transversals $\mathcal{S}$ such that $\nu|_S$ is σ-finite for each $S \in \mathcal{S}$ and $\nu|_S$ is quasi-invariant on G_S^S with modulus equal to Δ almost everywhere on G_S^S. If $\Delta = 1$, one says that ν is an *invariant transverse measure*.

A transverse measure allows one to talk consistently about what it means for a set L of equivalence classes of the equivalence relation $\mathcal{R}$ to have measure zero. The condition is that the intersection of the leaves in L with each Borel transversal S should be contained in some $\nu|_S$ Borel null set, or equivalently that this should happen for a single complete Borel transversal. Since the modulus of a quasi-invariant measure is constant on holonomy groups, we conclude from this discussion that Δ is constant on the holonomy groups of almost all leaves.

As an example of a transverse measure we consider the Kronecker foliation on the two-torus T^2 where the leaves are of the form

$$\{(e^{2\pi i(x+x_0)}, e^{2\pi i\lambda x}) | x \in \mathbb{R}\}$$

with λ irrational. Regard the two-torus as the square

$$\{(x, y) \mid 0 \le x < 1, 0 \le y < 1\},$$

and for each ρ with $-\lambda < \rho \le 1$ let ℓ_ρ be the part of the line $y = \lambda x + \rho$ inside the square described above. Any Borel transversal S must meet each ℓ_ρ in at most a countable set. If $n(\rho)$ is the cardinality of $S \cap \ell_\rho$, then n is obviously a Borel function. We define ν by the formula

$$\nu(S) = \int_{-\lambda}^{1} n(\rho)\, d\rho.$$

It is not difficult to verify that this produces an invariant transverse measure for the graph of this foliation. If instead one defined

$$\nu(S) = \int_{-\lambda}^{1} n(\rho) f(\rho)\, d\rho$$

for some positive Borel function f, the result would be a transverse measure with modular function

$$\Delta((x_1, y_1), (x_2, y_2)) = \frac{f(y_1 - \lambda x_1)}{f(y_2 - \lambda x_2)}.$$

Recall that given a diffeomorphism ϕ of F then one may form as in (2.3) its suspension $M = \mathbb{R} \times_{\mathbb{Z}} F$, which is foliated with leaves of dimension 1. An invariant transverse measure for M corresponds to a ϕ-invariant measure on F. More generally, in the situation (2.2) of a manifold with discrete structural group

$$M = \widetilde{B} \times_{\pi_1(B)} F$$

an invariant transverse measure on M corresponds to a measure on F which is invariant under the action $\pi_1(B) \to \mathrm{Homeo}(F)$.

Also let us consider the very special case when $G = \mathcal{R}$ is an equivalence relation coming from a Borel map p of X onto a standard Borel space B — in other words, a fibration. Here $x \sim y$ if and only if $p(x) = p(y)$. We let $\Delta = 1$ so we are looking for invariant transverse measures. If $\tilde{\nu}$ is a measure on the base B then if N is transversal we define

$$\nu(N) = \int \left| N \cap p^{-1}(b) \right| d\tilde{\nu}(b).$$

It is clear that ν so defined on the σ-ring of transversals is an invariant transverse measure. Conversely we claim every such ν is of this form. To see this, observe that the assumed existence of a complete transversal yields by Proposition 4.6 the existence of a Borel cross section S for the map p. It follows that p maps S bijectively onto B; by [Kuratowski 1966] it is therefore a Borel isomorphism. If ν is an invariant transverse measure on X, ν gives in particular an ordinary measure on S. This may be transported to B via $p \mid S$ to give a measure $\tilde{\nu}$ on B. Then it is an easy exercise to see that ν on any transversal N is given by the formula above in terms of $\tilde{\nu}$ and $|N \cap p^{-1}(b)|$.

It is well to extend the remarks above a bit to observe that ν is determined by what happens on any complete transversal.

Proposition 4.10. *For any standard Borel groupoid with countable holonomy and unit space X, a transverse measure ν of modulus Δ is completely determined by $\nu|_N$, where N is any complete transversal. Conversely, if ν_N is a transverse measure on N with modulus $\Delta|_N$, there exists a (unique) transverse measure on X with modulus Δ.*

Proof. By Proposition 4.6 we construct a Borel map t from X to N with $f(x) \sim x$. If S is any transversal, f restricted to S, $f|_S$, is a countable to one map of S to N; then assuming we know $\nu|_N = \nu_N$ for some transverse measure, we can immediately calculate ν on S given the invariance properties in terms of $\Delta(f(s), s)$ as follows:

$$\nu(S) = \int_N \left(\sum_s \Delta(t, s) \right) d\nu_N(t),$$

where for each t the sum is taken over all s with $f(s) = t$. This shows that ν on N determines ν altogether.

Conversely if we are given a transverse measure ν_N on N, we use the same formula to extend ν_N to all transversals. It is a simple calculation to show that the result is a transverse measure on X. □

If X is a foliated manifold with oriented transverse bundle, there is a canonical transverse measure class given by the volume element on q-dimensional transverse submanifolds. This may or may not be an invariant transverse measure (class).

A transverse measure on a general groupoid in this formulation is really an ordinary measure but is defined on a σ-ring $\mathcal{S}$ instead of a σ-field. The measure could of course be extended to the σ-field generated by $\mathcal{S}$ but this extension would in general be impossibly non-σ-finite as a measure on the entire space. (If the entire groupoid has countable orbits then a transverse measure is just an ordinary (σ-finite) measure on the unit space.) These facts make a huge difference in the type of object that can be integrated in general against a transverse measure.

We insert here several diverse examples of foliated spaces which yield interesting classes of (primarily Type III) von Neumann algebras. In Chapter VI we shall consider the question of exactly which von Neumann algebras may be realized as the von Neumann algebras of foliated spaces.

Let $G = \mathrm{SL}(2,\mathbb{R})$, let Γ be a discrete cocompact subgroup, and let $M = G/\Gamma$ be the resulting compact 3-dimensional manifold. Foliate M by the left action of the triangular subgroup

$$B = \begin{pmatrix} a & 0 \\ b & a^{-1} \end{pmatrix}, \quad a > 0.$$

The orbits are two-dimensional, hence this is a codimension 1 foliation of M. Each leaf is dense. In fact, if one lets

$$A = \begin{pmatrix} 1 & 0 \\ b & 1 \end{pmatrix}$$

act instead (this is called the horocycle flow), then each leaf is still dense. The foliation arising from A has an invariant transverse measure. However, there is *no* invariant transverse measure at all for the foliation which arises from the action of B. The associated von Neumann algebra is a III_1 factor [Bowen 1978].

Here is an example, due to Furstenberg [1961], of a 1-dimensional foliation of a 3-dimensional manifold. It is built by first defining a $\mathbb{Z}$ action on a 2-manifold and then suspending it to make an $\mathbb{R}$ action on a 3-manifold.

Let $M = \mathbb{T}\times\mathbb{T}$ be the 2-torus and let ζ be an irrational number. Let

$$\phi(x,y) = (e^{2\pi i\zeta}x, g(x)y),$$

where x, y are complex numbers of absolute value 1 and

$$g : \mathbb{T} \to \mathbb{T}$$

is a function at our disposal. We construct g by first defining

$$h(x) = \sum_{k\neq 0} \frac{1}{k} e^{2\pi i n_k \zeta},$$

where n_k is a sequence of integers tending to ∞ at our disposal. Observe that

$$k(x) = h(e^{2\pi i\zeta}x) - h(x) = \sum_{k\neq 0} \frac{1}{k}(e^{2\pi i n_k\zeta} - 1)e^{2\pi i n_k \zeta}.$$

Now pick ζ and n_k such that, say,

$$|e^{2\pi i n_k\zeta} - 1| < r^{n_k} \qquad \text{some } r < 1.$$

This is possible for suitable ζ, but such ζ's are not very common—they are highly Liouville; alternatively one could make

$$|e^{2\pi i n_k \zeta} - 1| = O(n_k^{-r}) \quad \text{for all } r > 0.$$

Then consider

$$g(x) = e^{it(h(e^{2\pi i\zeta}x) - h(x))}$$

for suitable t as our g. First of all, if $k(x) = h(\zeta x) - h(x)$, then k is real analytic under the stronger of the two conditions above ($|e^{2\pi i n_k \zeta} - 1| < r^{n_k}$) and C^∞ under the weaker condition. Hence $\phi(x, y)$ is real analytic or C^∞, respectively. It is a theorem of Furstenberg [1961], whose proof is not hard, that if we choose ϕ in this way, then

(1) ϕ is minimal if and only if one cannot factor any power of g as

$$g^m(x) = u(e^{2\pi i\zeta}x)/u(x)$$

for a continuous function $u : \mathbb{T} \to \mathbb{T}$, and

(2) ϕ is ergodic with respect to Lebesgue measure if one cannot factor any power of g as

$$g^m(x) = u(e^{2\pi i\zeta}x)/u(x)$$

for a measurable function $u : \mathbb{T} \to \mathbb{T}$.

Now the function g is cooked up so that

$$g(x) = e^{ith(e^{2\pi i\zeta}x)}/e^{ith(x)},$$

where t is at our choice. For all t the transformation is not ergodic, hence not uniquely ergodic. However, if one could factor as above, the factorization would be unique up to a constant, as ζ is irrational and rotation by ζ is ergodic on $\mathbb{T}$. So if one could factor g (or any power of g), the factorization would have the same form as above. Hence ϕ will be minimal for given t provided that we can be assured that $e^{ith(x)}$ is *not* continuous. If this is continuous for all t, it is easy enough to see that $h(x)$ is continuous (and conversely, of course). But h is *not* continuous because the Fourier series of $h(x)$ would then be Cesàro summable to h for every x. Then we would have

$$h(1) = \sum_{k \neq 0} \frac{1}{k} \quad \text{(Cesàro sum)},$$

which is nonsense, since this is a sum of positive terms.

So ϕ is minimal—each orbit is dense, but (for suitable choice of g and ζ) ϕ is not ergodic. Now form the suspension of ϕ to obtain a one-dimensional foliation of the 3-torus which has corresponding properties. A transversal is of course M with the equivalence relation induced by powers of ϕ. This is a real analytic foliation. There are a continuum of ergodic invariant transverse measures of this foliation — in fact they are indexed by the circle. Each is singular with respect to Lebesgue measure and in the foliation case live on a measurable *but not* topological 2-torus inside the manifold. Measure theoretically this foliation looks like a Kronecker foliation on the 2-torus with angle ζ crossed with a circle — nothing happening in the transverse direction here. The invariant ergodic transverse measures are just the measures on the copies of the Kronecker torus in this product structure.

Here is an example by Connes [1978, p. 150] of a foliation whose von Neumann algebra is of type III_λ for some fixed λ with $0 < \lambda < 1$. Let S be a circle of length s, let $X = \mathrm{SL}(2,\mathbb{R})/\Gamma$ for a discrete cocompact subgroup Γ, and let $Y = S \times X$. Act on Y by the group of matrices of the form

$$\begin{pmatrix} e^t & 0 \\ b & e^{-t} \end{pmatrix}$$

for $t, b \in \mathbb{R}$, where

$$\begin{pmatrix} 1 & 0 \\ b & 1 \end{pmatrix}$$

acts trivially on S and by the horocycle action on X, and

$$\begin{pmatrix} e^t & 0 \\ 0 & e^{-1} \end{pmatrix}$$

acts by a rotation of speed 1 on S and by the geodesic flow on X. The resulting foliation has a von Neumann algebra of type III_λ, where $\lambda = e^{-s}$. If S is replaced by a space K of dimension at least 2 with an ergodic action then a III_0 factor results.

With these examples in hand, we return to the general development. The next order of business is the introduction of appropriate integrands to pair with transverse measures.

By way of motivation to see what the appropriate integrands are, we consider the case when G is an equivalence relation on X with each equivalence class consisting of one point. As noted, a transverse measure ν is an ordinary measure; one uses a (nonnegative) Borel function f on X as integrand. Instead of looking at f as a function on X, we view f as an assignment to each equivalence class of G (i.e., each point of X), of a measure living on that equivalence class. The measure attached to $\{x\}$ is of course $f(x)\delta_x$, where δ_x is the Dirac measure at x. Moreover, we regard the process of integration as first passing from the integrand f to the measure $f \cdot \nu$ on X, where

$$(f \cdot \nu)(E) = \int_E f \, d\nu,$$

and then passing to the total mass of $f \cdot \nu$ to obtain a real number — the integral of f.

This point of view guides us in the general case: the proper integrand for a transverse measure ν on a standard Borel groupoid G will be a family of measures $\{\lambda^\ell\}$, one on each "leaf" of the groupoid. If G is an equivalence relation this is simply an assignment $\ell \to \lambda^\ell$ of a (nonnegative, σ-finite) measure λ^ℓ on each equivalence class ℓ of the equivalence relation. This map $\ell \to \lambda^\ell$ should be Borel in an obvious but tedious sense that we shall not write down.

If for example G has countable orbits, there is a very natural such family of measures; namely, λ^ℓ is counting measure on the (countable) set ℓ. For the Kronecker foliations discussed above, each orbit is an affine real line; that is, the real line without an origin specified. On such affine lines we can simultaneously normalize Haar measure to obtain a family $\{\lambda^\ell\}$ of the type described. Finally if $\mathcal{R}$ is any standard equivalence relation and if S if a Borel transversal, we can define a family $\{\lambda^\ell\}$ by letting λ^ℓ be the counting measure on the countable set $T \cap \ell$, viewed as a measure on ℓ.

Definition 4.11. A *tangential measure* $\lambda = \{\lambda^\ell\}$ for an equivalence relation $\mathcal{R}$ is an assignment of (nonnegative) measures $\lambda \mapsto \lambda^\ell$ as above.

This was all for a principal groupoid (an equivalence relation). The presence of holonomy complicates matters a bit, but the complication is largely notational. Recall that the inverse images of the range map r are denoted $G^x = r^{-1}(x)$. A tangential measure on G is first an assignment of a (σ-finite) measure λ^x on G^x for each x in a Borel fashion subject to an invariance condition. For equivalence relations, when $x \sim y$, $r^{-1}(x)$ is actually the same as $r^{-1}(y)$ and we demanded that $\lambda^x = \lambda^y$ $(= \lambda^\ell)$, where ℓ is the common equivalence class of x and y. In general the requirement is that

$$\int f(uu')\, d\lambda^x(u') = \int f(u')\, d\lambda^y(u')$$

for every $u \in G_x^y$ $(= r^{-1}(y) \cap s^{-1}(x))$ and every nonnegative Borel function f on G. Since the meaning of this formula is not immediately transparent, we rephrase it more geometrically. Each set G^x is acted upon by the group G_x^x which acts freely from the left by groupoid multiplication. The quotient space $G_x^x \backslash G^x$ is canonically identified to the equivalence class $\ell(x)$ of the corresponding principal groupoid (equivalence relation) associated to G. If $y \sim x$ with respect to $\mathcal{R}$, then each element of G_x^y defines a bijection of G^x onto G^y; moreover G_x^y is acted upon freely by G_x^x on the right and G_y^y on the left again using groupoid multiplication. By associativity, the transformations of G_x^y intertwine the actions of G_x^x on G^x and G_y^y on G^y so that the quotient spaces $G_x^x \backslash G^x$ and $G_y^y \backslash G^y$ can be identified. The identification is independent of the element in G_x^y and when these two sets are further identified with $\ell(x)$ and $\ell(y)$ respectively, the mapping becomes the identity map between $\ell = \ell(x)$ and $\ell = \ell(y)$, the common equivalence classes of x and y under $\mathcal{R}$.

The invariance condition expressed by the integral formula above says first of all that each λ^x on G^x is invariant under the left action of G_x^x for all x, and furthermore that elements of G_x^y, viewed as mappings from G^x to G^y, carry λ^x onto λ^y. We see now that the standing hypothesis of countability of G_x^x allows us to simplify the situation. By a choice of cross section, G^x can be viewed as the product $G_x^x \times \ell(x)$, and using counting measure on G_x^x, there is a bijection between measures on $\ell(x)$ and G_x^x-invariant measures on G^x which is independent of the cross section. Thus if λ^x is a choice of G_x^x invariant measures on G^x, $x \in X$, with corresponding measures $\tilde{\lambda}^x$ on $\ell(x)$, the further invariance under G_x^y for a tangential measure means that $\tilde{\lambda}^x = \tilde{\lambda}^y$ if $x \sim y$. Hence $\tilde{\lambda}^x = \tilde{\lambda}^\ell$ if $x \in \ell$ defines a tangential measure on $\mathcal{R}$, the associated principal groupoid. Summarizing, we obtain the following observation, which allows us better to understand tangential measures in general.

Proposition 4.12. *If G is a standard Borel groupoid with countable isotropy groups and $\mathcal{R}$ is the corresponding equivalence relation, then the map $\lambda \to \tilde{\lambda}$ defined above is a bijection from tangential measures on G to tangential measures on $\mathcal{R}$.*

To illustrate further the notion of a tangential measure when there is nontrivial holonomy present, consider the example of a groupoid G coming from the action of a locally compact group H on a Borel space X. Recall that elements of G are pairs (h, x) and that the range map is $r(h, x) = h \cdot x$. If we fix a point $x_0 \in X$, then $r^{-1}(x_0)$ can be represented as

$$r^{-1}(x_0) = \{(h, h^{-1}x_0) \mid h \in H\}$$

and we use the first coordinate to parametrize this set. If y_0 is equivalent to x_0, so that $y_0 = h_0 \cdot x_0$, then $r^{-1}(y_0)$ can be represented as the set

$$r^{-1}(y_0) = \{(k, k^{-1}y_0) \mid k \in H\}$$

and elements of $G_{x_0}^{y_0}$ are of the form $(h_0 h_1, x_0)$, where h_1 is in the isotropy group of x_0. Groupoid multiplication shows that the map from G^{x_0} to G^{y_0} is

$$(h, h^{-1}x_0) \mapsto (h_0 h_1 h, h^{-1}h_1^{-1}h_0^{-1}y_0).$$

Hence in terms of the parameters on these spaces, the map is left translation. Therefore a suitable choice of tangential measure would be λ^x equal to left Haar measure on H transported over to $r^{-1}(x)$ as indicated above. There are evidently many other choices also.

Ultimately we will want to consider tangential measures of mixed sign. In outline the notion is clear, but there are technical dificulties because generically the measures λ^ℓ (or λ^x) will be infinite measures. Indeed one sees easily that for an equivalence relation $\mathcal{R}$, the existence of a tangential measure with λ^ℓ finite for each ℓ implies that the equivalence relation $\mathcal{R}$ is smooth; that is, the quotient space $X/\mathcal{R}$ is an analytic Borel space [Arveson 1976, p. 71]. Since infinite signed measures cause problems in this general context, one would only want to discuss tangential measures of mixed sign in the presence of some topological assumptions.

Let us now turn to the integration process, which is related to the Ruelle–Sullivan pairing [1975]. Begin with a standard Borel groupoid G together with a transverse measure ν with modulus Δ and a tangential measure λ. The integration process is going to produce first a measure μ, written $d\mu = \lambda\, d\nu$, on the unit space X whose total volume

$$\mu(X) = \int \lambda\, d\nu$$

will be the integral of the tangential measure with respect to the transverse measure. To define these objects we first fix a complete Borel transversal S, which exists by our standing hypothesis. By Proposition 4.6 we find a Borel function f from X to S with $f(x) \sim x$. Next we observe by Proposition 4.12 that we may as well assume that $G = \mathcal{R}$ is principal. Then for each point $s \in S$ we define a measure ρ_s on $f^{-1}(s)$ as the restriction of $\lambda^{\ell(s)}$ to $f^{-1}(s) \subset \ell(s)$, the equivalence class of s. The modular function Δ of ν comes to us as a function on G_S^S, but we have observed that if we stay away from a ν-null set of equivalence classes of the relation $\mathcal{R}$, then Δ is constant on holonomy groups, and is almost everywhere really a function on $\mathcal{R}$. In the present context, this means that there is a saturated null set N of S so that $\Delta(s, x)$ is well defined whenever $s \notin N$. That is the meaning of the function appearing in the integral below, which defines the measure $\mu = \int \lambda\, d\nu$ on X, the result of integrating λ against the transverse measure ν:

$$\int_E \lambda\, d\nu = \mu(E) = \int \left(\int_{f^{-1}(s)} \Delta(s, x) \chi_E(x) d\rho_s(x) \right) d\nu(s)$$

for any Borel set E in X. The first remark is that this is independent of the choice of the complete transversal S and of the function f from X to S. The presence of the modular function Δ in the above formula is exactly what is needed to achieve this, and we omit the simple calculation.

The resulting measure μ on X is thus well defined and depends only on the data given, the transverse measure ν of modulus Δ and the tangential measure λ. Its total mass is written as

$$\mu(X) = \int_X \lambda\, d\nu.$$

In the most primitive special case of an equivalence relation on X given by a fibration p of a space X over a base space B, we have seen already that a transverse measure ν with modulus $\Delta = 1$ is exactly a measure on the base

B, and that a tangential measure is a family of measures $\{\lambda^b\}$, one on each fibre $p^{-1}(b)$. The integral $\lambda\, d\nu$ is the usual construction of a measure on the total space X from a measure on the base and measures on the fibres. The formula given above in the general case makes the general situation very similar intuitively to the fibration case. Indeed the total space X is fibred measure theoretically over the transversal S, instead of a base space B; the picture is quite similar:

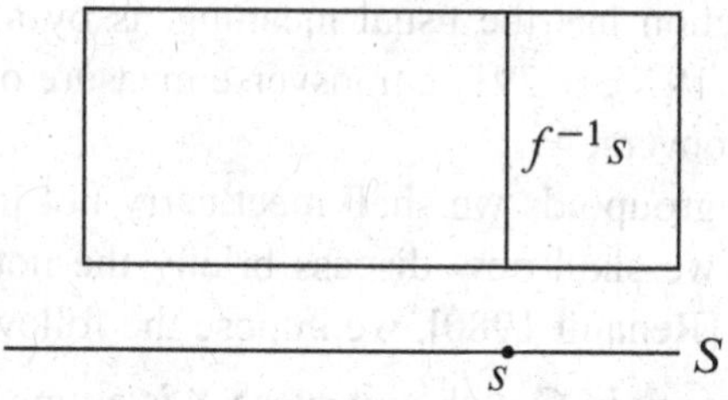

In accord with the notion that a transverse measure ν on G is in some sense a measure on the orbit space X/G, we have already remarked that it is possible to say what it means for a Borel set of orbits to be a null set of orbits. This is clear for a Borel set of orbits corresponds to a Borel set E in the unit space which is saturated or invariant with respect to the equivalence relation $\mathcal{R}$ of G.

Definition 4.13. An invariant Borel set E in X is a *ν-null set* if every transversal in E has ν measure zero.

Using this definition it is easy to define an ergodic transverse measure; a transverse measure is ergodic if whenever $X = E_1 \cup E_2$, where E_i are invariant Borel sets, then it follows that one of them is a ν-null set. In addition one has as usual a type classification of ergodic transverse measures into type I, II, and III. Indeed if N is a complete transversal then $(\mathcal{R}_N, N, \nu|_N)$ is an ergodic countable standard measured equivalence relation which has a type classification [Feldman and Moore 1977]. In the type II case, one may have different transversals, where one is type II_1 while another is type II_∞. Hence there is no meaningful distinction between these types and one has one class of type II transverse measures. As usual one may further divide the type III case into the III_λ $0 \le \lambda \le 1$ subtypes by the type classification of the discrete versions $(\mathcal{R}_N, N, \nu|_N)$. For some examples of type III_λ factors, see [Connes 1978, pp. 149–150].

Further, a general transverse measure ν can be displayed as a continuous sum of ergodic components. To see this, one makes an ergodic decomposition of $(N, \nu|_N)$ and then uses the projection map p of Proposition 4.6 of all of X on N to decompose ν itself. By construction, all of the groupoids appearing as disintegration products will have complete transversals.

Throughout this entire discussion the modular function Δ has remained fixed. If we change the modular function to a new one Δ' which is however in the same cohomology class, that is

$$\Delta'(u) = \Delta(u)b(r(u))b(s(u))^{-1},$$

where b is some Borel function on X into the strictly positive real numbers, then there is no essential difference between transverse measures of modulus Δ and transverse measures of modulus Δ'. Indeed if ν is a transverse measure of modulus Δ, then $b \cdot \nu$, where multiplication of a (transverse) measure by a positive Borel function has the usual meaning, is by a simple computation [Feldman and Moore 1977, p. 291] a transverse measure of modulus Δ', where Δ' is as above, and conversely.

Since most of the groupoids we shall meet carry not just a Borel structure, but also a topology, we shall now discuss briefly the notion of a topological groupoid. Following [Renault 1980], we impose the following conditions.

Definition 4.14. A groupoid G with unit space X is a *topological groupoid* if G and X are topological spaces and the following conditions hold.

(1) The set where the partially defined multiplication is defined is closed in $G \times G$ and multiplication is continuous.

(2) The range and source maps are open and continuous.

(3) The inversion map is a homeomorphism.

For our discussion G and X will be assumed to be locally compact, in which case we will say that G is a locally compact (topological) groupoid. Ordinarily one would automatically assume that G and X are Hausdorff and most of the time in the sequel we will have this as a standing assumption. However the reader should be aware that there are a number of interesting, natural, and significant examples where a non-Hausdorff structure is forced upon one. The graph of the Reeb foliation discussed in Chapter II is one such example. All interesting examples known to us satisfy the following condition that could be used in place of the Hausdorff condition:

(4) X is Hausdorff and G is *locally Hausdorff*, that is, it has a cover consisting of open sets each of which is Hausdorff.

We remark that if $G = \mathcal{R}$ is an equivalence relation, then $\mathcal{R}$ is a subset of $X \times X$; yet the topology of $\mathcal{R}$ will not be the relative topology from $X \times X$. For instance, if we consider the Kronecker equivalence relation $\mathcal{R}$ on the circle $\mathbb{T}^1$, given by

$$\xi \sim \xi e^{2\pi i n\lambda} \quad \text{for } n \in \mathbb{N},$$

with λ some fixed irrational number, then $\mathcal{R}$ as a subset of $\mathbb{T}^1 \times \mathbb{T}^1$ is a line of irrational slope in the two-torus. To make it a locally compact groupoid one has to give $\mathcal{R}$ the usual topology of the real line.

The prime example we have in mind is the graph of a foliation, at least when it is Hausdorff, as described in Chapter II. If H is a locally compact group acting as a topological transformation group on a locally compact Hausdorff space X, then the groupoid $H \times X$ described earlier in this chapter becomes a locally compact topological groupoid.

Finally, the following simple example displays for us in a discrete context the need for introducing the graph of a foliation. On the real line $\mathbb{R}$ consider the equivalence relation $\mathcal{R}$, where $x \sim 2^{-n}x$ for all $n \in \mathbb{Z}$. In spite of the simplicity of this, the equivalence relation $\mathcal{R}$ does not admit any reasonable locally compact topology. The trouble comes near $(0,0) = \rho_0$, where $\mathcal{R}$ appears to have an infinite number of line segments all passing through this point:

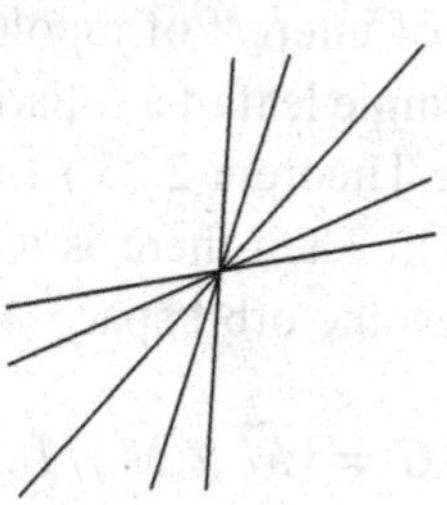

If however we introduce points p_n which are formally the limits of $(x, 2^{-n}x)$ as $x \to 0$ with n fixed, we can visualize this new object G as an infinite set of (parallel) real lines:

$$\vdots$$

$$\underline{\hspace{4cm}}_{p_1} = \{(x, x/2)\}$$

$$\underline{\hspace{4cm}}_{p_0} = \{(x, x)\}$$

$$\underline{\hspace{4cm}}_{p_{-1}} = \{(x, 2x)\}$$

$$\vdots$$

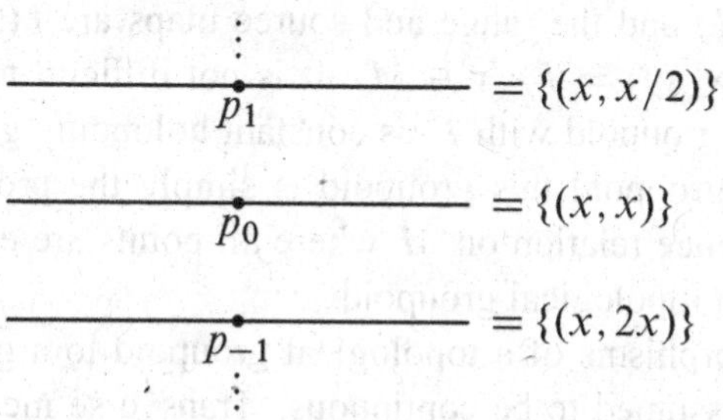

It is easy to see that G may be turned into a locally compact topological groupoid. Indeed it is a discrete version of the graph construction for a foliation. We remark that if we modify the equivalence relation $\mathcal{R}$ by saying that $x \sim x$ for $x < 0$ and $x \sim 2^{-n}x$ all n, for $x \geq 0$, then this construction leads to a non-Hausdorff graph-like object

$$\overline{\hspace{3cm}}_{p_1}$$

$$\underline{\hspace{4cm}}_{p_0} = \{(x, x)\}$$

$$p_{-1} \underline{\hspace{3cm}}$$

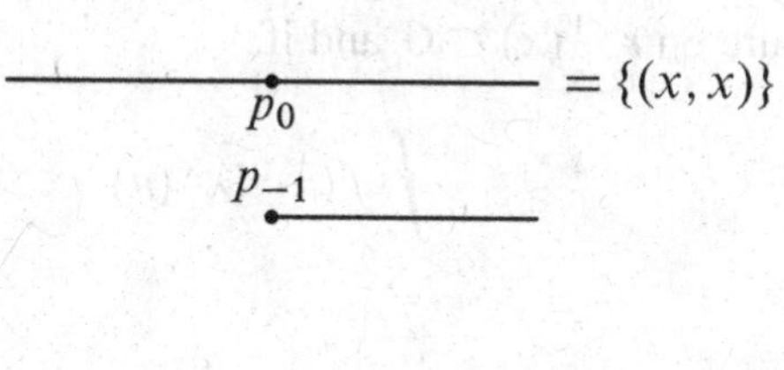

where a neighborhood of p_1 is a small interval containing p_1 and extending to the right of p_1 plus a small interval to the left of p_0 (but not including p_0) which has already arisen in Chapter II.

In both examples it is clear that Lebesgue measure is a quasi-invariant measure. It would be natural to hope that the modular function Δ could be fixed up to be continuous. A simple calculation shows that on the n-th horizontal line in these examples Δ is almost everywhere equal to 2^n. Hence in the first example we can make Δ continuous, but then over the point 0 it is nonconstant on the holonomy group G_0^0. This happens only on a null set (namely, one point!), in accord with our earlier discussion. In the second example we see that Δ cannot be constructed so as to be continuous.

Another class of examples of interest of topological groupoids are ones that arise from the holonomy of a single leaf of a foliation. (Compare with the bundle construction in Chapter II; see Theorem 2.25.) Let M be a manifold and let Γ be a quotient group of $\pi_1(M)$. Then there is a covering $\widetilde{M}$ of M with deck group Γ, and we identify M as the orbit space $\widetilde{M}/\Gamma$. We form

$$G = (\widetilde{M} \times \widetilde{M})/\Gamma,$$

where Γ is acting diagonally. Two Γ-orbits $\Gamma \cdot (x, y)$ and $\Gamma \cdot (z, w)$ are multipliable if $\Gamma \cdot y = \Gamma \cdot z$; we define their product to be $\Gamma \cdot (\gamma_1 \cdot x, \gamma_2 \cdot w)$, where γ_1 and γ_2 are elements of Γ so that $\gamma_1 \cdot y = \gamma_2 \cdot z$. The unit space is the original manifold M, and the range and source maps are $r(\Gamma \cdot (x, y)) = \Gamma \cdot x \in M$, and $s(\Gamma \cdot (x, y)) = \Gamma \cdot y \in M$. It is not difficult to see that this produces a topological groupoid with Γ as constant holonomy group. One easily sees that as a Borel groupoid this groupoid is simply the product of the group Γ and the equivalence relation on M where all points are equivalent, but it is *not* the product as a topological groupoid.

Homomorphisms of a topological groupoid to a group or another groupoid should be assumed to be continuous. Transverse measures will be assumed to have continuous modular functions.

In the context of topological groupoids there is a special kind of tangential measure of interest. If we recall that tangential measures are objects to be integrated against transverse measures and hence are analogues of functions, it makes sense to try to define, in analogy with a continuous function, a continuous tangential measure.

Definition 4.15. We say that a tangential measure λ is *continuous* if each λ^x is a Radon measure on $r^{-1}(x) \subset G$ and if

$$\int f(u)\, d\lambda^x(u)$$

is continuous in x for every continuous function f of compact support in G. This is appropriate if G is Hausdorff. If G is only locally Hausdorff we demand instead that the integral above be continuous in x when f is compactly supported inside some Hausdorff open set and is continuous there. Such a function f need not be even continuous on all of G.

As an example consider the case of a G arising from a locally compact group H acting topologically on a locally compact space X. We saw earlier in this chapter that the assignment $x \to \lambda^x$, where λ^x is Haar measure on H, carried over to $r^{-1}(x) = \{(h, h^{-1}x)\}$ by the map $h \to (h, h^{-1}x)$ is a tangential measure. Evidently this is also a continuous tangential measure.

An obvious item of concern is to find conditions on a transverse measure ν and a tangential measure λ so that the integral $\lambda\, d\nu$ produces a *finite* measure on X. Rather than taking this question up in this general context we shall take it up in the more special context of primary interest when G is the graph of a foliation. We turn to that case now.

So assume that X is a locally compact foliated space with G the graph of the foliation, which we assume is Hausdorff. Then G is itself a foliated space as described in Chapter II with leaves equal to the holonomy groupoids of the leaves of the original foliation. All homomorphisms θ of G to a Lie group and in particular to $\mathbb{R}^+$ will be assumed to be tangentially smooth on the foliated space G in the sense of Chapter II.

Now suppose that ν is a transverse measure on X of modulus Δ. As suggested previously, the notion of ν being a Radon measure, to the extent that this can be defined in general, would be a condition demanding that ν be finite on some distinguished set of compact transversals. But in a foliated space there is a distinguished set of compact transversals given by the foliation structure.

Definition 4.16. Call a transversal C *open-regular* if there is an open set L in $\mathbb{R}^p$, where p is the dimension of the foliation, and an isomorphism ϕ of foliated spaces of $L \times C$ onto an open subset of X, which is the identity on C. A transversal C is *regular* if it is contained in an open-regular transversal.

If U_x is one of the coordinate patches in the definition of the foliation so that $U_x \cong L_x \times N_x$, with L_x open in $\mathbb{R}^p$, then any compact subset of N_x is a compact *regular* transversal. Our definition of a Radon transverse measure involves finiteness of these transversals.

Definition 4.17. A transverse measure ν on a topological groupoid is *Radon* if $\nu(C)$ is finite for every compact regular transversal.

We observe that in order to check this condition, it will suffice to check finiteness on a much smaller family of compact regular transversals. For instance, let C_i be a family of such transversals with maps ϕ_i of $L_i \times C_i$ into X, and suppose that there are relatively open subsets of C_i, $U_i \subset \overline{T}_i \subset V_i \subset C_i$ so that the open sets $\phi_i(L_i \times U_i)$ cover X.

Proposition 4.18. *If $\nu(C_i)$ is finite for each i for such a family, then ν is Radon.*

Proof. Let B be any compact regular transversal with a map ϕ of $L \times D$ into X with $D \supset B$. By covering argument and by shrinking L if necessary we may assume that $\phi(L \times B)$ lies inside some $\phi_i(L_i \times V_i)$ and has compact closure there. The projection mapping to the second coordinate of $L_i \times V_i$ gives rise to a continuous map f of B to V_i so that b and $f(b)$ lie in the same plaque of the coordinate neighborhood $L_i \times V_i$. Using the geometry of this situation, we easily show that there is an integer n so that $f^{-1}(b)$ has at most cardinality n. Now using the quasi-invariance properties of transverse measures, we can calculate $\nu(B)$ by the formula

$$\nu(B) = \int_{f(b)} \left(\sum_{f(b)=x} \Delta(b, x) \right) d\nu(x).$$

Since the modulus Δ is a continuous function, it is bounded; and because

$$\{(b, f(b)) : b \in B\}$$

is compact, the integrand is bounded. Since $f(B) \subset V_i \subset C_i$, the value of $\nu(f(B))$ is finite and we are done. □

It is evident of course that a Radon transverse measure is completely determined by what it does on regular transversals. For instance, the union $C = \bigcup_i C_i$ in the proposition above is a complete transversal and if ν is known on C_i, it is known on the union C and then knowledge of ν on a complete transversal determines the transverse measure entirely.

Up to now transverse measures have always been positive measures. However at this point we are in a position to consider signed or even complex transverse measures. We simply take differences or complex linear combinations of (positive) *Radon* transverse measures. Such an object cannot be defined on all transversals, but clearly it can be defined on regular transversals.

Definition 4.19. *A signed or complex transverse Radon measure of modulus Δ is a real or complex linear combination of positive Radon transverse measures of modulus Δ defined on all finite unions of regular transversals.*

By our remarks above to the effect that a positive Radon transversal measure, viewed as a measure on all transversals, is completely determined by what it is on regular transversals, the domain we have specified for signed or complex Radon transverse measures is surely large enough. They can be expanded of course to a somewhat larger class of transversals without confronting expressions like $\infty - \infty$, but not in general to all transversals. We shall make use of these objects only briefly in connection with the Riesz Representation Theorem (4.27) for compact foliated spaces.

On the graph of a foliation of X we can construct tangential measures of particular interest. Each set $r^{-1}(x)$ is itself a C^∞ manifold, and so has a unique equivalence class of measures, those equivalent to nonvanishing densities. As each set $r^{-1}(x)$ is a covering space of the leaf ℓ_x of x in the foliation, and as tangential measures are invariant under the deck group, giving a tangential measure λ^x (as we have already noted in Proposition 4.11) is the same as giving measures $\tilde{\lambda}^\ell$, one for each leaf ℓ.

To construct such measures, cover X by coordinate charts of the form $L_i \times N_i$, where L_i is an open ball in $\mathbb{R}^p$ and let λ_i be tangential measure on the foliated space $L_i \times N_i$, where λ_i^n is for $n \in N_i$, normalized Legesgue measure on (L_i, n). Now choose a partition of unity θ_i subordinate to the covering and define $\tilde{\lambda}$ to be the sum $\sum \theta_i \lambda_i$. Then we lift $\tilde{\lambda}^\ell$ on each leaf ℓ to a unique measure λ^x on $r^{-1}(x)$ using counting measure on the fibres of the covering map. Proposition 4.12 implies that $\lambda = \{\lambda^x\}$ satisfies the invariance properties required and thus is a tangential measure.

Proposition 4.20. *The tangential measure just constructed is a continuous tangential measure (with G Hausdorff or locally Hausdorff).*

Proof. We have to check the continuity of

$$x \mapsto \int f(u)\, d\lambda^x(u)$$

for each f of compact support on G for G Hausdorff. Using partitions of unity we may localize the support of f so that it lies within a subset K of G on which the map (r, s) is injective into a subset of $X \times X$ contained in $\mathrm{Supp}(\theta_i) \times \mathrm{Supp}(\theta_j)$ for suitable (i, j), where θ_i is the original partition of unity used to define λ. One easily verifies the continuity of the integral as a function of x for such f. One proceeds similarly in the locally Hausdorff case. □

If we perform the construction using different coordinate charts, or using different partitions of unity, we obtain a tangential measure λ_1 which is equivalent to λ in the sense that λ_1^x is mutually absolutely continuous with respect to λ^x on $r^{-1}(x)$. The Radon–Nikodým derivative $d\lambda_1/d\lambda$ is a continuous nonvanishing function on G which one can check is bounded from 0 and ∞ not just on compact subsets of G but also on any set $r^{-1}(C)$, C compact in X. In terms of this we may define local boundedness of a tangential measure.

Definition 4.21. A tangential measure λ' is *locally bounded* (*Lebesgue*) if $(\lambda')^x$ has a Borel density on $r^{-1}(x)$ for each x and if $d\lambda'/d\lambda$ is bounded on any set $r^{-1}(C)$, C compact, for one (and hence any) tangential measure λ of the kind constructed above by partitions of unity. If the unit space is compact, we will for simplicity call such a measure a *bounded tangential measure.*

With these definitions the desired finiteness result is quite straightforward.

Proposition 4.22. *If ν is a Radon transverse measure on the graph G of a foliated space X, and if λ is a locally bounded (Lebesgue) tangential measure, then for any compact set K of X the integral $\mu(K) = \int_K \lambda\, d\nu$ is finite.*

Proof. We consider coordinate patches U_i isomorphic as foliated spaces via ψ_i to $L_i \times N_i$ so that ψ_i extends to $L_i' \times N_i'$, where N_i' is compact and contains N_i in its interior and where L_i is a relatively compact open ball in the ball L_i'. The compact set K can be covered by a finite number of such sets U_i so it suffices to show that $\mu(U_i)$ is finite. But by the definition of μ we can evaluate $\mu(U_i)$ by the formula

$$\mu(U_i) = \int_{N_i} \left(\int_{L_i} \Delta((x_0, n), (x, n))\, d\lambda^n(x) \right) d\nu_0(n),$$

where x_0 is a fixed point of L_i and ν_0 is the transverse measure ν restricted to the transversal $\psi_i(x_0, N_i)$. As this transversal is contained in a compact regular transversal, ν_0 is a finite measure. Moreover the measure λ^n on the plaques $\psi_i(L_i, n)$ have smooth densities which extend uniformly in n to a slightly larger "ball" and hence are bounded uniformly in n. The modular function Δ is continuous, and hence its values entering into the integrand are bounded. (Note that strictly speaking Δ is a function on the graph. It can be transported locally down to the equivalence relation $\mathcal{R}$ as we have done, since we are operating in coordinate patches with the plaques contractible). It now follows at once that the integral above is finite, and we are done. □

We remark that one could easily obtain finiteness results for tangential measures which do not have densities by imposing similar local boundedness conditions.

Our final goal now is to relate the previous discussion, which has been mostly analytic, to more geometric and topological aspects of the foliation. We begin with a tangentially smooth homomorphism Δ of G into $\mathbb{R}^+$, such as the modular function of a transverse measure on X. Tangential smoothness is with respect to the foliation of G by the holonomy groupoids of the leaves of the original foliation. We consider $\log \Delta$ as a real-valued function on G and form its differential. On each set $G^x = r^{-1}(x)$, the homomorphism property of Δ implies that

$$(\log \Delta)(\gamma u) = (\log \Delta)(\gamma) + (\log \Delta)(u)$$

for γ in the holonomy group G_x^x. Hence the differential of the function $\log(\Delta)$ becomes in a natural way a differential on the quotient $G_x^x \backslash G^x$, or in other words the leaf ℓ_x of x. Again by the homomorphism property of Δ, this differential on ℓ_x is independent of x, and hence one has an intrinsically defined differential 1-form on each leaf ℓ. Moreover the tangential smoothness of Δ implies immediately that these 1-forms on the leaves fit together continuously to what we have called in Chapter III a tangentially smooth 1-form for the foliation; recall that this is a tangentially smooth section of the dual F^*X of the foliation bundle. We denote this 1-form by α (or α_Δ if there is confusion). Summarizing:

Proposition 4.23. *For a tangentially smooth homomorphism Δ on G, the construction above yields a tangentially smooth 1-form α_Δ on X. The map $\Delta \to \alpha_\Delta$ is injective.*

Proof. If $U \cong L \times N$ is a coordinate patch with L a p-ball with coordinates $(\bar{x}, u) = (x_1, \ldots, x_p, n)$, where $n \in N$, then locally Δ can be written as a function of pairs $(\bar{x}, n)$, $(\bar{y}, n)$, with $\bar{x}, \bar{y} \in L$:

$$\Delta((\bar{x}, n), (\bar{y}, n)) = f(\bar{x}, \bar{y}, n).$$

Then the procedure for calculating α gives

$$\alpha = \sum \frac{\partial}{\partial y_i} (\log f)(\bar{x}_0, \bar{y}, n)\, dy_i.$$

This expression is seen to be independent of $\bar{x}_0$. The desired properties of α follow from this explicit local formula.

To see the final statement, we observe that for a point $(x, y, [\gamma])$ in G, we can obtain the value of Δ by integrating α_Δ along a smooth version of the path γ. Recall that γ is totally on a leaf so integration of tangential 1-forms makes sense. □

Now suppose that Δ is the modular function of a transverse measure ν, and suppose for simplicity that the bundle of the foliation FX is oriented. If o is the orientation, and if σ is a tangentially smooth p-form on FX ($p =$ leaf dimension) , then $\sigma_1 = o \cdot \sigma$ is a tangentially smooth volume form on FX. Then σ_1 restricted to any leaf ℓ defines a signed measure with a C^∞ density, and hence a (signed) tangential measure λ. We can write $\sigma_1 = \sigma_1^+ - \sigma_1^-$, where $\sigma_1^\pm$ have corresponding positive (negative) measures $\lambda_1^\pm$. Then assuming that ν is a Radon transverse measure, we define the integral $\mu = \int \lambda\, d\nu$ to be

$$\mu = \int \lambda\, d\nu \equiv \int \lambda_1\, d\nu - \int \lambda_2\, d\nu$$

which by Proposition 4.22 is the difference of two Radon measures on X, and is therefore a signed Radon measure defined on bounded Borel sets in X. If we further assume that the form σ has compact support in X, then evidently μ has compact support and is a Radon measure.

The integral can therefore be viewed as a linear functional

$$C_\nu : \Omega^p_{\tau c}(X) \longrightarrow \mathbb{R}$$

on the space $\Omega^p_{\tau c}(X)$ of compactly-supported tangentially smooth p-forms on X, where

$$C_\nu(\sigma) = \int_X \lambda\, d\nu.$$

Such an object is what we have called a tangential p-dimensional current in Chapter III. This was first defined in [Ruelle and Sullivan 1975] and is called the *Ruelle–Sullivan current*. The point of this discussion is to determine the boundary of this current. The boundary is a $(p-1)$-dimensional current defined by

$$d_* C_\nu(\sigma) = (-1)^p C_\nu(d\sigma),$$

where d is the differential on tangential forms.

Proposition 4.24. *For a compactly supported $p-1$ tangential form σ, we have*

$$C_\nu(d\sigma) = C_\nu(\sigma \wedge \alpha),$$

where α is the tangential 1-form associated to the modulus of the transverse measure ν.

It follows that if $\alpha = 0$, or equivalently $\Delta = 1$, then C_ν is a closed current. Conversely if C_ν is closed, we can deduce that $\alpha = 0$. Thus, whenever ν is an invariant transverse measure, C_ν defines a class in the tangential homology group $H^\tau_p(X, \mathbb{R})$ of Chapter III (Proposition 3.35) because the map $\sigma \to C_\nu(\sigma)$ is continuous with respect to the natural topology on $\Omega^p_{\tau c}(X)$. We denote this class by $[C_\nu]$. Summarizing:

Theorem 4.25. *For a Radon transverse measure ν with tangentially smooth modular function Δ, the following are equivalent:*

(1) *The Ruelle–Sullivan current C_ν is closed and so defines $[C_\nu] \in H^\tau_p(X, \mathbb{R})$.*

(2) *The 1-form α vanishes.*

(3) *The modular function Δ is identically 1.*

(4) *The transverse measure ν is an invariant transverse measure.*

Proof of Proposition 4.24. This is a straightforward calculation: first we may assume that σ is supported inside of some coordinate patch $U \cong L \times N$, where we use coordinates

$$(\bar{x}, n) = (x_1, x_2, \ldots, x_p, n).$$

The form σ can be written as

$$\sigma = \sum a_i(\bar{x}, n) dx_1 \wedge \cdots \wedge d\check{x}_i \wedge \cdots \wedge dx_p,$$

and we can represent the modular function locally as

$$\Delta((x', u), (x, u)) = f(x', x, u).$$

The 1-form α is

$$\sum \frac{\partial}{\partial x_i} \log(f(x_0, x, n))\, dx_i,$$

which does not depend on x_0. Now if ν_0 is the transverse measure on the transversal given by $x = x_0$, $h(x,n)dx_1 \wedge \cdots \wedge dx_p$ is a p-form, and λ_p the corresponding tangential measure, the definitions yield

$$\int_U \lambda\, d\nu = \int_N \left(\int_L h(x,n) f(x_0, x, n)\, dx \right) d\nu_0(n).$$

Thus for our $p-1$ form σ,

$$C_\nu(d\sigma) = \int_N \left(\int_L \left(\sum (-1)^i \frac{\partial a_i}{\partial x_i} \right) f(x_0, x, n)\, dx \right) d\nu_0(n).$$

On the other hand, we see that

$$C_\nu(\sigma \wedge \alpha) = \int_N \left(\int_L \sum (-1)^{i-p} n_i \frac{\partial f}{\partial x_i}(x_0, x, n)\, dx \right) d\nu_0(n).$$

Integration by parts on L gives the desired result, since the functions a_i vanish in a neighborhood of the boundary of L. □

Corollary 4.26. *If X is a compact oriented foliated space which has a nonzero invariant Radon transverse measure then $H_\tau^p(X) \neq 0$.*

This is the case, for instance, when X has a closed leaf. We improve this result significantly in Theorem 4.27 below.

Haefliger [1980] has used tangential transversely smooth cohomology in connection with the question of the existence of a Riemannian metric on M for which all the leaves are minimal (in the sense of area-minimizing) submanifolds. One consequence of his work is that the group $C_\tau^\infty(N)_H$ of compactly supported functions on some competely transverse submanifold N modulo holonomy maps onto the group $H_\tau^p(M)$. The map fails to be an isomorphism (e.g., for the Liouville-irrational flow on the torus).

Recalling the definition of a signed (or complex) Radon measure from 4.19 we see from Theorem 4.25 and Corollary 4.26 that any signed Radon invariant transverse measure will define a continuous linear functional on $H_\tau^p(X)$ or equivalently $\overline{H}_\tau^p(X)$—the topology on these spaces was defined in connection with Proposition 3.7. In the special case of a compact space X foliated by points, so $p = 0$, $H_\tau^0(X) = \overline{H}_\tau^0(X)$ is the Banach space of continuous functions on X. An invariant Radon (signed) transverse measure is just a Radon (signed) measure on X and the Riesz Representation Theorem says that these measures provide all the continuous linear functionals on $\overline{H}_\tau^0(X)$. More generally, if the foliation on X arises from a fibre bundle structure on X as total space, a base B and fibre L which we take to be a p-dimensional oriented manifold, then as we have already remarked (Proposition 4.11), invariant transverse Radon measures for this foliated space can be viewed simply as Radon measures on B. On the other hand, we have seen in Chapter III that in that case $H_\tau^p(X) = \overline{H}_\tau^p(X)$ can be identified topologically as $C(B)$, the set of continuous functions on B. Again the usual Riesz Representation Theorem tells us that all continuous linear functionals on $\overline{H}_\tau^p(X)$ are given by invariant transverse measures. We show that this is true in general. This result is clearly closely related to, but distinct from, [Haefliger 1980, Section 3.3, Corollary] and [Sullivan 1976, Proposition I.8].

Let $MT(X)$ denote the vector space of Radon invariant transverse measures on X.

Theorem 4.27 (Riesz Representation Theorem). *If X is a compact oriented foliated space with leaf dimension p, then the continuous linear functionals on $\overline{H}_\tau^p(X)$ can be identified as the Radon invariant transverse measures. More precisely, the Ruelle–Sullivan map*

$$MT(X) \to \mathrm{Hom}_{\mathrm{cont}}(H_\tau^p(X), \mathbb{R})$$

is an isomorphism of vector spaces.

For X compact, $\mathrm{Hom}_{\mathrm{cont}}(H_\tau^p(X), \mathbb{R})$ is isomorphic to $H_p^\tau(X)$ by Proposition 3.35.

Given the theorem it is easy sometimes to compute the top tangential cohomology group. For example, an invariant transverse measure on the Kronecker flow on the torus corresponds by (4.10) to a measure on a transverse circle which is invariant under rotation by an irrational angle, hence a multiple of Haar measure. Hence

$$MT(\text{Kronecker flow}) \cong \mathbb{R}$$

and so

$$\overline{H}_\tau^1(\text{Kronecker flow}) \cong \mathbb{R}.$$

A more interesting case arises from the Reeb foliation of S^3. The only holonomy invariant measures are multiples of the counting measure associated to the unique closed leaf. Thus

$$MT(\text{Reeb}) \cong \mathbb{R}$$

and so

$$\overline{H}_\tau^2(\text{Reeb}) \cong \mathbb{R}.$$

Proof of Theorem 4.27. Let Φ be a continuous linear functional on $\overline{H}_\tau^p(X)$. Now choose an open "coordinate" chart U around $x \in X$ with $U \cong B \times N$, where $B = B^p$ is an open ball in $\mathbb{R}^p$ and where N is locally compact. Then the set

$$N_\lambda = \{(\lambda, n) \mid n \in N,\ \lambda \text{ fixed in } B\}$$

is a transversal and if D is a compact subset of N, then

$$D_\lambda = \{(\lambda, n) \mid n \in D\}$$

is a regular transversal in the sense of Proposition 4.12. We fix a tangentially smooth p-form σ which has compact support in B. Now if f is any compactly supported real valued function on N, $f \in C_c(N)$, the formula

$$f\sigma(\lambda, n) = f(n)\sigma(\lambda)$$

defines a tangentially smooth p form of compact support on the foliated space $U \cong B \times N$. If we extend it by zero outside U to X, it yields a tangentially smooth p-form on X, which we also denote by $f\sigma$.

We now consider the map

$$\phi : f \mapsto \Phi(f\sigma)$$

for fixed σ. By the definition of the topology on $\Omega_\tau^p(X)$, it is evident that φ is norm continuous on $C_c(N)$. By the usual Riesz representation theorem, it must be represented by a finite Radon measure μ_σ on N.

The orientation on leaves of X gives by restriction an orientation on the ball B which is an open subset of a leaf of X, and hence we may integrate the forms σ on B. By the Poincaré lemma two compactly supported forms σ_1 and σ_2 on B are cohomologous, that is, $\sigma_1 - \sigma_2 = dp$ on B if and only if their integrals are the same. It follows that $f\sigma_1$ and $f\sigma_2$ as elements of $\Omega_\tau^p(X)$ differ by a coboundary if σ_1 and σ_2 have the same integral. Now define μ on N to be μ_σ for any σ of integral one. Then clearly

$$\Phi(f\sigma) = \int_N \left(\int_B \sigma \right) f(n)\, d\mu(n).$$

Moreover for any λ we can identify N with N_λ by $n \to (\lambda, n)$ and can transport μ onto N_λ, calling it μ^λ. Then we can rewrite the above as

$$\Phi(f\sigma) = \int_{N_\lambda} \left(\int_B (f\sigma)(\lambda, n) \right) d\mu^\lambda(n).$$

Finally if σ is any tangentially smooth p-form on X with compact support inside $U \cong B \times N$, it may by a kind of Stone–Weierstrass theorem be approximated in the topology of $\Omega_\tau^p(X)$ by linear combinations of forms of the type $f\sigma$. By continuity of both sides of the formula above,

$$\Phi(\sigma) = \int_{N_\lambda} \left(\int_B \sigma(\lambda, n) \right) d\mu^\lambda(n)$$

holds for any λ.

Now each N_λ is a transversal and μ^λ is a measure on it; we have to see now that we can piece these together to construct a transverse measure. First we observe that our compact space X can be covered by a finite number of open sets of the form $U \cong B \times N$, say $U^1, \ldots, U^n$ with $U^i \cong B \times N^i$. We identify each N^i with say N_b^i $(b \in B)$ and then $N = \bigcup N^i$ is a complete transversal; we can also arrange for simplicity that the N^i are all disjoint as subsets of X. Each N^i carries a Radon signed measure denoted by μ^i from the construction above and we fit them together to give a (signed) measure on N. As we have observed before, the foliated structure on N gives rise to a countable standard equivalence relation on N in the sense of [Feldman and Moore 1977]. We want to show that μ is invariant under this equivalence relation. To see this, we observe that if U^i and U^j intersect, then the projection of their intersection onto the respective transversals N^i and N^j are open subsets N^{ij} and N^{ji} respectively of N^i and N^j. Clearly for each $n \in N^{ij}$ there is a unique x' in N^{ji} which lies on the same leaf and it is evident that the map φ^{ij} taking x to x' is a homeomorphism of N^{ij} onto N^{ji}.

It is further evident that these partial homeomorphisms generate the equivalence relation on N in the obvious sense. To see that μ is invariant under this equivalence relation, it suffices by [Feldman and Moore 1977] to see that each φ^{ij} is measure preserving. (The fact that here we have signed measures, while Feldman and Moore use positive measures, is of course irrelevant.) However the formulas above for $\Phi(\sigma)$ when σ is supported in U^i or U^j in terms of μ^i and μ^j show immediately that φ^{ij} is measure preserving, for we apply these formulas to σ's which are supported in $U^i \cap U^j$.

Thus we have an invariant measure μ on the complete transversal N. To get transverse measures in the usual sense, we should first split $\mu = \mu^+ - \mu^-$ into its positive and negative parts, each of which is automatically invariant because $\mu^\pm$ are canonically defined. Then $\mu^\pm$ is extended to all transversals as in 4.10. Thus finally μ is a signed Radon transverse measure in the sense of our definition.

Let Φ_μ be the corresponding linear functional on $\overline{H}^p_\tau(X)$. Then the integral formulas above when compared to the formulas of Proposition 4.19 show that $\Phi_\mu(\sigma) = \Phi(\sigma)$ for σ supported in U^i. But then a partition of unity argument shows that these span and so $\Phi = \Phi_\mu$ and we are done. □

This result identifies the dual of the topological vector space $\overline{H}^p_\tau(X)$ in an explicit fashion as the set of invariant Radon transverse measures $MT(X)$. Then of course by duality, any $\sigma \in \overline{H}^p_\tau(X)$ defines a linear functional $F\sigma$ on $MT(X)$ by

$$(F\sigma)(\nu) = \int \sigma \, d\nu.$$

It will be of considerable interest to us at several points to know which linear functionals F on $MT(X)$ can be so represented. Of course there is no problem in those cases when $MT(X)$ and $\overline{H}^p_\tau(X)$ are finite-dimensional, but it is a problem in general. Following standard techniques, we introduce a "weak" topology on $MT(X)$ with the result that those linear functionals representable as $F\sigma$ are just the ones continuous in this topology. For each open-regular transversal N

(cf. 4.16) and each continuous real valued function on N of compact support, and for each $\nu \in MT(X)$, the integral $\int f \, d\nu_N$ is well defined, where ν_N is the transverse measure on ν on the transversal N: this defines a linear functional I_f on $MT(X)$.

Definition 4.28. The *weak topology* on $MT(X)$ is the smallest topology making these linear functions continuous.

Proposition 4.29. *The weak topology thus defined coincides with the weak-$*$ topology on $MT(X)$ as the dual of $\overline{H}^p_\tau(X)$ and consequently a linear function F on $MT(X)$ is representable as $F\sigma$, with $\sigma \in \overline{H}^p_\tau(X)$, if and only if it is continuous in the weak topology.*

Proof. If N is an open-regular transversal, let B be a ball in $\mathbb{R}^p$; then there is a tangentially smooth homeomorphism of $B \times N$ onto an open set U in X; we shall think of $U = B \times N$ as sitting inside X. If f is a compactly supported function on N, we can easily construct a tangentially smooth p-form σ on X supported on $U = B \times N$ so that

$$\int_B \sigma(b, r) = f(n).$$

Then from our formulas for integration it is immediate that

$$I_f(\nu) = \int f \, d\nu_N = \int \sigma \, d\nu = \nu([\sigma]),$$

where $[\sigma]$ is the class of σ in $\overline{H}^p_\tau(X)$. Hence the weak topology defined by the I_f is contained in the weak$-*$ topology on $MT(X)$ as the dual of $\overline{H}^p_\tau(X)$. Conversely we see, using a partition of unity argument, that a linear functional $\nu \to \nu([\sigma])$ for any σ can be represented as a finite linear combination for I_f's. Hence the two topologies coincide and the result follows. □

We note that it would suffice in defining the weak topology to restrict to any finite set of open-regular transversals N_i so that there are corresponding coordinate charts $N_i \times B$, B a ball in $\mathbb{R}^p$, which cover X.

We close Chapter IV with two examples which illustrate the Riesz Representation Theorem 4.27.

Suppose that T is a homeomorphism of a separable metrizable space N and that f is a positive continuous function on N. Then we may form the space X_T obtained as the quotient of the space

$$\{(t, n) \in \mathbb{R} \times N \mid 0 \le t \le f(n)\}$$

by the relation $(f(n), n) \sim (0, T(n))$. If $f \equiv 1$ then X_T is simply the suspension of the homeomorphism T (cf. 2.3). The space X_T has a natural oriented foliation of dimension one corresponding to the action of $\mathbb{R}$ on the first factor of $R \times N$. As f changes, the topological foliated conjugacy class of X_T remains the same; so in that sense at least the dependence of X_T on f is minimal. Invariant transverse measures on X_T correspond to T-invariant measures on N, denoted $M(N)^T$. Theorem 4.27 implies that $\overline{H}^1_\tau(X_T)^* \cong M(N)^T$.

Let us look at this example in more detail. The general tangential 1-form $a(t,n)dt$ is a tangential cocycle, since it is in the top degree. The function a must satisfy

$$a(f(n),n) = a(0,T(n)) \tag{4.30}$$

in order to be defined on X_T. If $a(t,n)dt = (\partial b/\partial t)(t,n)$, then b must also satisfy the counterpart of (4.30). Set $b(0,n) = b_0(n)$. Then

$$b(t,n) = \int_0^t a(t,n)\,dt + b_0(n)$$

and hence

$$b(f(n),n) = \int_0^{f(n)} a(t,n)\,dt + b_0(n).$$

Now

$$\int_0^{f(n)} a(t,n)\,dt = b_0(T(n)) - b_0(n)$$

and so any tangential 1-coboundary must be of the form

$$(b_0(T(n)) - b_0(n))\,dt.$$

Thus

$$H^1_\tau(X_T) \cong \frac{C(N)}{(T-1)C(N)}$$

and

$$\overline{H}^1_\tau(X_T) \cong \frac{C(N)}{\overline{(T-1)C(N)}}.$$

It is clear then that

$$\overline{H}^1_\tau(X_T)^* \cong M(N)^T,$$

as predicted by Theorem 4.27.

This example generalizes to the case of bundles with discrete structural group, as follows. Let B be an oriented compact manifold of dimension p with $\Gamma = \pi_1(B)$ and $\widetilde{B} \to B$ the universal cover. Suppose that Γ acts on a space F. Then the space

$$X = \widetilde{B} \times_\Gamma F$$

is foliated by leaves of dimension p which are the images of $\widetilde{B} \times \{x\}$ for $x \in F$; see (2.2). We may regard differential forms on X as forms $\omega(b,x)$ defined on $\widetilde{B} \times F$ satisfying the invariance condition

$$\omega(\gamma b, \gamma x) = \omega(b,x) \quad \text{for } \gamma \in \Gamma.$$

Fix a fundamental domain U in $\widetilde{B}$. Let ω be a p-form (necessarily closed) and define

$$f_\omega(x) = \int_U \omega(b, x).$$

If ν is an invariant transverse measure on X, then $\int f_\omega \, d\nu$ is independent of choice of U. If ω is a coboundary, say $\omega = d\sigma$, then

$$f_\omega(x) = \int_U \omega(b, x) = \int_{\partial U} \sigma(b, x)$$

(by Stokes' theorem) and

$$\int f_\omega \, d\nu = \int \int_{\partial U} \sigma(b, x) \, d\nu = \int_{\partial U} \left(\int \sigma(b, x) \right) d\nu = 0.$$

for any invariant transverse measure $d\nu$, since $\int \sigma(b, x)$ is a periodic function and $\int_{\partial U}(\text{periodic}) \, d\nu = 0$.

Suppose that U is sufficiently well-behaved so that ∂U consists of $2k$ piecewise smooth hypersurfaces

$$\partial U = H_1^+ \cup H_1^- \cup \cdots \cup H_k^+ \cup H_k^-$$

and there are elements $\gamma_i \in \Gamma$ which reflect H_i^+ and with H_i^- and general Γ.[1] Then

$$\int_{\partial U} \sigma(b, x) = \sum_1^k \int_{H_i^+} \sigma(b, x) + \int_{-H_i^-} \sigma(b, x),$$

where $-H_i^-$ indicates H_i^- with the orientation reserved. Let

$$g_i(x) = \int_{H_i^+} \sigma(b, x).$$

Then

$$\int_{\partial U} \sigma(b, x) = \int \sum_l^k g_i(x) - g_i(\gamma_i x),$$

[1] This sort of decomposition is quite familiar in the theory of Riemann surfaces. In general one may assume that Γ acts by isometries. Let D be an open dense PL disk in B and let $\widetilde{V}$ be one component of its preimage. Then $U = \text{int}(\text{closure}(\widetilde{V}))$ is an open disk in $\widetilde{B}$ with PL boundary ∂U. The deck group Γ acts in PL fashion on ∂U which decomposes into smooth hypersurfaces. However, to ensure that Γ is generated by $\{\gamma_i\}$ which act as reflections on these hypersurfaces is a very delicate (and sometimes impossible) matter. The interested reader is referred to [Davis 1983] for a taste of the difficulty.

so that terms cancel in pairs under integration with respect to $d\nu$. We see from this analysis that the p-coboundaries correspond to the algebraic sum in $C(X)$

$$\sum_{1}^{k}(\gamma_i - 1)C(X),$$

which is also

$$(\Gamma - 1)C(X) = \sum_{\gamma \in \Gamma}(\gamma - 1)C(X).$$

Thus

$$H_\tau^p(X) \cong \frac{C(X)}{(\Gamma - 1)C(X)} \cong \frac{C(X)}{\sum_1^k(\gamma_i - 1)C(X)}$$

and

$$\overline{H}_\tau^p(X) \cong \frac{C(X)}{\overline{(\Gamma - 1)C(X)}} \cong \frac{C(X)}{\overline{\sum_1^k(\gamma_i - 1)C(X)}},$$

which is the predual of $MT(X)$.

□ □□□□□ □□□□

In the course of this book, we always assumed that isotropy groups of the groupoids were discrete. It is now very clear why that assumption is necessary; indeed, Crainic and Moerdijk [2001] (see also [Muhly et al. 1987] for definitions) prove that for a smooth groupoid G, the following are equivalent:

(1) G is Morita equivalent to a smooth étale groupoid;

(2) All isotropy Lie groups of G are discrete.

They refer to such groupoids as *foliation groupoids* and observe that any foliation groupoid defines a foliation on the unit space G^0. (These are foliated manifolds; we don't know if the analogous theorem for foliated spaces is true.) They then prove that if G and H are Morita equivalent foliation groupoids then

$$HC_*(C_c^\infty(G)) \cong HC_*(C_c^\infty(H)),$$

where HC_* denotes cyclic homology, and similarly for Hochschild and periodic cyclic homology, and this result is established via explicit formulas. This is a very nice complement to the work of Brylinski and Nistor [1994] on the cyclic cohomology of étale groupoids.

CHAPTER V

Characteristic Classes

In this chapter we mimic as closely as possible [Milnor and Stasheff 1974], itself an exposé of the Chern–Weil construction of characteristic classes in terms of curvature forms. See also [Dupont 1978; Husemoller 1975; Lawson and Michelsohn 1989; de Rham 1955].

The Chern–Weil procedure begins with a vector bundle with a certain structural group G. In our situation we consider complex (tangentially smooth) bundles with structural group $\mathrm{GL}(n, \mathbb{C})$, real vector bundles with structural group $\mathrm{GL}(n, \mathbb{R})$, and oriented real even-dimensional vector bundles with structural group $\mathrm{SO}(2n)$. Choose a tangential connection ∇, see below, that respects the structure. The associated curvature form K determines a closed tangential 2-form whose tangential cohomology class is independent of choice of the connection. Then any polynomial or formal power series P which is G-invariant determines a characteristic form. In the case $X = M$ is a manifold with $FX = TM$ then this yields the usual characteristic classes in de Rham cohomology $H^*(M)$.

We shall assume throughout that all bundles over foliated spaces are tangentially smooth and that leaf-preserving maps between foliated spaces are also tangentially smooth; this is not a real restriction, in view of our smoothing results (Proposition 2.16). We use Milnor and Stasheff's sign conventions for characteristic classes.

Let $E \to X$ be a (tangentially smooth) complex n-plane bundle over the foliated space X, and let $F^*_{\mathbb{C}} = \mathrm{Hom}_{\mathbb{R}}(F, \mathbb{C})$ be the complexified dual tangent bundle of the foliated space X.

Definition 5.1. A *tangential connection* on $E \to X$ is a $\mathbb{C}$-linear mapping

$$\nabla : \Gamma_\tau(E) \to \Gamma_\tau(F^*_{\mathbb{C}} \otimes E)$$

which satisfies the Leibnitz formula

$$\nabla(fs) = df \otimes s + f\nabla(s)$$

for every $s \in \Gamma_\tau(E)$ and every $f \in C^\infty_\tau(X, \mathbb{C})$. The image $\nabla(s)$ is called the *tangential covariant derivative* of s.

Equivalently, we may regard ∇ as a bilinear map

$$\Gamma_\tau(F_{\mathbb{C}}) \times \Gamma_\tau(E) \to \Gamma_\tau(E)$$

with

$$\nabla_{fv}(s) = f\nabla_v(s) \quad \text{for } v \in F_{\mathbb{C}}$$

and

$$\nabla_v(gs) = v_g \cdot s + g\nabla_v(s) \quad \text{for } f, g \in C_\tau^\infty(X) \text{ and } s \in \Gamma_\tau(E).$$

One may regard ∇ as a map between the Lie algebras $\Gamma_\tau(F_{\mathbb{C}})$ (with Lie bracket) and $\mathrm{Hom}(\Gamma_\tau(E), \Gamma_\tau(E))$ (with bracket corresponding to $AB - BA$ for matrices). Thus

$$\nabla : \Gamma_\tau(F_{\mathbb{C}}) \to \mathrm{Hom}(\Gamma_\tau(E), \Gamma_\tau(E)).$$

Note that ∇ is not generally a Lie algebra homomorphism.

The correspondence $s \mapsto \nabla(s)$ *decreases supports*; that is, if the section s vanishes throughout an open subset $U \subset X$, then $\nabla(s)$ vanishes throughout U also. For given $x \in U$ we can choose a tangentially smooth function f which vanishes outside U and is identically 1 near x. The identity

$$df \otimes s + f\nabla(s) = \nabla(fs) = 0$$

evaluated at x shows that $\nabla(s)$ vanishes at x.

Since a connection is a local operator (i.e., it decreases supports), it makes sense to talk about the restriction of ∇ to an open subset of X. If a collection of open sets U_α covers X, then a global tangential connection is uniquely determined by its restrictions to the various U_α.

If the open set is small enough that $E|_U$ is trivial, $\Gamma(E|_U)$ is a free $C_\tau^\infty(X)$-module with basis $s_1, \ldots, s_n$, say. Tangential connections may be constructed as follows.

Proposition 5.2. *Let $[\omega_{ij}]_{1 \le i,j \le n}$ be an arbitrary $n \times n$ matrix of tangentially smooth complex 1-forms on U. Then there is a unique tangential connection ∇ on the trivial bundle $E|_U$ such that*

$$\nabla(s_i) = \sum \omega_{ij} \otimes s_j.$$

Proof. The connection ∇ is determined uniquely by the formula

$$\nabla\left(\sum_i f_i s_i\right) = \sum_i (df_i \otimes s_i + f_i \nabla(s_i)). \qquad \square$$

Henceforth, we assume that *all tangential connections are given locally as differential operators*, as in the preceding proposition.

There is exactly one tangential connection on a coordinate patch such that the tangential covariant derivatives of the s_i are all zero; or in other words so that the connection matrix is zero. It is given by

$$\nabla\left(\sum_i f_i s_i\right) = \sum_i df_i \otimes s_i.$$

This particular "flat" connection depends of course on the choice of basis $\{s_i\}$.

If ∇_1 and ∇_2 are tangential connections on E and g is a tangentially smooth complex-valued function on X, then the linear combination $g\nabla_1 + (1-g)\nabla_2$ is again a well defined tangential connection on E.

Proposition 5.3. *Every tangentially smooth vector bundle*

$$\pi \colon E \to X$$

with paracompact foliated base space possesses a tangential connection.

Proof. Choose open sets U_α covering X with $E \mid U_\alpha$ trivial, and choose a tangentially smooth partition of unity $\{r_\alpha\}$ subordinate to $\{U_\alpha\}$. Each restriction $E|_{U_\alpha}$ possesses a connection ∇_α by Proposition 5.2. The linear combination $\sum_\alpha r_\alpha \nabla_\alpha$ is now a well defined global tangential connection. □

Given a tangentially smooth map $g : X' \to X$ we can form the induced vector bundle $E' = g^*E$. Note that there is a canonical $C_\tau^\infty(X, \mathbb{C})$-linear map

$$g^* \colon \Gamma_\tau(E) \to \Gamma_\tau(E').$$

Similarly, any tangentially smooth 1-form on X pulls back to a 1-form on X', so there is a canonical $C_\tau^\infty(X, \mathbb{C})$-linear mapping

$$g^* : \Gamma_\tau(F_{\mathbb{C}}^* \otimes E) \to \Gamma_\tau(F_{\mathbb{C}}'^* \otimes E').$$

Proposition 5.4. *To each tangential connection ∇ on E there corresponds one and only one tangential connection $\nabla' = g^*\nabla$ on $g^*E = E'$ so that the diagram*

$$\begin{array}{ccc} \Gamma_\tau(E) & \xrightarrow{\nabla} & \Gamma_\tau(F_{\mathbb{C}}^* \otimes E) \\ \downarrow g^* & & \downarrow g^* \\ \Gamma_\tau(E') & \xrightarrow{\nabla'} & \Gamma_\tau(F_{\mathbb{C}}'^* \otimes E') \end{array}$$

is commutative.

Proof. Let $\{U_\alpha\}$ be an open cover and $\{r_\alpha\}$ a tangentially smooth partition of unity subordinate to a locally finite refinement of the cover $\{g^{-1}(U_\alpha)\}$. On a typical set U_α, pick sections $s_1, \ldots, s_n$ with $\nabla(s_i) = \sum_j \omega_{ij} \otimes s_j$. Lift the 1-forms ω_{ij} to $\omega'_{ij} = g^*\omega_{ij}$ and lift the sections s_i to $s'_i = g^*s_i$ over $g^{-1}(U_\alpha)$. If ∇' exists then

$$\nabla'|_{g^{-1}(U_\alpha)} = \sum_j \omega'_{ij} \otimes s'_j,$$

which shows uniqueness for ∇'. For existence, use the preceding equality to define the connection $\nabla'|_{g^{-1}(U_\alpha)}$ locally, and then define ∇' globally by

$$\nabla' = \sum r_\alpha (\nabla'|_{g^{-1}(U_\alpha)}).$$ □

Given a tangential connection ∇, we proceed to construct its curvature.

Proposition 5.5. *Given a tangential connection ∇, there is one and only one $\mathbb{C}$-linear mapping*

$$\widehat{\nabla} : \Gamma_\tau(F_{\mathbb{C}}^* \otimes E) \to \Gamma_\tau(\Lambda^2 F_{\mathbb{C}}^* \otimes E)$$

which satisfies the Leibnitz formula

$$\widehat{\nabla}(\zeta \otimes s) = d\zeta \otimes s - \zeta \wedge \nabla(s)$$

for every 1-form ζ and every section $s \in \Gamma_\tau(E)$. Furthermore, $\widehat{\nabla}$ satisfies the identity

$$\widehat{\nabla}(f(\zeta \otimes s)) = df \wedge (\zeta \otimes s) + f\widehat{\nabla}(\zeta \otimes s).$$

Proof. In terms of a local basis $s_1, \ldots, s_n$ for the sections, we must have

$$\widehat{\nabla}\Big(\sum_i \zeta_i \otimes s_i\Big) = \sum_i \big(d\zeta_i \otimes s_i - \zeta_i \wedge \nabla(s_i)\big).$$

This formula specifies $\widehat{\nabla}$ uniquely. Existence follows from an argument involving a (tangentially smooth) partition of unity. □

The *tangential curvature tensor* of the tangential connection ∇ is defined by

$$K = \widehat{\nabla} \circ \nabla : \Gamma_\tau(E) \to \Gamma_\tau(\Lambda^2 F_{\mathbb{C}}^* \otimes E).$$

Proposition 5.6. *The value of the section $K(s)$ at $x \in X$ depends only upon $s(x)$, not on the values of s at other points of X. Hence the correspondence*

$$s(x) \mapsto K(s)(x)$$

defines a tangentially smooth section of the complex vector bundle

$$\mathrm{Hom}(E, \Lambda^2 F_{\mathbb{C}}^* \otimes E) \cong \Lambda^2 F_{\mathbb{C}}^* \otimes \mathrm{Hom}(E, E).$$

Proof. Clearly K is a local operator, and $Kf(s) = fK(s)$ by direct computation; K is $C_\tau^\infty(X, \mathbb{C})$-linear. Suppose that $s(x) = s'(x)$. In terms of a local basis $s_1, ., s_n$ for sections we have

$$s' - s = \sum_i f_i s_i$$

near x, where $f_1(x) = \cdots = f_n(x) = 0$. Hence

$$K(s') - K(s) = \sum_i f_i K(s_i)$$

vanishes at x. This completes the proof. □

In terms of a basis $s_1, \ldots, s_n$ for the sections $E|_U$, with

$$\nabla(s_i) = \sum_j \omega_{ij} \otimes s_j,$$

we have

$$K(s_i) = \hat{\nabla}\left(\sum_j \omega_{ij} \otimes s_j\right) = \sum_j \Omega_{ij} \otimes s_j,$$

where Ω is the $n \times n$ matrix of 2-forms given by

$$\Omega_{ij} = d\omega_{ij} - \sum_\alpha \omega_{i\alpha} \wedge \omega_{\alpha j},$$

or

$$\Omega = d\omega - \omega \wedge \omega$$

in matrix form.

Recall that ∇ may be regarded as a linear map

$$\nabla : \Gamma(F_{\mathbb{C}}) \to \mathrm{Hom}(\Gamma_\tau(E), \Gamma_\tau(E)).$$

Then the curvature K may be regarded as

$$K = K_\nabla : \Gamma_\tau(F_{\mathbb{C}}) \times \Gamma_\tau(F_{\mathbb{C}}) \to \mathrm{Hom}(\Gamma_\tau(E), \Gamma_\tau(E)),$$

where K_∇ is given by the formula

$$K_\nabla = \nabla_v \nabla_w - \nabla_w \nabla_v - \nabla_{[v,w]}.$$

Thus the curvature is the obstruction to ∇ being a Lie algebra homomorphism: if the connection is flat then ∇ is a Lie algebra homomorphism and $K \equiv 0$.

Starting with the tangential curvature tensor K, we construct tangential characteristic classes as follows. Recall that $M_n(\mathbb{C})$ denotes the algebra consisting of all $n \times n$ complex matrices.

Definition 5.7. An *invariant polynomial* on $M_n(\mathbb{C})$ is a function

$$P : M_n(\mathbb{C}) \to \mathbb{C}$$

which may be expressed as a complex polynomial in the entries of the matrix and satisfies

$$P(XY) = P(YX)$$

for all matrices X, Y, or equivalently

$$P(TXT^{-1}) = P(X)$$

for all X and for all nonsingular matrices T. (The structure group is, of course, $\mathrm{GL}(n, \mathbb{C})$.)

The trace and determinant functions are well-known examples of invariant polynomials on $M_n(\mathbb{C})$.

If P is an invariant polynomial, then an exterior form

$$P(K) \in \Gamma_\tau(\Lambda^* F_{\mathbb{C}}^*) = \bigoplus_m \Gamma_\tau(\Lambda^m F_{\mathbb{C}}^*)$$

is defined as follows. Choose a local basis $s_1, \dots, s_n$ for the sections in a neighborhood U of x, so that

$$K(s_i) = \sum_j \Omega_{ij} \otimes s_j.$$

The matrix $\Omega = [\Omega_{ij}]$ has entries in the commutative algebra over $\mathbb{C}$ consisting of all exterior forms of even degree. It makes good sense to form $P(\Omega)$. This lies a priori in $\Omega^*_\tau(U)$ but patches together to form $P(K) \in \Omega^*_\tau(X)$, since a change of basis will replace Ω by a matrix $T\Omega T^{-1}$ and $P(T\Omega T^{-1}) = P(\Omega)$.

If P is a homogeneous polynomial of degree r then $P(K) \in \Omega^{2r}_\tau(X)$. If P is an invariant formal power series of the form

$$P = P_0 + P_1 + \cdots,$$

where each P_r is an invariant homogeneous polynomial of degree r, then $P(K)$ is still well-defined since $P_r(K) = 0$ for $2r > p$ (the leaf dimension).

Lemma 5.8 (Fundamental Lemma). *For any invariant polynomial (or invariant formal power series) P, the exterior form $P(K)$ is closed; that is, $dP(K) = 0$. Thus $P(K)$ represents an element $[P(K)]$ in the tangential de Rham cohomology group $H^*_\tau(X; \mathbb{C})$.*

Proof. We summarize the proof found in [Milnor and Stasheff 1974, p. 296–298]. Given any invariant polynomial or formal power series $P(A) = P([A_{ij}])$ form the matrix $[\partial P/\partial A_{ij}]$ of formal first derivatives and let $P'(A)$ denote the transpose of this matrix. Let $\Omega = [\Omega_{ij}]$ be the curvature matrix with respect to some basis for the restriction of the bundle to U. Then

$$dP(\Omega) = \sum \frac{\partial P}{\partial \Omega_{ij}} d\Omega_{ij} = \operatorname{Trace}(P'(\Omega) d\Omega).$$

Since $\Omega = d\omega - \omega \wedge \omega$, taking exterior derivatives yields the Bianchi identity

$$d\Omega = \omega \wedge \Omega - \Omega \wedge \omega.$$

The matrix $P'(A)$ commutes with A, and hence

$$\Omega \wedge P'(\Omega) = P'(\Omega) \wedge \Omega.$$

Now

$$\begin{aligned} dP(\Omega) &= \operatorname{trace}((P'(\Omega) \wedge \omega) \wedge \Omega - \Omega \wedge (P'(\Omega) \wedge \omega)) \\ &= \sum (P'(\Omega) \wedge \omega)_{ij} \wedge \Omega_{ji} - \Omega_{ji} \wedge (P'(\Omega) \wedge \omega)_{ij}. \end{aligned}$$

Since each $(P'(\Omega) \wedge \omega)_{ij}$ commutes with the 2-form Ω_{ji}, this sum is zero, which proves the lemma. □

Corollary 5.9. *The cohomology class $[P(K)] \in H^*_\tau(X)$ is independent of the choice of tangential connection ∇.*

Proof. Let ∇_0 and ∇_1 be two different tangential connections on E. Map $X \times \mathbb{R}$ to X by the projection $(x,t) \mapsto x$ and form the induced bundle E' over $X \times \mathbb{R}$, the induced tangential connections ∇'_0 and ∇'_1 and the linear combination

$$\nabla = t\nabla'_1 + (1-t)\nabla'_0.$$

Thus $P(K_\nabla)$ is a tangential de Rham cocycle on $X \times \mathbb{R}$ (foliated of dimension $p+1$).

Consider the map $i_\epsilon : x \mapsto (x,\epsilon)$ from X to $X \times \mathbb{R}$, where ϵ equals 0 or 1. Evidently the induced tangential connection $(i_\epsilon)^*\nabla$ on $(i_\epsilon^*)E'$ may be identified with the tangential connections ∇_ϵ on E. Therefore

$$(i_\epsilon^*)(P(K_\nabla)) = P(K_{\nabla_\epsilon}).$$

But the mappings i_0 and i_1 are homotopic and hence

$$[P(K_{\nabla_0})] = [P(K_{\nabla_1})]. \qquad \square$$

The polynomial P determines a tangential characteristic cohomology class in the group $H^*_\tau(X;\mathbb{C})$, which depends only upon the isomorphism class of the vector bundle E. If a tangentially smooth map $g : X' \to X$ induces a bundle $E' = g^*E$ with induced tangential connection ∇', then clearly

$$P(K_{\nabla'}) = g^* P(K_\nabla).$$

Thus these characteristics classes are well behaved with respect to induced bundles.

The entire treatment may be repeated for real vector bundles, and one obtains characteristic cohomology classes $[P(K)] \in H^*_\tau(X;\mathbb{R})$ for any $\mathrm{GL}(n,\mathbb{R})$-invariant polynomial P on $M_n(\mathbb{R})$.

For any square matrix A, let $\sigma_k(A)$ denote the k-th elementary symmetric function of the eigenvalues of A, so that

$$\det(I + tA) = 1 + t\sigma_1(A) + \cdots + t^n\sigma_n(A).$$

Newton's Theorem [Milnor and Stasheff 1974, p. 299] asserts that any invariant polynomial on $M_n(\mathbb{C})$ can be expressed as a polynomial function of $\sigma_1, \ldots \sigma_n$.

Definition 5.10. Let E be a tangentially smooth complex vector bundle with tangential connection ∇. The *tangential Chern classes* $c^\tau_m(E)$ are defined for $m = 1, 2, \ldots$ by

$$c^\tau_m(E) = (2\pi i)^{-m}[\sigma_m(K_\nabla)] \in H^{2m}_\tau(X;\mathbb{C}).$$

The tangential Chern classes do not depend on the choice of tangential connection, by Corollary 5.9. The fact that any invariant polynomial on $M_n(\mathbb{C})$ can be expressed as a polynomial function of $\sigma_1, \ldots, \sigma_n$ implies that any characteristic class $c = [Q(K)]$ can be expressed as a polynomial in the Chern classes.

If $g : X' \to X$ is a tangentially smooth map, then

$$g^* c^\tau_m(E) = c^\tau_m(g^* E)$$

by Proposition 5.4. If E has a flat tangential connection, all characteristic classes vanish and in particular $c^\tau_m(E) = 0$.

If $X = M$ is a compact smooth manifold foliated by one leaf, then a tangential connection *is* a connection, tangential curvature *is* curvature, and

$$c^\tau_m(E) = c_m(E) \in H^{2m}(M; \mathbb{C});$$

the tangential Chern classes *are* Chern classes. In general, however, this cannot be the case. If X is a compact foliated space with leaves of dimension p, then $H^m_\tau(X; \mathbb{C}) = 0$ for $m > p$, so $c^\tau_m(E) = 0$ for $2m > p$. On the other hand, the ordinary Chern classes $c_m(E)$ (defined topologically, since we do not assume that X is a manifold) need not vanish. The following proposition explains the relation between the c_m and the c^τ_m.

Proposition 5.11. *Let E be a tangentially smooth complex vector bundle over a compact foliated space X. Then*

$$c^\tau_m(E) = r_* c_m(E),$$

where $r_* : H^*(X; \mathbb{C}) \to H^*_\tau(X; \mathbb{C})$ is the canonical map.

Proof. Since X is compact there is a compact Grassmann manifold $G_k(\mathbb{C}^{n+k})$ with universal n-plane bundle E^n and a continuous map $g : X \to G_k(\mathbb{C}^{n+k})$ (which we may assume to be tangentially smooth) such that $E = g^* E^n$. Let ∇ be a connection on E^n, so that

$$c_m(E^n) = (2\pi i)^{-m}[\sigma_m(K_\nabla)] \in H^{2m}(G_k(\mathbb{C}^{n+k}); \mathbb{C}).$$

If $\nabla' = g^* \nabla$ is the induced tangential connection on X, then

$$c_m(E) = g^* c_m(E^n) = (2\pi i)^{-m} g^*[\sigma_m(K_\nabla)].$$

To complete the proof, then, we need only show that the diagram

$$\begin{array}{ccc} H^{2m}(G_k(\mathbb{C}^{n+k}); \mathbb{C}) & \xrightarrow[\cong]{r_*} & H^{2m}_\tau(G_k(\mathbb{C}^{n+k}); \mathbb{C}) \\ \Big\downarrow g^* & & \Big\downarrow g^* \\ H^{2m}(X; \mathbb{C}) & \xrightarrow{r_*} & H^{2m}_\tau(X; \mathbb{C}) \end{array}$$

commutes; this follows from the naturality of r. □

Corollary 5.12. *The tangential Chern classes satisfy the following properties*:

(1) *If $g : X' \to X$ is tangentially smooth, then*

$$g^* c^\tau_m(E) = c^\tau_m(g^* E).$$

(2) $c^\tau_m(E \oplus E') = \sum_{i=0}^m c^\tau_i(E) c^\tau_{m-i}(E')$.

(3) *If E is a line bundle, then* $c^\tau_0(E) = 1$ *and*

$$c^\tau_m(E) = 0 \text{ for } m > 1.$$

(4) *If E is of dimension n, then* $c^\tau_m(E) = 0$ *for* $m > n$.

(5) *If E has a tangentially flat connection, then* $c^\tau_m(E) = 0$ *for all* m.

Proof. We have observed (1) and (5) previously. The rest follows from the analogous properties of Chern classes and the fact that $r_* : H^*(X; \mathbb{C}) \to H^*_\tau(X; \mathbb{C})$ is a ring map. □

There are several important combinations of Chern classes. Here are two of them. The *tangential Chern character*

$$\mathrm{ch}^\tau(E) \in \bigoplus_m H^{2m}_\tau(X; \mathbb{C})$$

is the characteristic class associated to the invariant formal power series

$$\mathrm{ch}^\tau(A) = \mathrm{trace}(e^{A/2\pi i}). \tag{5.13}$$

The *tangential total Chern class* of E is the formal sum

$$c^\tau(E) = 1 + c^\tau_1(E) + c^\tau_2(E) + \cdots, \tag{5.14}$$

which lies in $\oplus H^{2m}_\tau(X; \mathbb{C})$, and satisfies

$$c^\tau(E \oplus E') = c^\tau(E) c^\tau(E').$$

It corresponds to the invariant polynomial $\det(I + A/2\pi i)$.

Let σ_i be the elementary symmetric polynomials and let s_i be the universal polynomials determined inductively by Newton's formula

$$\sigma_n - \sigma_1 s_{n-1} + \sigma_2 s_{n-2} - \cdots \mp \sigma_{n-1} s_1 \pm n\sigma_n = 0.$$

For example,

$$s_1(\sigma_1) = \sigma_1, \qquad s_2(\sigma_1, \sigma_2) = \sigma_1^2 - 2\sigma_2, \qquad s_3(\sigma_1, \sigma_2, \sigma_3) = \sigma_1^3 - 3\sigma_1\sigma_2 + 3\sigma_3.$$

Proposition 5.15. *The tangential Chern character has the following properties*:

(1) $\mathrm{ch}^\tau(E) = n + \displaystyle\sum_{k=1}^{\infty} \frac{s_k(c^\tau(E))}{k!}$, *where* $n = \dim E$. *In particular, if E is a*

line bundle, then

$$\mathrm{ch}^\tau(E) = \sum_{k=0}^{\infty} \frac{c_1^\tau(E)^k}{k!} = \exp(c_1^\tau(E)).$$

(2) $\mathrm{ch}^\tau(E \oplus E') = \mathrm{ch}^\tau(E) + \mathrm{ch}^\tau(E')$.

(3) $\mathrm{ch}^\tau(E \otimes E') = \mathrm{ch}^\tau(E)\,\mathrm{ch}^\tau(E')$.

(4) $\mathrm{ch}^\tau : K^0(X) \to \oplus_m H_\tau^{2m}(X;\mathbb{C})$ *is a ring map.*

In anticipation of index theory needs, we extend the tangential Chern character to $K^1(X)$ by defining

$$\mathrm{ch}^\tau : K^1(X) \longrightarrow \bigoplus\nolimits_m H_\tau^{2m-1}(X;\mathbb{C})$$

to be the composite

$$\mathrm{ch}^\tau : K^1(X) \cong K^0(SX) \xrightarrow{\mathrm{ch}_\tau} \bigoplus\nolimits_m H_\tau^{2m}(SX;\mathbb{C}) \xrightarrow{\cong} \bigoplus\nolimits_m H_\tau^{2m-1}(X;\mathbb{C}),$$

where SX is the suspension of X. Then we note:

Proposition 5.16. *The tangential Chern character commutes with coboundary maps. Specifically, if (X, A) is a cofibration pair and ∂ represents the coboundary homomorphism in the associated long exact sequences in K-theory and tangential cohomology, then there is a commutative diagram*

$$\begin{array}{ccc}
K^1(A) & \xrightarrow{\quad\partial\quad} & K^0(X/A) \\
\Big\downarrow{\scriptstyle \mathrm{ch}_\tau} & & \Big\downarrow{\scriptstyle \mathrm{ch}_\tau} \\
\bigoplus_m H_\tau^{2m-1}(A;\mathbb{C}) & \xrightarrow{\partial} & \bigoplus_m H_\tau^{2m}(X/A;\mathbb{C})
\end{array}$$

Proof. The map ch_τ commutes with the suspension isomorphism, essentially by definition, and this is equivalent to commuting with coboundary maps [May 1999, p. 144]. □

As an example we compute the Chern classes of the canonical bundles of $\mathbb{C}\mathrm{P}^n$ (regarded as a foliated space with one leaf). Let E be the canonical complex line bundle over $\mathbb{C}\mathrm{P}^n$ and D its orthogonal complement, so that $E \oplus D = \mathbb{C}\mathrm{P}^n \times \mathbb{C}^{n+1}$ (the trivial complex $(n+1)$-plane bundle). A geometric argument, which we omit, implies that the tangent bundle of $\mathbb{C}\mathrm{P}^n$ (a complex n-plane bundle, as $\mathbb{C}\mathrm{P}^n$ is a complex manifold) satisfies $T(\mathbb{C}\mathrm{P}^n) \cong \mathrm{Hom}(E, D)$. Then

$$\begin{aligned}
T(\mathbb{C}\mathrm{P}^n) \oplus (\mathbb{C}\mathrm{P}^n \times \mathbb{C}) &\cong \mathrm{Hom}(E, D \oplus (\mathbb{C}\mathrm{P}^n \times \mathbb{C})) \\
&\cong \mathrm{Hom}(E, \mathbb{C}\mathrm{P}^n \times \mathbb{C}^{n+1}) \\
&\cong \bar{E} \oplus \cdots \oplus \bar{E},
\end{aligned}$$

where $\bar{E}$ is the conjugate bundle of E. In general we have

$$c_k(\bar{E}) = (-1)^k c_k(E)$$

for any bundle E. Thus

$$\begin{aligned} c(T(\mathbb{C}P^n)) &= c(T(\mathbb{C}P^n) \oplus (\mathbb{C}P^n \times C)) \\ &= c(\bar{E} \oplus \cdots \oplus \bar{E}) \quad (n+1 \text{ times}) \\ &= c(\bar{E})^{n+1} \\ &= \left(1 + c_1(\bar{E})\right)^{n+1} \\ &= \left(1 - c_1(E)\right)^{n+1}. \end{aligned}$$

For example, if $n = 1$ so that $\mathbb{C}P^n = \mathbb{C}P^1 = S^2$ then

$$c(T(S^2)) = \left(1 - c_1(E)\right)^2 = 1 - 2c_1(E).$$

The classes $c_1(E)^k$ vanish for $k > 1$ since $H^{2k}(S^2) = 0$ for $k > 1$. Thus $c_1(T(S^2)) = -2c_1(E)$. Similarly,

$$c(T(\mathbb{C}P^2)) = 1 - 3c_1(E) + 3c_1(E)^2.$$

For real vector bundles we may use real tangential connections or else complexify. If E is a real tangentially smooth n-plane vector bundle with complexification $E_{\mathbb{C}}$, then $c_i(E_{\mathbb{C}}) = 0$ in $H^{2i}(X;\mathbb{C})$ for i odd (see [Milnor and Stasheff 1974, p. 174]), and hence $c_i^\tau(E_{\mathbb{C}}) = 0$ for i odd. Define the *tangential Pontryagin classes* $p_i^\tau(E)$ by

$$p_i^\tau(E) = (-1)^i c_{2i}^\tau(E_{\mathbb{C}}) \in H_\tau^{4i}(X;\mathbb{C}).$$

Define the *tangential total Pontryagin class* to be the unit

$$p^\tau(E) = 1 + p_1^\tau(E) + t_2^\tau(E) + \cdots$$

We may regard $p_i^\tau(E) \in H_\tau^{4i}(X)$ as the image of $(-1)^i c_{2i}(E) \in H^{4i}(X;\mathbb{Z})$ via the topological definition. The following properties of the tangential Pontryagin classes follow immediately from the corresponding properties of tangential Chern classes.

Proposition 5.17. *For each tangentially smooth real vector bundle E over a compact foliated space X there are tangential Pontryagin classes $p_i^\tau(E) \in H_\tau^{4i}(X)$ satisfying the following properties:*

(1) *If $g : X' \to X$ is tangentially smooth then $g^* p_i^\tau(E) = p_i^\tau(g^* E)$.*

(2) $p_m^\tau(E \oplus E') = \sum_{i=0}^{m} p_i^\tau(E) p_{m-i}^\tau(E') \quad (p_0^\tau = 1)$.

(3) *If E is of real dimension n then $p_i^\tau(E) = 0$ for $i > n/2$.*

(4) *The total tangential Pontryagin class*

$$p^\tau(E) = 1 + p_1^\tau(E) + p_2^\tau(E) + \cdots$$

corresponds to the invariant polynomial $\det\Big(I + \dfrac{A}{2\pi}\Big)$.

To complete our discussion of characteristic classes it remains to define the tangential Euler class. For this we need to assume given a *tangential Riemannian metric*; that is, each leaf of X is given a smooth Riemannian metric which varies continuously in the transverse direction. Recall that a tangential connection on F^* is if the composition

$$\Gamma_\tau(F^*) \xrightarrow{\nabla} \Gamma_\tau(F^* \otimes F^*) \xrightarrow{\wedge} \Gamma_\tau(\Lambda^2 F^*)$$

is equal to the exterior derivative d.

Proposition 5.18. *The dual tangent bundle F^* possesses one and only one symmetric tangential connection which is compatible with its tangential Riemannian metric.*

This preferred tangential connection ∇ is called the *Riemannian or Levi–Civita tangential connection.*

Proof. Let $s_1, \dots, s_n$ be an orthonormal basis for $\Gamma_\tau(F^* |_U)$. There is one and only one skew-symmetric matrix $[\omega_{kj}]$ of 1-forms such that

$$ds_k = \sum_j \omega_{kj} \wedge s_j.$$

(See [Milnor and Stasheff 1974, p. 302–303]). Define the tangential connection ∇ over U by

$$\nabla(s_k) = \sum_j \omega_{kj} \otimes s_j$$

and extend by partitions of unity to all of X. □

Let E be an *oriented* tangentially smooth real $2n$-plane bundle with a tangential Riemannian metric. Choose an oriented orthonormal basis for the sections $\Gamma_\tau(E|_U)$ for some coordinate patch U. Then the tangential curvature matrix Ω obtained from a symmetric tangentially smooth connection is skew-symmetric. There is a unique polynomial with integer coefficients on skew-symmetric matrices, called the *Pfaffian* and written Pf, with the property that

$$\operatorname{Pf}(A)^2 = \det A$$

and

$$\operatorname{Pf}(\operatorname{diag}(S, S, \dots, S)) = 1.$$

The Pfaffian satisfies the invariance condition

$$\operatorname{Pf}(BAB^t) = \operatorname{Pf}(A) \det B$$

and is hence SO($2n$)-invariant. (See [Milnor and Stasheff 1974, p. 309–310] for the linear algebra we omit.) Thus $\mathrm{Pf}(\Omega) \in \Omega_\tau^{2n}(U)$ makes sense. Choosing a different oriented orthonormal basis for the sections over U, this exterior form will be replaced by $\mathrm{Pf}(B\Omega B^t)$, where the matrix B is orthogonal ($B^{-1} = B^t$) and orientation-preserving ($\det(B) = 1$). Thus these local forms coalesce to create a global $2n$-form

$$\mathrm{Pf}(K) \in \Omega_\tau^{2n}(X).$$

As before, this class is a cocycle and hence represents a tangential characteristic cohomology class. It is convenient to normalize. Define the *tangential Euler class* $e^\tau(E)$ by

$$e^\tau(E) = [\mathrm{Pf}(K/2\pi)] \in H_\tau^{2n}(X; \mathbb{R}) \tag{5.19}$$

The tangential Euler class is well-defined and independent of choice of symmetric tangential connection. Here are its elementary properties.

Proposition 5.20. *Each $2n$-dimensional oriented tangentially smooth real vector bundle E with a tangential Riemannian metric over a compact foliated space X has an associated tangential Euler class*

$$e^\tau(E) \in H_\tau^{2n}(X; \mathbb{R}),$$

which is of the form $e^\tau(E) = [\mathrm{Pf}(K)/2\pi]$ and is independent of choice of symmetric connection. Further:

(1) *If $g : X' \to X$ is tangentially smooth then $g^* e^\tau(E) = e^\tau(g^* E)$.*

(2) $e^\tau(E \oplus E') = e^\tau(E) e^\tau(E')$.

(3) *If E has a nowhere zero tangentially smooth section then*

$$e^\tau(E) = 0.$$

(4) *The tangential Pontryagin class $p_n^\tau(E)$ is equal to the square of the tangential Euler class $e^\tau(E)$*:

$$p_n^\tau(E) = e^\tau(E)^2.$$

(In topological treatments of characteristic classes matters are somewhat different. Classes take values in *integral* cohomology and may very well be torsion classes. The resulting formulas are more complicated. Our classes are the images of those under

$$H^*(\cdot\,; \mathbb{Z}) \to H_\tau^*(\cdot).$$

In the Chern–Weil approach the classes take values in cohomology with *real* or *complex* coefficients, so torsion has been destroyed. There is apparently no way known of showing directly from the Chern–Weil approach that Chern classes are integral cohomology classes; proofs known to us rely on the topological construction or on Hodge theory.)

Recall that for any compact foliated space X we have defined the tangential Chern character

$$\mathrm{ch}^\tau : K^0(X) \to \bigoplus_m H_\tau^{2m}(X;\mathbb{C})$$

to be that map which, in the Chern–Weil setting, arises from the invariant polynomial $\mathrm{Trace}(e^{A/2\pi i})$. The map ch^τ is a ring map and it extends to a natural transformation of $\mathbb{Z}/2$-graded functors

$$\mathrm{ch}^\tau : K^*(X) \to H_\tau^{**}(X;\mathbb{C}),$$

where H_τ^{**} is the $\mathbb{Z}/2$-graded functor

$$H_\tau^{**} = H_\tau^{\mathrm{even}} \oplus H_\tau^{\mathrm{odd}} = \left(\bigoplus_m H_\tau^{2m}\right) \oplus \left(\bigoplus_m H_\tau^{2m+1}\right)$$

We recall a fact from classical algebraic topology about compact spaces that are not foliated and the classical Chern character. The cohomology groups being used are ordinary Čech cohomology.

Proposition 5.21. *If X is a compact space then*

$$\mathrm{ch} \otimes 1 : K^*(X) \otimes \mathbb{Q} \to H^{**}(X;\mathbb{Q})$$

is an isomorphism of $\mathbb{Q}$-algebras.

Proof. This theorem is established for X a finite complex by Atiyah and Hirzebruch [1961] in one of the very first papers on topological K-theory. The generalization to compact spaces is routine: write the space as an inverse limit of finite complexes [Eilenberg and Steenrod 1952] and observe that both sides take inverse limits to direct limits. □

Rationalizing is essential: the natural map $\mathrm{ch} : K^0(S^{2n}) \to H^{2n}(S^{2n};\mathbb{Z})$ is one-to-one but not onto.

Lest the reader fall into an obvious trap, we note that the natural map

$$\mathrm{ch}^\tau \otimes 1 : K^*(X) \otimes \mathbb{C} \to H_\tau^{**}(X;\mathbb{C})$$

is *not* an isomorphism in general for foliated spaces, or even for foliated manifolds. In the diagram

$$\begin{array}{ccc} K^*(X)\otimes\mathbb{C} & \xrightarrow[\cong]{\ \mathrm{ch}\otimes 1\ } & H^{**}(X;\mathbb{C}) \\ & {}_{ch^\tau \otimes 1}\searrow & \downarrow r_* \\ & & H_\tau^{**}(X;\mathbb{C}) \end{array}$$

only $\mathrm{ch} \otimes 1$ is an isomorphism, since r_* is neither injective nor surjective in general.

Next we consider Thom isomorphisms. Recall (Theorem 3.30) that if X is a compact foliated space and if $E \to X$ is a tangentially smooth oriented real n-plane bundle then there is a unique Thom class

$$u_E \in H^n_{\tau c}(E)$$

and a Thom isomorphism

$$\Phi_\tau : H^k_\tau(X) \xrightarrow{\cong} H^{k+n}_{\tau c}(E)$$

given by

$$\Phi_\tau(\omega) = u_E \omega.$$

The same result holds in ordinary cohomology. Precisely, there is a Thom class $\tilde{u}_E \in H^n_c(E)$ and a Thom isomorphism

$$\Phi : H^k(X) \xrightarrow{\cong} H^{k+n}_c(E) \tag{5.22}$$

given by

$$\Phi(\omega) = \tilde{u}_E \omega.$$

The proof of this is essentially identical to that of the tangential Thom isomorphism [Bott 1969, §§6 and 7]. Further, the restriction map $r_* : H^*_c(E) \to H^*_{\tau c}(E)$ respects Thom classes:

$$r_*(\tilde{u}_E) = u_E$$

and hence there is a commutative diagram

$$\begin{array}{ccc} H^k(X) & \xrightarrow{r_*} & H^k_\tau(X) \\ \Phi \downarrow & & \downarrow \Phi_\tau \\ H^{k+n}_c(E) & \xrightarrow{r_*} & H^{k+n}_{\tau c}(E). \end{array}$$

There is also a Thom isomorphism in K-theory. To obtain it, however, it is necessary to assume that the structural group of the bundle reduces to the group spin^c. (This is slightly more than orientability.) For instance, it suffices to assume that $E \to X$ is a complex vector bundle (which is all we shall require).

If $E \to X$ is indeed a spin^c-bundle of even real dimension then there is a K-theory Thom class

$$u^K_E \in K^0(E).$$

(This means K-theory with compact supports: $K^0(E) = \widetilde{K}^0(E^+)$.) Further, multiplication by this class induces an isomorphism

$$\Phi_K : K^0(X) \to K^0(E) \tag{5.23}$$

given by

$$\Phi_K(x) = u^K_E x.$$

(For the proof of this theorem the reader may consult [Atiyah et al. 1964], [Atiyah 1967] and [Karoubi 1978].) All three Thom isomorphisms extend to the case X locally compact; see [Karoubi 1978].

It would be natural to suppose that Thom isomorphisms commute with the Chern character, i.e., that the diagram

$$\begin{array}{ccc} K^0(X) & \xrightarrow{\mathrm{ch}_\tau} & H^{**}_{\tau c}(X) \\ \downarrow \Phi_K & & \downarrow \Phi_\tau \\ K^0(E) & \xrightarrow{\mathrm{ch}_\tau} & H^{**}_{\tau c}(E) \end{array}$$

would commute. Denote by $1 \in K^0(X)$ the class of the complex one-dimensional trivial bundle over X, which is the identity of $K^0(X)$. Then

$$\mathrm{ch}_\tau \Phi_K(1) = \mathrm{ch}_\tau(u^K_E), \qquad \Phi_\tau \,\mathrm{ch}_\tau(1) = \Phi_\tau(1) = u_E.$$

Thus commutativity boils down to the relation between the cohomology Thom class u_E and the Chern character of the K-theory Thom class $\mathrm{ch}_\tau(u^K_E)$: the diagram commutes if and only if

$$u_E = \mathrm{ch}_\tau(u^K_E).$$

Generally these classes are *not* equal. Define the *tangential Todd class*

$$\mathrm{Td}_\tau(E) \in H^{**}_\tau(X)$$

by the formula

$$\mathrm{Td}_\tau(E) = [\Phi_\tau^{-1}(\mathrm{ch}_\tau(u^K_E))]^{-1}. \tag{5.24}$$

Thus

$$\mathrm{Td}_\tau(E) = 1 \Leftrightarrow u^\tau_E = \mathrm{ch}(u^K_E).$$

Our definition is of course modeled after the classical Todd class which is defined by

$$\mathrm{Td}(E) = [\Phi^{-1}(\mathrm{ch}(u^K_E))]^{-1} \in H^{**}(X)$$

so that

$$\mathrm{Td}(E) = 1 \Leftrightarrow \tilde{u}_E = \mathrm{ch}(u^K_E).$$

We list the elementary properties of the tangential Todd class. Recall that

$$r_* : H^*(X) \to H^*_\tau(X)$$

is the restriction map.

Proposition 5.25. *The tangential Todd class has the following properties*:

(1) $r_* \,\mathrm{Td}(E) = \mathrm{Td}_\tau(E)$.

(2) $\mathrm{Td}_\tau(E \oplus E') = \mathrm{Td}_\tau(E)\,\mathrm{Td}_\tau(E')$.

(3) *If $f : X \to Y$ is a tangentially smooth map and $E \to Y$ is a tangentially smooth bundle then*

$$\mathrm{Td}_\tau(f^* E) = f^* \mathrm{Td}(E).$$

(4) Td_τ *is the tangential characteristic class associated with the invariant power series*

$$\frac{x}{1-e^{-x}}.$$

Proof. The first property follows from the fact that $r_* \tilde{u}_E = u_E$. The remaining properties may be proved directly or deduced form the analogous properties of the classical Todd class as in [Karoubi 1978, p. 285]. □

Note that $\mathrm{Td}(E)$ is a unit in the ring $H^{**}(X)$. Let E' be a real bundle such that $E \oplus E'$ is a trivial bundle. Then

$$\begin{aligned} 1 &= \mathrm{Td}(E \oplus E') && \text{since } \mathrm{Td}(1) = 1 \\ &= \mathrm{Td}(E)\,\mathrm{Td}(E') && \text{by (1).} \end{aligned}$$

It is customary to define the *Todd genus* of a smooth manifold M by

$$\mathrm{Td}(M) = \mathrm{Td}(TM \otimes \mathbb{C})$$

and following custom we define the *tangential Todd genus* of a foliated space X by

(5.26) $$\mathrm{Td}_\tau(X) = \mathrm{Td}_\tau(FX \otimes \mathbb{C}).$$

We emphasize that we may regard classes such as $\mathrm{Td}_\tau(X)$ as tangential *forms* in $\Omega_\tau^*(X)$ given by certain universal polynomials in the tangential curvature form K_E. Given a tangential connection, these forms are uniquely defined (not just up to cohomology class). Changing the tangential connection changes the form but preserves the cohomology class of the form.

We may see the Todd class very explicitly. The power series $x/(1-e^{-x})$ expands as

$$\frac{x}{1-e^{-x}} = 1 + \frac{1}{2}x + \sum_{s=1}^{\infty}(-1)^{s-1}\frac{B_s}{(2s)!}x^{2s},$$

where $B_s \in \mathbb{Q}$ is the s-th Bernoulli number (see [Milnor and Stasheff 1974, Appendix]):

$$\begin{aligned} B_1 &= 1/6, & B_5 &= 5/66, \\ B_2 &= 1/30, & B_6 &= 691/2730, \\ B_3 &= 1/42, & B_7 &= 7/6, \\ B_4 &= 1/30, & B_8 &= 3617/510. \end{aligned}$$

For example, if X is a foliated space with leaf dimension $p \leq 8$ then $H_\tau^k(X) = 0$ for $k > 8$ and the polynomial has the form

$$1 + \frac{1}{2}x + \frac{B_1}{2}x^2 - \frac{B_2}{24}x^4 == 1 + \frac{x}{2} + \frac{1}{12}x^2 - \frac{1}{720}x^4.$$

Thus if E is a complex line bundle over X then

$$\mathrm{Td}_\tau(E) = 1 + \tfrac{1}{2}c_1^\tau(E) + \tfrac{1}{12}c_1^\tau(E)^2 - \tfrac{1}{720}c_1^\tau(E)^4.$$

This is a nonhomogeneous class, sitting as is usual in the group

$$H_\tau^{\mathrm{even}}(X) = \bigoplus_m H_\tau^{2m}(X).$$

For instance, let $X = M = \mathbb{C}\mathrm{P}^2$ with canonical complex line bundle E^1 and write $\omega = K/(2\pi i)$. Then

$$c(T\mathbb{C}\mathrm{P}^2) = 1 - 3\omega + 3\omega^2.$$

The Chern character and Todd class are given at the form level by

$$\mathrm{ch}(T\mathbb{C}\mathrm{P}^2) = 2 - 3\omega + \tfrac{3}{2}\omega^2 \qquad \text{and} \qquad \mathrm{Td}(T\mathbb{C}\mathrm{P}^2) = 1 - \tfrac{3}{2}\omega + \omega^2.$$

We follow the usual convention in interpreting expressions of the type $\int \omega \, d\nu$, where ω is a nonhomogeneous form; take the part of ω which lies in Ω^p and ignore the rest. For instance,

$$\int \mathrm{Td}_\tau(E)\, d\nu$$

is to be understood as follows: write $\mathrm{Td}_\tau(E) = \sum \mathrm{Td}_\tau^m(E)$, where $\mathrm{Td}_\tau^m(E) \in H_\tau^m(X)$, and define

$$\int \mathrm{Td}_\tau(E)\, d\nu \equiv \int \mathrm{Td}_\tau^p(E)\, d\nu.$$

Finally, note that if M is a foliated manifold with tangent bundle TM and foliation bundle FM then the normal bundle to the foliation $NM = TM/FM$ has a flat connection in the leaf direction and so its relevant characteristic classes vanish. Thus if ω is any tangential cohomology class, then

$$\int \omega\, \mathrm{Td}(M)\, d\nu \equiv \int \omega\, \mathrm{Td}(TM)\, d\nu = \int \omega\, \mathrm{Td}(FM)\, d\nu$$

and so we may use $\mathrm{Td}(M)$ and $\mathrm{Td}(FM)$ interchangeably in index formulas.

□ □□□□□ □□□□

Were we to be writing the book afresh we would have to talk about cyclic cohomology at some length, even though strictly speaking it is not necessary for the presentation of this Index Theorem. For a recent elementary introduction showing cyclic theory in context, we recommend [Khalkhali 2004]. There are several books on the subject; we recommend [Loday 1998] for a very detailed and explicit exposition. However, it is probably better to learn as you go.

CHAPTER VI

Operator Algebras

We turn now to the discussion of operator algebras that can be associated with groupoids and in particular to the groupoid of a foliated space. For this discussion we start with a locally compact second countable topological groupoid G and we assume given a continuous tangential measure λ (see Chapter IV for the definition). Thus for each x in the unit space X of G we have a measure λ^x on $G^x = r^{-1}(x)$ with certain invariance and continuity properties as described in Chapter IV. For the moment we do not need to assume that the groupoid has discrete holonomy groups as in Chapter IV, but all the examples and all the applications will satisfy this condition. If in addition the support of the measure λ^x is equal to $r^{-1}(x)$, as is usual in our examples, then λ is called a Haar system.

In this chapter we construct the C^*-algebra of the groupoid and we determine this algebra in several important special cases. (As general references for C^*-algebras, we recommend [Davidson 1996; Fillmore 1996; Arveson 1976; Pedersen 1979].) We describe the Hilsum–Skandalis stability theorem. Assuming a transverse measure, we construct the associated von Neumann algebra and develop its basic properties and important subalgebras. This leads us to the construction of the weight associated to the transverse measure; it is a trace if and only if the transverse measure is invariant. Finally, we introduce the K-theory index group $K_0(C_r^*(G))$ and construct a partial Chern character

$$c : K_0\big(C_r^*(G(X))\big) \to MT(X)^* \cong \overline{H}_\tau^p(X),$$

given explicitly as follows. If $[u] \in K_0\big(C_r^*(G(X))\big)$ and ν is an invariant transverse measure with associated trace ϕ_ν then

$$c([u])(\nu) = \phi_\nu^n(e - f),$$

where e and f are suitably chosen projections in $C_r^*(G(X))^+ \otimes M_n$ whose difference represents u and $\phi_\nu^n = \phi_\nu \times \mathrm{Tr}$. The partial Chern character applied to the symbol of a tangential, tangentially elliptic operator D yields the cohomology analytic index class $[\iota_D] \in \overline{H}_\tau^p(X)$.

We shall first review the construction of a C^*-algebra associated to the pair (G, λ) [Connes 1979; Renault 1980]. Suppose first that G is Hausdorff. On the space $C_c(G)$ of continuous compactly supported functions on G one defines a multiplication and an involution:

$$(6.1)\qquad \begin{aligned} (f * g)(u) &= \int f(v)g(v^{-1}u)\,d\lambda^{r(u)}(v), \\ f^*(u) &= \overline{f(u^{-1})}. \end{aligned}$$

That these define an associative algebra with involution on $C_c(G)$ is a straightforward calculation paralleling the case when G is a locally compact group, [Pedersen 1979, p. 233]. The invariance property of tangential measures allows one to rewrite the convolution as

$$(f * g)(u) = \int f(uv)g(v^{-1})\,d\lambda^{s(u)}(v).$$

In the case when G is an equivalence relation $\mathcal{R}$ on a space X, then a tangential measure is simply a measure λ^x for each $x \in X$ such that $\lambda^x = \lambda^y$ if $x \sim y$. Functions on $G = \mathcal{R}$ are viewed as partially defined functions of two variables, and the formulas become

$$\begin{aligned} (f * g)(x, z) &= \int f(x, y)g(y, z)\,d\lambda^x(y), \\ f^*(x, y) &= \overline{f(y, x)}, \end{aligned}$$

where in the first formula λ^x could be λ^y or λ^z as x, y, and z in the formula are all in the same equivalence class.

There are two ways to norm the involutive algebra $C_c(G)$. The first norm is constructed as follows. For each $x \in X$ there is a natural homomorphism

$$\pi_x : C_c(G) \longrightarrow \mathcal{B}(L^2(G^x, \lambda^x_{G(X)}))$$

into the algebra of bounded operators on the Hilbert space $L^2(G^x, \lambda^x_{G(X)})$ defined essentially by convolution:

$$(6.2)\qquad (\pi_x(f)\phi)(u) = \int f(u^{-1}v)\phi(v)\,d\lambda^x(v).$$

The integral is clearly well defined for $\phi \in L^2(G^x, \lambda^x_{G(X)})$ and $f \in C_c(G)$, and it yields a bounded operator $\pi_x(f)$ on $L^2(G^x, \lambda^x_{G(X)})$. That π_x defines a $*$-homomorphism is likewise easily checked. Note that formula (6.2) displays $\pi_x(f)$ in effect as right convolution by f' $(= \bar{f}^*)$, where $f'(u) = f(u^{-1})$.

One norms $C_c(G)$ by

$$|f| = \sup_x |\pi_x(f)|.$$

The completion of $C_c(G)$ under this norm is virtually by construction a C^*-algebra, for we obtain it by embedding $C_c(G)$ into bounded operators on a Hilbert space (the sum of the $L^2(G^x, \lambda^x_{G(X)})$) and closing up the image.

Definition 6.3. The *reduced C^*-algebra of the groupoid G* is the completion of $C_c(G)$ with respect to the norm $|f|$ above; it is denoted $C_r^*(G)$.

This construction is analogous to the construction of the reduced C^*-algebra of a locally compact group by closing up the image of the regular representation. Connes and his students write this algebra as $C^*(V, F)$ or $C^*(V/F)$ when G is the graph of a foliated manifold (V, F).

The second norm on $C_c(G)$ corresponds to the full C^*-algebra of a group. Namely we first put a kind of an L_1 norm on $C_c(G)$

$$|f|_1 = \max\{\sup_x \int |f(u)|\, d\lambda^x(u),\ \sup_x \int |f(u^{-1})|\, d\lambda^x(u)\},$$

so that it becomes a normed $*$-algebra. Then we form the C^*-completion of this algebra using all bounded $*$-representations. This is denoted $C^*(G)$ and is called the *full* or *unreduced* C^*-algebra of the groupoid. As the representations π_x are among all bounded representations, it is evident that the reduced C^*-algebra $C_r^*(G)$ is a quotient of $C^*(G)$.

As our concern here will be with analysis and differential operators on foliated spaces where the representations π_x play the central role, it is evident that it is the reduced C^*-algebra $C_r^*(G)$ rather than the full C^*-algebra that will be the focus of attention. Of course the construction of both $C_r^*(G)$ and $C^*(G)$ presupposes a tangential measure or a Haar system on the groupoid G. These algebras can depend on this choice, and if one is being absolutely precise, the underlying Haar system should be included in the notation. The reader is referred to [Renault 1980] for a more extended discussion on this point. This will not be an issue for us because in the first place if λ is a tangential measure (resp. Haar system) and if $\lambda' = f\lambda$, where f is a continuous everywhere positive function on G that is constant on the fibres of the map $u \to (r(u), s(u))$ of G into $X \times X$, then λ' is also a tangential measure (resp. Haar system). In this case it is easy to check that the C^*-algebras $C_r^*(G)$ and $C^*(G)$ do not depend on whether one uses λ or λ'. Secondly, in the case of the graph of a foliated space, there is as we have already pointed out in Chapter IV (4.20 and remarks following) a choice of a class of Haar systems (each λ^x should have a continuous, or even tangentially C^∞, density on the leaves in local coordinates), any two of which differ like λ and λ' above. If the total space of the foliated space is compact one can also choose the function relating λ and λ' to be bounded above and below.

At all events when we speak about $C_r^*(G)$ or $C^*(G)$ in the context of the graphs of foliated spaces, we shall always understand that standard choice of Haar system. It is evident that the hypothesis that G be second countable makes the C^*-algebra $C_r^*(G)$ separable.

All of this discussion has assumed that the groupoid G is Hausdorff, but we know that the groupoid of a foliated space need not be Hausdorff. At all events the groupoid is locally Hausdorff, so it may be covered by a family of open sets each one of which is Hausdorff. We still assume that the space is second countable. Then as one can take this family to be a countable family $\{U_i\}$, it is straightforward using standard techniques to see that G is at least a standard Borel groupoid. (A set E is Borel if and only if $E \cap U_i$ is Borel for each i.) This will be useful later when we introduce von Neumann algebras associated with these groupoids.

It is still quite straightforward to introduce the C^*-algebra in the locally Hausdorff case. We gave a definition in (4.15) of what was meant by a continuous tangential measure $\lambda = \{\lambda^\ell\}$ in this situation. Now instead of considering all continuous compactly supported functions on G, let us consider instead the set of finite linear combinations of functions $f = \sum f_i$, where each f_i is a compactly supported function continuous on some open Hausdorff subset U_i of G extended to be zero on the rest of G. (Note that while f_i is continuous on U_i its extension to G is not in general a continuous function on G.) These functions can be convolved using the same formulas as in the Hausdorff case to give an $*$-algebra. Then one follows the same recipe for norming it and constructing a separable C^*-algebra $C_r^*(G)$.

The C^*-algebra associated to the groupoid of a foliated space X plays a key role in the analysis and geometry of X as we shall see. In particular its K-theory group $K_0(C_r^*(G))$ is the natural place where indices for operators live; see [Connes and Skandalis 1981; 1984]. One may also think of $C_r^*(G)$ as a noncommutative replacement for the algebra of functions on the quotient space $X/\mathcal{R}$, where X is the unit space of G and $\mathcal{R}$ is the equivalence relation on X defined by $\mathcal{R}$. For a foliated space this is the space of leaves. Indeed when $X/\mathcal{R}$ is a "good" space such as when G is the groupoid of a foliated space which is a fibration, then $C_r^*(G)$ looks very much like $C(X/\mathcal{R})$, as we shall see presently; they are in fact stably isomorphic. The interpretation of $C_r^*(G)$ as functions on the leaf space is enhanced by the following result from [Fack and Skandalis 1982].

Theorem 6.4. *If G is the groupoid of a foliated space, then $C_r^*(G)$ is simple as a C^*-algebra if and only if every leaf of the foliated space is dense.*

We shall not prove this result except to remark that if ℓ is a proper closed leaf, then the representation π_x above for any x in ℓ has a nontrivial kernel so that $C_r^*(G)$ is not simple.

One of the most important classes of examples of topological groupoids comes from group actions. Suppose that a locally compact group H acts as a topological transformation group on a space X with $h \in H$ acting on a point $x \in X$ denoted $h \cdot x$. The product space

$$G = X \times H$$

becomes in a natural way a groupoid where the product in G, say of (x, g) and (y, h), is defined if and only if $g \cdot y = x$ and then

$$(x, g) \cdot (y, h) = (x, gh).$$

X is the space of units and the range and source maps are given by $r(x, h) = x$, $s(x, h) = h^{-1} \cdot x$. Then

$$G^x = \{(h, x) \mid x \text{ fixed, } h \text{ arbitrary in } H\} \cong H.$$

If $u = (g, y)$ is an element of G which can multiply G^x on the left, that is $s(u) = s(y, g) = g^{-1}y = x$, then left multiplication by u maps G^x onto G^y, $y = g \cdot x$ and the map is $(x, h) \mapsto (y, gh)$. Now giving a tangential measure or a Haar system on the groupoid G is giving a measure λ^x on each G^x which is invariant under these left multiplications. There is a natural choice in this case, namely take for λ^x on $G^x \simeq H$, a fixed left Haar measure on H. Evidently this tangential measure is continuous in the sense of Definition 4.15. This example is of course the reason one calls such objects Haar systems. Of course, for the groupoid just defined to fall strictly within the context of Chapter IV, where we assume discrete holonomy groups, the various isotropy groups $H_x = \{h \mid h \cdot x = x\}$ of the action of H on X must be discrete. If for instance H is a Lie group acting on a manifold X, the action of H will give rise to a foliated space structure on X only in this case.

In the case of a group H acting on a space X as above, one may form a C^*-algebra, the *reduced crossed product* algebra of $C(X)$ by H, written

$$C(X)_r \rtimes H;$$

see [Pedersen 1979]. It is clear that the general construction for groupoids should and does yield the reduced crossed product construction in this case.

Proposition 6.5. *If $G = X \times H$ for an action of H on X (no assumptions on isotropy) then*

$$C_r^*(G) \cong C(X)_r \rtimes H.$$

Proof. One checks that there are dense subalgebras of both sides that are algebraically identical. The algebra $C_r^*(G)$ is obtained by completing in the norm defined by the family of representations π_x, for $x \in X$. Each of these comes from a covariant representation of the pair $(C(X), G)$ and one has to prove that these give the same norm as the subfamily of all covariant representations of the pair used to define the reduced crossed product. We omit the details. □

Another, somewhat trivial case, is of interest; let X be locally compact and let $G = X \times X$ be the equivalence relation (principal groupoid) with all points equivalent. If X is a manifold foliated by one leaf, G is its groupoid. A Haar system is simply a measure λ on X whose support is all of X. Evidently elements of the dense subalgebra of the definition can be realized as integral kernel operators on $L^2(X, \lambda)$ with compactly supported kernels. The completion is obviously all compact operators $\mathcal{K}$ on $L^2(X, \lambda)$.

Proposition 6.6. *In this case* $C_r^*(G) \cong \mathcal{K}$.

An important theme in [Feldman and Moore 1977], [Feldman et al. 1978], and [Ramsay 1982] is that for measured groupoids or equivalence relations, the special case when the orbits are discrete is much easier to handle and that in some sense the general case could be reduced to this special case. We want to see that the same is true in this context. First of all we need a definition.

Definition 6.7. The (locally Hausdorff) topological groupoid G has *discrete orbits* if the range and source maps are local homeomorphisms.

It follows that each equivalence class (or leaf) of the associated equivalence relation is countable and discrete in the relative topology from G (although not in the relative topology from X). In this case there is a natural choice of tangential measure, namely the counting measure on each leaf. It follows from the definition of discreteness that this is a continuous tangential measure, and so we can define the C^*-algebra $C_r^*(G)$.

It is useful to point out that in the case of a principal groupoid, where G is simply an equivalence relation, that G can be covered by sets of a very simple kind. For each open set O in X and b be a homeomorphism onto an open subset of X and then define

$$U(b, O) = \{(x, b(x)) \mid x \in O\}.$$

Proposition 6.8. *If the groupoid G is discrete and principal, the sets* $\{U(b, O)\}$ *are open sets and form a cover of G.*

The dense subalgebra A of compactly supported functions (or its substitute in the non-Hausdorff case) can be thought of as generalized matrices especially if there is no holonomy so that G is a principal groupoid, i.e., an equivalence relation $\mathcal{R}$. Then as we have already seen the formulas simplify and the product of two functions on $\mathcal{R} \subset X \times X$ is given by

$$(f * g)(x, z) = \sum f(x, y) g(y, z),$$

where the sum is extended over all y which lie in the same class as x and z. The condition that f and g be compactly supported implies that the sum is finite. Written this way the product really does look like matrix multiplication. When there is holonomy, multiplication is still given by a sum rather than an integral, but the sum must include summation (convolution) on the discrete holonomy groups.

For general groupoids, the process of completing the dense subalgebra A of functions to obtain $C_r^*(G)$ leads to elements in the C^* algebra which cannot be represented as functions on G. One of the nice features of discrete groupoids is that an element of the C^*-algebra can be represented by a continuous function on G, at least if G is Hausdorff.

Proposition 6.9. *For $f \in A$ and $u \in G$,*

$$|f(u)| \leq |f|,$$

where $|f| = \sup_x |\pi_x(f)|$ is the C^*-norm.

Proof. The representation π_x of A in $L^2(G^x, \lambda^x_{G(X)})$ in the definition of $C^*_r(G)$ is a representation by matrices since G^x is a countable discrete set and λ^x is counting measure. It is evident moreover that $f(u)$ is just one of the matrix coefficients of $\pi_x(f)$, and so the inequality is obvious. □

Thus, any sequence f_n in A with a limit in $C^*_r(G)$ must converge uniformly as continuous functions on G to a limit f, and we have the desired result when G is Hausdorff. Moreover multiplication of elements of $C^*_r(G)$ is given by the same "matrix multiplication" formulas for the functions which represent them. The sums are no longer finite but are absolutely convergent, as is easily seen using the argument of Proposition 6.9. The situation for non-Hausdorff G can be handed by localization to Hausdorff subsets.

Another feature of the discrete case is that the set of units X is an open subset of G because r and s are local homeomorphisms. Hence the set of compactly supported functions $C_c(X)$ is a subset of the algebra A used to define $C^*(G)$. Moreover it is a subalgebra; elements of $C_c(X)$ correspond to diagonal matrices in the description above of A as generalized matrices. Hence the C^*-algebra $C_0(X)$ becomes a subalgebra of $C^*_r(G)$. If X is compact, as it will be in most cases, then $C_0(X) = C(X)$ has a unit which is also a unit for $C^*_r(G)$.

Finally, suppose that G is discrete and principal—that is, an equivalence relation and Hausdorff (note that it would be Hausdorff automatically if X itself is Hausdorff since G can be mapped continuously into $X \times X$). In this case the subalgebra $C_0(X)$ of $C^*_r(G)$ has a very special property—namely it is a diagonal subalgebra of $C^*_r(G)$ in the language of [Kumjian 1986] (and a Cartan subalgebra in the language of [Renault 1980]). We are inclined to change terminology and call Kumjian's diagonal subalgebras Cartan subalgebras.

Definition 6.10 [Kumjian 1986]. A *Cartan subalgebra B* of a unital C^*-algebra A is an abelian subalgebra (that contains the unit of A) with a faithful conditional expectation $P : A \to B$ with the property that the kernel of P is spanned by all elements a of A such that

(i) $aBa^* \subset B$,

(ii) $a^*Ba \subset B$,

(iii) $a^2 = 0$.

(Kumjian calls these free normalizers of B.) If A is not unital, a Cartan subalgebra of A is a subalgebra B such that B^+ is a Cartan subalgebra of A^+, where $(\cdot)^+$ is the operation of appending a unit.

To see that $C_0(X)$ is a Cartan subalgebra of $C_r^*(G)$ [Kumjian 1986], one has to define first a conditional expectation P. If $m \in C_r^*(G)$, it is represented by a function on G by Proposition 6.9 and then one restricts the function to the diagonal to get an element in $C_0(X)$. Next note that free centralizers can be obtained by taking a function a supported on a set of the form $U(f, O)$ in G, where f has no fixed points and such that

$$a(x, f(x))a(f(x), f^2(x)) = 0$$

An easy localization argument shows that any compactly supported function on $G - \Delta X$ can be written as a finite sum of such functions, and hence that there are enough normalizers to span the kernel of P. Conversely it is evident from the condition $a^2 = 0$ that any such a viewed as a function on G must vanish on the diagonal and so is in the kernel of P.

Kumjian proves a powerful converse to this exercise. complementing an earlier result of Renault [1980]. Roughly stated it says that every pair (A, B), where B is a Cartan subalgebra (diagonal subalgebra in the language of [Kumjian 1986]) arises uniquely from a discrete equivalence relation but with a "twist" coming from a kind of two cocycle as in [Feldman and Moore 1977; Renault 1980]. In fact the topological objects which classify the pairs (A, B) are called twists. We shall not pursue this topic further here as it would take us afield.

If G_1 and G_2 are topological groupoids, their product

$$G = G_1 \times G_2$$

is also one. If λ_i is a Haar system on G_i, for $i = 1, 2$, clearly we can define a Haar system $\lambda_1 \times \lambda_2$ on $G = G_1 \times G_2$ for if X_i is the unit space of G_i, $X = X_1 \times X_2$ is the unit space of G and the range map r of G is $r_1 \times r_2$. Hence $r^{-1}(x_1, x_2) = r_1^{-1}(x_1) \times r_2^{-1}(x_2)$ and $(\lambda_1 \times \lambda_2)^{(x_1, x_2)}$ is defined to be the product measure. The following is then straightforward.

Proposition 6.11. *$C_r^*(G_1 \times G_2) \cong C_r^*(G_1) \otimes C_r^*(G_2)$, where $\otimes$ denotes the minimal or spatial tensor product.*

Proof. If A_i, A are the algebras of functions on G_i, G used to define these C^*-algebras, it is evident that the algebraic tensor product $A_1 \otimes A_2$ can be identified as a dense subalgebra of A. The completions $C_r^*(G_i)$ are defined by a family of $*$ representations $\pi_{x_{ij}}$ $(x_{ij} \in X_i)$ and it is clear that the completion $C_r^*(G)$ can be defined exactly by the family of tensor products $\pi_{x_{1,j}} \otimes \pi_{x_{2,j}}$. The result follows. □

As a corollary of this, suppose that G_1 is a groupoid and that $G_2 = X_2 \times X_2$ is a groupoid of the type in Proposition 6.6, for instance the groupoid of a manifold

X_2 foliated by a single leaf. Then form $G = G_1 \times G_2$. If for instance G_1 is the groupoid of a foliated space X_1 and X_2 is a fixed manifold foliated as a single leaf, then G is the groupoid of the foliated space $X = X_1 \times X_2$, where the leaves of X are $\ell \times X_2$, where ℓ is a leaf in X_1. In other words we have fattened up the leaves of X_1 by crossing with a fixed manifold. The foliated spaces X_1 and X have the same transversal structure. As a consequence of 6.6 and 6.11 we have for any G_1 and any X_2 the following:

Proposition 6.12. $C_r^*(G) \cong C_r^*(G_1) \otimes \mathcal{K}$, *where* $\mathcal{K}$ *is the algebra of compact operators.*

As a further example let us consider the groupoid arising from a fibration[1] $p : X \to B$ with standard fibre F. We let G be the equivalence relation on X, where $x \sim y$ if $p(x) = p(y)$. If the fibration is locally trivial and the standard fibre is a manifold, then X is a foliated space with leaves equal to the fibre of the fibration. We note an important fact for future use: if $X \to B$ is a fibre bundle with fibre H some Hilbert space and structural group the unitary group $\mathcal{U}H$, then $X \to B$ is a trivial bundle, since $\mathcal{U}H$ is contractible in the strong operator topology.

If $U \subset B$ is an open set over which the fibration is trivial, then U defines an open subfoliated space which is the product of U foliated by points with F foliated by one leaf. Hence "locally" the C^*-algebra is a product $C^*(U) \otimes \mathcal{K}$ by above. But this works globally at the algebra level, at least if B is finite-dimensional. In order to avoid degenerate cases we assume in the following that the standard fibre is not a finite set. The algebra is formed with respect to any given continuous Haar system.

Proposition 6.13. *If* G *is the groupoid of a locally trivial fibration with base* B, *then* $C_r^*(G)$ *is Morita equivalent to* $C(B) \otimes \mathcal{K}$. *If* B *is finite-dimensional then*

$$C_r^*(G) \cong C(B) \otimes \mathcal{K}.$$

See [Rieffel 1976] for the definition of Morita equivalence in the context of C^*-algebras.

(A related result is proved in [Candel and Conlon 2003, p. 34]: If G is the groupoid of a locally trivial fibration with base B, the fibre F is a smooth manifold, and the structural group of the fibration is Diff(F) then $C_r^*(G) \cong C(B) \otimes \mathcal{K}$.)

---

[1] A fibration $p : X \to B$ is a continuous map that has the homotopy lifting property: if $g_t : Y \to B$ is a continuous path of maps, and $f_0 : Y \to X$ is continuous with $pf_0 = g_0$ then there exists a continuous family $f_t : Y \to X$ extending f_0, and $pf_t = g_t$ for $0 \le t \le 1$. See [Steenrod 1951]. If B is path-connected then all fibres $F_b = p^{-1}(b)$ are of the same homotopy type. If we assume that the fibration is locally trivial then we may use any of these and we write F for the *standard fibre*. For example, by a theorem of Hurewicz (see [Dugundji 1965]), every fibre bundle over a paracompact space B is a fibration.

Proof. For each $b \in B$, let $p^{-1}(b)$ be the fibre over b. A Haar system is simply the assignment in a "smooth" fashion of a measure λ^b on $p^{-1}(b) \cong F$, where smoothness means that in each local trivialization of $p^{-1}(U) \cong U \times F$, the λ^b for b in U viewed as measures on F vary continuously. The Hilbert spaces $L^2(p^{-1}(b), \lambda^b)$ then form a continuous field of Hilbert spaces over B [Dixmier 1969b] and it is evident from Proposition 6.12 that $C_r^*(G)$ consists of the sections of the corresponding field of operator algebras $\mathcal{K}(L^2(p^{-1}(b), \lambda^b))$. The Dixmier–Douady invariant [1963] is trivial and hence $C_r^*(G)$ is Morita equivalent to $C(B) \otimes \mathcal{K}$. If B is finite-dimensional then the field of Hilbert spaces is trivial and so $C_r^*(G) \cong C(B) \otimes \mathcal{K}$. □

If in this example, the fibration $X \to B$ has a cross section s, then $s(B)$ is a complete transversal homeomorphic to B. Then $s(B)$ is a groupoid of a trivial sort—equivalence classes are points. Thus $C_r^*(s(B)) = C(B)$ and so $C_r^*(G) \cong C_r^*(s(B)) \otimes \mathcal{K}$. This is in fact quite a general phenomenon at least for groupoids of foliated spaces as is shown in [Hilsum and Skandalis 1983]. We describe this result, which will be of considerable use to us, in some more detail.

In Chapter IV we discussed regular transversals for foliated spaces. These were locally compact subsets N of the foliated space X so that $N \subset N'$ with $\overline{N} \subset N'$ and $\overline{N}$ compact, and such that there exists an open ball B in $\mathbb{R}^p$, p the leaf dimension, with a homeomorphism of $N' \times B$ onto an open subset U of X with the map an isomorphism of foliated spaces. For this discussion, we shall also assume that there is a larger ball B' containing B with an extension of the homeomorphism of $N' \times B$ to $N' \times B'$ onto some U'; we shall also assume that N is open in N' so that $N \times B$ corresponds to an open set. To simplify notation, let us take the $N \times B$ to be subsets of X. If X is compact one can clearly find a finite number of such N_i so that the union is a complete transversal. If X is locally compact, then as in [Fack and Skandalis 1982] one can find a locally finite such family and can also arrange that the $N_i \times B$ are disjoint from each other. At all events if $N = \bigcup N_i$, finite or infinite, then there is a ball B in $\mathbb{R}^p$ so that $N \times B = U$ is an open subset of X. We can also arrange that U^c contains a set of exactly the same form $N \times B$ using the fact that for the original N_i we had $N_i \times B' \supset N_i \times B$.

Let G be the groupoid of the foliated space (Hausdorff or not) and let G_N^N be the groupoid relativized to N;

$$G_N^N = \{u \in G \mid r(u), s(u) \in N\}.$$

Then G_N^N is a topological groupoid in its own right and it has discrete orbits. Then $C_r^*(G_N^N)$ is an algebra of the kind discussed earlier in the chapter. If we form $U = N \times B$ then G_U^U is an open subgroupoid of G and is clearly the product

$$G_U^U \cong G_N^N \times (B \times B),$$

where $B \times B$ is the principal groupoid (equivalence relation) with unit space B and with all points equivalent. It follows from Proposition 6.12 that

$$C_r^*(G_U^U) \cong C_r^*(G_N^N) \otimes \mathcal{K},$$

where $\mathcal{K}$ is the algebra of compact operators.

Further, as G_U^U is an open subgroupoid of G, we can extend functions in the dense subalgebra defining $C_r^*(G_U^U)$ to functions on G. Moreover the choice of Haar system for defining $C_r^*(G_U^U)$ and $C_r^*(G)$ are compatible. It follows now that the natural injection of the dense algebra of compactly supported functions on G_U^U into functions on G produces a map i on the C^*-algebra level of $C_r^*(G_U^U)$ into $C_r^*(G)$. The result of Hilsum and Skandalis [1983], in a slightly strengthened version, is the following, which shows in some sense that $C_r^*(G)$ is no more complicated than $C_r^*(G_U^U)$ and also that the complete transversal N controls the structure of these algebras.

Theorem 6.14 [Hilsum and Skandalis 1983]. *The algebra $C_r^*(G)$ is isomorphic to the algebra $M_2(C_r^*(G_U^U))$ of 2×2 matrices over $C_r^*(G_U^U)$ and the injection map i above corresponds to the natural inclusion of $C_r^*(G_U^U)$ into 2×2 matrices*

$$a \to \begin{pmatrix} a & 0 \\ 0 & 0 \end{pmatrix}.$$

Hence $C_r^*(G)$ is also isomorphic to $C_r^*(G_N^N) \otimes \mathcal{K}$, where $\mathcal{K}$ is the algebra of compact operators.

We shall not reproduce the details of the argument but will note some highlights. Fixing the complete transversal N as above, they define for each open set V of the unit space X, a C^*-module (see [Kasparov 1980]) $H(V)$ over $C_r^*(G_N^N)$. These add for disjoint U's and $H(V) = H(W)$ if $V = W - F$, where F is closed in X and meets each leaf in a null set. They also establish that the algebra of "compact operators" (in Kasparov's terminology) on $H(V)$ is $C_r^*(G_V^V)$. For the particular choice of $U = N \times B$, the "tube" around the transversal N which was constructed above, it is easy to see that $H(U) = H_\infty \otimes C_r^*(G_N^N)$, where H_∞ is an infinite-dimensional Hilbert space. Since by construction we can find another transversal N' which looks just like N and a "tube" around it, $N' \times B$ inside of $\overline{T}^c$, one may use the above to argue that $H(X) = H(U) \oplus H(\overline{T}^c)$ and that $H(\overline{T}^c)$ contains a submodule $H(U')$ isomorphic to $H(U)$. The Kasparov stabilization theorem [1980] says that $H(\overline{T}^c)$ is isomorphic to $H(U)$ which establishes the result. □

We note that there is another interesting approach to the isomorphism 6.14 due to Haefliger (see Theorem A5.1 on page 243) and Renault, Muhly and Williams [Renault 1982; Muhly et al. 1987]. One shows that G is equivalent to G_N^N as topological groupoids. Then one shows that under mild hypotheses, the C^*-algebras associated to equivalent groupoids are strongly Morita equivalent (see [Rieffel 1976] for the definition) and hence (by [Brown et al. 1977]) stably isomorphic.

Suppose that X is a compact foliated space with associated groupoid $G(X)$ which we assume for the moment to be Hausdorff. Suppose that E is a locally trivial tangentially smooth Hermitian vector bundle over X. In applications in Chapter VII, E will be finite-dimensional and we will be considering tangential pseudodifferential operators from sections of E to sections of E. For now we allow E to be finite- or infinite-dimensional. We wish to introduce the C^*-algebra $C_r^*(G(X), \mathrm{End}_\tau(E))$. □

The range and source maps may be used to pull back the bundle E to bundles E_s and E_r over $G(X)$ respectively. Given some $u \in G(X)$ we denote the fibres over u by $E_{s(u)}$ and $E_{r(u)}$ respectively. We define a bundle $\mathrm{Hom}_G(E_s, E_r)$ over $G(X)$ as follows. For each $u \in G(X)$, let $\mathrm{Hom}_G(E_s, E_r)_u$ denote the space of bounded linear operators $E_{s(u)} \to E_{r(u)}$. We topologize this bundle in the obvious way using local trivializations of the bundle E to obtain a tangentially smooth bundle over $G(X)$.

Define $\Gamma_c\big(G(X), \mathrm{Hom}_G(E_s, E_r)\big)$ to be the space of compactly supported continuous sections

$$f : G(X) \longrightarrow \mathrm{Hom}_G(E_s, E_r)$$

such that each $f(u)$ is a compact, or, better, a finite rank operator $E_{s(u)} \to E_{r(u)}$. This is obviously a linear space. We define convolution and involution exactly as in (6.1). Just as in the scalar case, we obtain an associative algebra with involution.

For each $x \in X$ there is a natural Hilbert space

$$L^2\big(G^x, \mathrm{Hom}_G(E_s, E_r)|_{G^x}, \lambda^x_{G(X)}\big)$$

and hence a natural $*$-homomorphism

$$\pi_x : \Gamma_c\big(G(X), \mathrm{Hom}_G(E_s, E_r)\big) \longrightarrow \mathcal{B}\big(L^2\big(G^x, \mathrm{Hom}_G(E_s, E_r)|_{G^x}, \lambda^x_{G(X)}\big)\big)$$

defined by (6.2) exactly as in the scalar case. We complete with respect to these representations to obtain a C^*-algebra which we denote $C_r^*(G(X), \mathrm{End}_\tau(E))$.

All this has been for $G(X)$ Hausdorff. In the locally Hausdorff case we modify just as in the scalar situation—there is really nothing to check.

If E is a trivial bundle, say $E \cong X \times V$ for some fixed (finite or infinite-dimensional) Hilbert space V, then there are natural isomorphisms

$$E_s \cong E_r \cong G(X) \times V$$

and a bundle isomorphism

$$\mathrm{Hom}(E_{s(u)}, E_{r(u)}) \cong G(X) \times \mathcal{B}(V)$$

so

$$\Gamma_c\big(G(X), \mathrm{Hom}_G(E_s, E_r)\big) \cong \Gamma_c\big(G(X), G(X) \times \mathcal{B}(V)\big) \cong C_c(G(X), \mathcal{F}(V))$$

(where $\mathcal{F}(V)$ denotes the finite rank operators $V \to V$), and it follows that

$$C_r^*(G(X), \mathrm{End}_\tau(E)) \cong C_r^*(G(X)) \otimes \mathcal{K}(V).$$

The following theorem is essentially folklore. It follows directly from [Renault 1987, Corollaire 5.4].

Theorem 6.15. *Suppose that X is a compact foliated space and that E_1, E_2 are tangentially smooth Hermitian bundles over X. Then $C_r^*(G(X), \mathrm{End}_\tau(E_1))$ is stably isomorphic to $C_r^*(G(X), \mathrm{End}_\tau(E_2))$.*

Proof. Tensor the vector bundles E_1 and E_2 with a fixed infinite-dimensional Hilbert space H_∞. Since the E_i were locally trivial, so are $E_i \otimes H_\infty$.

By [Dixmier and Douady 1963, Theorem 1], $E_{i,\infty} = E_i \otimes H_\infty$ are trivial (and hence isomorphic) bundles. Thus we have

$$\begin{aligned} C_r^*\big(G(X), \mathrm{End}_\tau(E_1)\big) \otimes \mathcal{K}(H_\infty) &\cong C_r^*\big(G(X), \mathrm{End}_\tau(E_{1,\infty})\big) \\ &\cong C_r^*\big(G(X), \mathrm{End}_\tau(E_{2,\infty})\big) \\ &\cong C_r^*\big(G(X), \mathrm{End}_\tau(E_2)\big) \otimes \mathcal{K}(H_\infty). \qquad \square \end{aligned}$$

We now turn our attention to another and closely related operator algebra that one can construct. Let G be a locally compact groupoid with discrete holonomy groups together with a given Haar system λ. We also assume that the underlying Borel groupoid has a complete transversal — a condition that is *a fortiori* satisfied for the groupoid of a foliated space. We also assume given on this Borel groupoid a positive transverse measure ν, not necessarily invariant — see Chapter IV. Indeed for the coming discussion we can and shall neglect any topological structure and simply work as in Chapter IV with a standard Borel groupoid with a complete transversal, a fixed tangential measure and with countable holonomy groups G_x^x.

The integration process of Chapter IV where we integrate the tangential measure λ with respect to the transverse measure ν produces a measure $\mu = \int \lambda \, d\nu$ on the unit space X. Then as noted in Chapter IV one may turn G into a *measured groupoid* [Mackey 1966; Ramsay 1971] by defining a measure $\tilde{\mu}$ on G

by

$$\tilde{\mu}(E) = \int_X \lambda^x(E \cap G^x)\, d\mu(x)$$

(i.e., $\tilde{\mu} = \mu_r$ in the terminology of Chapter IV). We note that conversely if G is a standard measured groupoid, then by a result from [Hahn 1978] there is a Haar measure λ (= tangential measure $\sim$ Haar system) on G and a measure ν on X so that the original measure on G is given by the formula above.

Now any measured groupoid has a regular representation [Hahn 1978; Connes and Takesaki 1977] which in form looks just like the construction defining $C_r^*(G)$. We form the Hilbert space $L^2(G, \tilde{\mu})$, which is decomposed as a direct integral

$$L^2(G, \tilde{\mu}) = \int L^2(G^x, \lambda^x_{G(X)}).$$

If $\phi = (\phi^x)$ is an element of H and if f is a suitable function (see below) on G one defines just as in (6.2):

$$(\pi(f)\phi)(u) = \int f(u^{-1}v)\phi(v)\, d\lambda^x(v).$$

In order for this to define a bounded operator f has to satisfy conditions as in [Hahn 1978].

Definition. A measurable function f on G equipped with a Haar system λ and a transverse measure ν is *left integrable* with respect to the Haar system λ if

$$\operatorname*{ess\,sup}_u \int |f(u^{-1}v)|\, d\lambda^{r(u)}(v) < \infty,$$

the essential sup taken with respect to $\tilde{\mu}$; f is *right integrable* if f^* is left integrable, $f^*(u) = \overline{f(u^{-1})}$, and *integrable* if left and right integrable. A function is *left* (*right, two-sided*) *square-integrable* if $|f|^2$ is left (right, two-sided) integrable.

It is not hard to see that the integrable functions form a $*$-algebra which we denote $\widetilde{L}^1(G, \tilde{\mu})$ under the same operations (6.1) we used to define $C_r^*(G)$. Note that the integrability conditions are not the same as f being in $L^2(G, \tilde{\mu})$, and that the condition depends only on the equivalence class, i.e., the null sets, of the transverse measure ν, and not on ν itself.

We observe that if f is integrable with respect to λ then the operator

$$\pi_x(f) : L^2(G^x, \lambda^x_{G(X)}) \longrightarrow L^2(G^x, \lambda^x_{G(X)})$$

is given by a kernel function which, when we unravel the respective definitions, is integrable in the sense of Proposition 1.14. Hence $\pi_x(f)$ defines a bounded operator with a norm that is essentially bounded in x by Proposition 1.14 and so defines a bounded operator

$$\pi(f) : L^2(G, \tilde{\mu}) \longrightarrow L^2(G, \tilde{\mu}).$$

Further, $f \to \pi(f)$ is a $*$-homomorphism

$$\pi : \widetilde{L}^1(G, \tilde{\mu}) \longrightarrow \mathcal{B}(L^2(G, \tilde{\mu})).$$

We note parenthetically that if $f \in C_c(G)$, the continuous compactly supported functions on a locally compact topological groupoid with Haar system λ (or the replacement for $C_c(G)$ in the non-Hausdorff case), then the integrability conditions are satisfied with ordinary suprema instead of essential suprema.

Definition. Let $(G, \tilde{\mu})$ be a measured groupoid. The *von Neumann algebra* $W^*(G, \tilde{\mu})$ associated to $(G, \tilde{\mu})$ is the weak closure of the $*$-algebra

$$\pi(\widetilde{L}^1(G, \tilde{\mu})) \subset \mathcal{B}(L^2(G, \tilde{\mu}))$$

generated by the operators $\pi(f)$, for all integrable functions f.

The algebra $W^*(G, \tilde{\mu})$ quite evidently commutes with the abelian algebra A_r of multiplication operators generated by all bounded measurable functions on G which depend only on the range $r(u)$ of a point u in G.

The fact that elements of $W^*(G, \tilde{\mu})$ commute with A_r means, by direct integral theory [Takesaki 1979, IV, §8], that any $m \in W^*(G, \tilde{\mu})$ may be decomposed as a direct integral. Specifically the abelian algebra A_r on $L^2(G, \tilde{\mu})$ decomposes $L^2(G, \tilde{\mu})$ as a direct integral

$$L^2(G, \tilde{\mu}) = \int_X L^2(G^x, \lambda^x_{G(X)})\, d\nu.$$

Then any operator m commuting with A_r, and in particular any m in $W^*(G, \tilde{\mu})$ has a direct integral decomposition

$$m = \int m^x\, d\nu,$$

where m^x is an operator on $L^2(G^x, \lambda^x_{G(X)})$. Conversely every bounded Borel field of operators $x \to m^x$ on the Borel field of Hilbert spaces $\{L^2(G^x, \lambda^x_{G(X)})\}$ defines an operator that commutes with A_r.

Moreover for each $u \in G$, left translation L_u by u defines a bijection from $G^{s(u)}$ to $G^{r(u)}$ which maps $\lambda^{s(u)}$ to $\lambda^{r(u)}$. (This is the definition of invariance for λ.) Consequently left multiplication by u^{-1} gives rise to a unitary operator U_u which is a unitary equivalence

$$U_u : L^2(G^{s(u)}, \lambda^{s(u)}) \xrightarrow{\cong} L^2(G^{r(u)}, \lambda^{r(u)})$$

and these evidently satisfy $U_u U_v = U_{uv}$. It is further easily verified that the convolution operators $\pi(f)$ which are dense in $W^*(G, \tilde{\mu})$ have the further property that their disintegration products above $\pi(f)^x$ satisfy

$$U_u \pi(f)^{s(u)} = \pi(f)^{r(u)} U_u \quad \text{for almost all } u.$$

Consequently the same holds for any $m \in W^*(G, \tilde{\mu})$, namely

$$(6.16) \qquad U_u m^{s(u)} = m^{r(u)} U_u \quad \text{for almost all } u.$$

The intuitive reason for this is that the m's are a kind of right convolution operator on the groupoid and so a sum of right translations. The U_u are left translation operators and right translations always commute with left translations. Finally it is true that $W^*(G, \tilde{\mu})$ is exactly the set of operators which commute with A_r and whose disintegration products satisfy (6.16).

There are some important subalgebras of $W^*(G, \tilde{\mu})$ that will occur. First of all, if ϕ is a bounded measurable function on $(G, \tilde{\mu})$ with the property that $\phi(u)$ depends only on the source $s(u)$ of u (so $\phi(u) = \phi'(s(u))$, then m_ϕ, multiplication by ϕ on $L^2(G)$, defines a bounded operator which evidently commutes with A_r and whose direct integral disintegration products m_ϕ^x on $L^2(G^x, \lambda^x_{G(X)})$ are multiplication operators by the function $\phi'(s(v)) v \in G^x$. This field of operators evidently satisfies (6.16), because left translation by u^{-1} maps G_y^x to G_y^z, where $u^{-1} \in G_z^x$. Hence m_ϕ defines an element of $W^*(G, \tilde{\mu})$. The set of such is evidently a von Neumann subalgebra of $W^*(G, \tilde{\mu})$, denoted A_s and isomorphic to $L^\infty(X)$. In case G is principal — that is, an equivalence relation — this is the usual diagonal subalgebra, and if the equivalence relation is countable, it is a Cartan subalgebra [Feldman and Moore 1977] that plays a key role in the structure of $W^*(G, \tilde{\mu})$.

Another slightly larger subalgebra of $W^*(G, \tilde{\mu})$ which takes account of the holonomy is also useful. Let

$$E = \{u \in G \mid r(u) = s(u)\}.$$

Then E can be viewed as the union

$$E = \bigcup_y G_y^y$$

of the (discrete) holonomy groups. If f is any Borel function on E which is not only bounded, but for which

$$\sum_{u \in G_y^y} |f(u)|$$

is bounded in y, then right convolution by f restricted to G_y^y defines an operator $R(f)_y^x$ on $L^2(G_y^x)$ for any x because G_y^x is a principal homogeneous space on the right for G_y^y. Then as $L^2(G^x, \lambda^x_{G(X)})$ can be regarded as the direct integral

$$L^2(G^x, \lambda^x) = \int L^2(G_y^x)\, d\lambda^x(y).$$

The operators $R(f)_y^x$ integrate to give an operator $R(f)^x$ on $L^2(G^x, \lambda^x_{G(X)})$. For exactly the same reasons as above, this field satisfies (6.16) and so defines an element $R(f)$ of $W^*(G, \tilde{\mu})$. Suppose that f happens to be supported on the subset of $E = \bigcup G_y^y$ consisting of the identity elements of the (discrete) groups G_y^y. Then f is in effect a function on the unit space X, and $\phi(u) = f(s(u))$ defines a function on $\widetilde{G}$ depending only on $s(u)$ that in turn defines an element m_ϕ of the algebra A_s. A moment's thought shows that $m_\phi = R(f)$. The closure D_s of the set of operators $R(f)$, which is evidently a von Neumann subalgebra of $W^*(G, \tilde{\mu})$ contains A_s. This generalized diagonal subalgebra D_s has a readily apparent structure.

Proposition 6.17. *The algebra D_s is a direct integral*

$$D_s = \int_X R^x\, d\nu(x)$$

of the right group von Neumann algebras R^x of the discrete groups G_x^x with $A_s \cong L^\infty(X)$ the obvious subalgebra.

The algebra $W^*(G, \tilde{\mu})$ on the Hilbert space $\widetilde{H}$ is in standard form [Takesaki 1983] in the sense that there exists a conjugate linear isometry J of $\widetilde{H}$ such that $J^2 = \mathrm{id}$, and

$$J W^*(G, \tilde{\mu}) J = W^*(G, \tilde{\mu})',$$

where N' denotes the commutant of N in $\mathcal{B}(\widetilde{H})$. In fact the J that works is quite easy to write down. Recall from Chapter IV that the transverse measure ν, which we started with here, has a modular function, or modulus, Δ which is a positive function on the groupoid G satisfying $\Delta(u)\Delta(v) = \Delta(uv)$ whenever uv is defined. This function measures the extent that ν is not an invariant transverse measure. This modular function has the further property that if $i(v) = v^{-1}$ is the inversion map on G, then i transforms the measure $\tilde{\mu}$ on G into a measure $i_*(\tilde{\mu})$ (where $i_*(\tilde{\mu}) = \mu_s$ in the language of Chapter IV) which is equivalent to $\tilde{\mu}$ with Radon–Nikodým derivative given by

$$\frac{d\tilde{\mu}}{d(i_*(\tilde{\mu}))}(v) = \Delta(v).$$

It follows then that for $\phi \in \widetilde{H} = L^2(G, \tilde{\mu})$,

$$(J\phi)(u) = \bar{\phi}(u^{-1})\Delta(u^{-1})^{1/2}$$

defines a conjugate linear involutive isometry. The following summarizes results from [Hahn 1978] and [Connes and Takesaki 1977]; but also see [Takesaki 1983].

Theorem 6.18. *With the preceding notation we have*

$$JW^*(G,\tilde{\mu})J = W^*(G,\tilde{\mu})'$$

and $W^*(G,\tilde{\mu})$ is the algebra of all operators m commuting with A_r so that the corresponding disintegration products m^x satisfy

$$U^u m^{s(u)} = m^{r(u)} U^u$$

for almost all $u \in G$. Moreover $JA_sJ = A_r$.

We shall not go into the somewhat tedious details of the proof; the idea is that what works for groups works for groupoids. The algebra $W^*(G,\tilde{\mu})$ consists of right convolutions and conjugation by J makes them into left convolutions which at the von Neumann algebra level are each others commutants. As to the second part, A_r is clearly in the commutant of $W^*(G,\tilde{\mu})$ and A_r together with "smoothed" versions of the U^u suffice to generate this commutant. □

It is evident from the definitions that once we fix a Haar system λ, the C^*-algebra $C_r^*(G)$ has a natural representation into $W^*(G,\tilde{\mu})$ for any choice of transverse measure ν and corresponding $\tilde{\mu}$. Recall that $C_r^*(G)$ is defined by representations π_x of a dense subalgebra A. These representations π_x take place on $L^2(G^x,\lambda^x_{G(X)})$ and so the direct integral π of the π_x gives a representation

$$\beta : C_r^*(G) \to W^*(G,\tilde{\mu}),$$

which of course depends on the measures involved. The following is clear.

Proposition 6.19. *The image of $C_r^*(G)$ is dense in $W^*(G,\tilde{\mu})$ and the representation is faithful if the support of the transverse measure ν is all of X in the sense that the measure $\int \lambda\, d\nu$ has support equal to X.*

It is well to reflect for a moment on the geometric meaning of these algebras for a topological groupoid G. First of all each orbit or leaf ℓ of the equivalence relation on X associated to G has a "holonomy covering" $\tilde{\ell}$ which we can take to be G^x for any $x \in \ell$. The left translations

$$L_u : G^{s(u)} \longrightarrow G^{r(u)}$$

provide canonical identifications between these models of $\tilde{\ell}$ when $x = s(u)$, and $y = r(u)$ are points of ℓ. In addition the "holonomy group" G^x_x operates by left translation freely on $G^x \simeq \tilde{\ell}$, and the quotient $G^x_x \backslash \tilde{\ell}$ is exactly the original leaf ℓ. Each leaf ℓ and its covering $\tilde{\ell}$ come equipped with a measure so we have Hilbert spaces $L^2(\tilde{\ell})$ which are just $L^2(G^x,\lambda^x_{G(X)})$ for any $x \in \ell$.

Then elements of $W^*(G, \tilde{\mu})$ can be thought of as providing for almost all holonomy coverings $\tilde{\ell}$ an operator

$$m(\tilde{\ell}) : L^2(\tilde{\ell}) \longrightarrow L^2(\tilde{\ell}).$$

These operators are supposed to be bounded and to vary in a Borel way with $\tilde{\ell}$. The exact meaning of the last statement is that when we identify $L^2(\tilde{\ell})$ with $L^2(G^x, \lambda^x_{G(X)})$ for any $x \in \ell$ and get a field of operators $\{m^x\}$, then the m^x are Borel sections of the Borel field of Hilbert spaces $\{L^2(G^x, \lambda^x_{G(X)})\}$ over X. The commuting relations in the second part of Theorem 6.18 say in part that whether we identify $L^2(\tilde{\ell})$ with $L^2(G^x, \lambda^x)$ or with $L^2(G^y, \lambda^y)$ with $x, y \in \ell$, we get the same operator on $L^2(\tilde{\ell})$. Finally $m(\tilde{\ell})$ is not an arbitrary operator on $L^2(\tilde{\ell})$ but the commuting relations in Theorem 6.18 say also that $m(\tilde{\ell})$ must commute with left translation by G^x_x, and that these are the only restrictions.

Elements of the groupoid C^*-algebra $C^*_r(G)$ have a very similar interpretation. Each m in this algebra defines an operator $m(\tilde{\ell})$ on all (not almost all) holonomy coverings of the leaves which commutes with left translation by G^x_x and which is further restricted to be a uniform limit of such operators that can be defined by convolution with suitable continuous kernel functions. Finally the $m(\tilde{\ell})$ have to vary continuously as $\tilde{\ell}$ varies in a manner that is fairly clear heuristically.

It is evident that the von Neumann algebra $W^*(G, \tilde{\mu})$ depends only on the equivalence class, in the sense of absolute continuity, of the measure μ on the unit space X of G because of its definition in terms of fields of operators. In turn the equivalence class of μ depends only on the equivalence class of the transverse measure ν from which it is constructed (regarding of course the Haar system $\{\lambda^x\}$ as fixed once and for all). The Hilbert space $L^2(G, \tilde{\mu})$ upon which we have realized $W^*(G, \tilde{\mu})$ of course depends on μ itself but for two equivalent μ's there is a natural unitary equivalence of the two spatial realizations of the algebra. For simplicity we sometimes write $W^*(G)$, where the Haar system and the equivalence class of transverse measures entering into the definition are understood.

If N is a complete transversal for the equivalence relation on X defined by the groupoid G, then as in Chapter IV, the transverse measure ν defines a measure on N, and the part of G over N, G^N_N becomes a measured groupoid $(G^N_N, \tilde{\mu}_N)$ whose orbits are countable. There should be a close relation between $W^*(G, \tilde{\mu})$ and $W^*(G^N_N, \tilde{\mu}_N)$ paralleling Theorem 6.14 and indeed there is. For convenience we assume that the tangential measure $\{\lambda^x_{G(X)}\}$ on G^x that we are given at the very beginning of the discussion has the property that all (or almost all) the measures $\lambda^x_{G(X)}$ have no atoms. This will surely be the case for the groupoid of a foliated space with the usual choice of tangential measures. In this case, the arguments of [Feldman et al. 1978, Theorem 5.6], trivially modified to cover the case of nonprincipal groupoids, shows that there is an isomorphism of measured groupoids

$$(G, \tilde{\mu}) \cong (G_N^N, \tilde{\mu}_N) \times \mathcal{I},$$

where $\mathcal{I}$ is the principal groupoid (equivalence relation) with unit space the interval $I = [0, 1]$ with all points equivalent and with the measure μ on I Lebesgue measure, the measure on each leaf also Lebesgue measure. With this structural result for G the following is clear.

Proposition 6.20. *Under the conditions above there is an isomorphism*

$$W^*(G, \tilde{\mu}) \cong W^*(G_N^N, \tilde{\mu}_N) \otimes \mathcal{B}(L^2(I)).$$

The importance and usefulness of this result is that it allows most questions about $W^*(G, \tilde{\mu})$ to be reduced to questions about $W^*(G_N^N, \tilde{\mu}_N)$. Since G_N^N has countable orbits, the structure and properties of the algebra built on it is far more understandable and transparent, and there are far fewer technical details to wrestle with. In particular an operator in the algebra is represented by a "matrix" over G_N^N (that is, formally it is of the form $\pi(f)$ for a function f on G_N^N), and the study of unbounded weights on $W^*(G, \tilde{\mu})$ will often reduce to the study of (bounded) states on $W^*(G_N^N, \tilde{\mu}_N)$.

It is evident that the abelian and diagonal subalgebras A_s and D_s of $W^*(G, \tilde{\mu})$ introduced above decompose naturally with respect to the tensor product decomposition. Let A_s^N and D_s^N be the corresponding abelian and diagonal subalgebras of $W^*(G_N^N, \tilde{\mu}_N)$.

Proposition 6.21. *In the decomposition of Proposition 6.20 we have isomorphisms*

$$A_s \simeq A_s^N \otimes L^\infty(I),$$
$$D_x \simeq D_s^N \otimes L^\infty(I),$$

where $L^\infty(I)$ is the subalgebra of $\mathcal{B}(L^2(I))$ consisting of multiplications by bounded measurable functions.

One example of the usefulness of the reduction to a cross section is the following which of course could be established directly but less transparently.

Proposition 6.22. *The relative commutant of A_s in $W^*(G, \tilde{\mu})$ is D_s, and the relative commutant of D_s is the center of D_s, which in the direct integral decomposition of Proposition 6.17 is the direct integral of the centers Z^x of the right group von Neumann algebras R^x of the holonomy groups G_x^x. In particular if almost all of the holonomy groups are infinite conjugacy class (i.c.c.) groups then the relative centralizer of D_s is A_s.*

Proof. By the previous proposition, the question is reduced to A_s^N and D_s^N. All operators are given by "matrices" as in [Feldman and Moore 1977]; then easy computation in this discrete case does the trick. As to the final statement, recall that a discrete group H is i.c.c. (all nontrivial conjugacy classes are infinite) if and only if the center of the group von Neumann algebra is trivial. □

The next step begins with the crucial observation that the algebra $W^*(G)$ comes with a natural family of normal semifinite weights. Indeed each (positive) transverse measure ν in the fixed equivalence class will define in a natural way a weight ϕ_ν on $W^*(G)$; this weight will be a trace if and only if ν is an *invariant* transverse measure. There are several different ways to define these weights; one way starts by utilizing the natural Hilbert algebra structure that is implicit in the construction of $W^*(G, \tilde{\mu})$ and uses the basic Tomita–Takesaki construction of weights from a Hilbert algebra [Takesaki 1983]. We will rather approach the matter through the ideas developed in Chapter I of locally traceable operators; we can give a very simple and direct definition as follows.

Suppose given a transverse measure ν with its associated von Neumann algebra $W^*(G, \tilde{\mu})$. We wish to define ϕ_ν on the positive part $W^*(G, \tilde{\mu})^+$ and taking values in $[0, \infty]$. Here is a rough idea of the construction of the weight. To each $m \in W^*(G, \tilde{\mu})^+$ we shall associate a tangential measure λ_m which has the property that if one decomposes m to a field of operators m^x on $L^2(G^x, \lambda^x_{G(X)})$, then the local trace of m^x determines the measure λ^x_m on $G^x_x \backslash G^x \equiv \ell(x)$ uniquely. Then the weight ϕ_ν corresponding to the transverse measure ν is given by

$$\phi_\nu(m) = \int \lambda_m(\ell)\, d\nu(\ell),$$

where the integral is taken in the sense of Chapter IV. Now here are the details.

Any $m \in W^*(G, \tilde{\mu})^+$ corresponds to a field of positive operators $\{m(\tilde{\ell})\}$, one for almost all holonomy coverings $\tilde{\ell}$ or equivalently a field m^x of positive operators on $L^2(G^x, \lambda^x_{G(X)})$ for almost all x. Then since m^x is positive we can define its local trace as a positive measure $\mathrm{Tr}(m^x)$ on G^x. This measure may be identically plus infinity. At all events it is defined even in this degenerate sense and recall that our definition of m^x being locally traceable was that this measure should be σ-finite (or Radon if G^x comes with a locally compact topology). These measures are always absolutely continuous with respect to $\lambda^x_{G(X)}$ by their definition. The invariance properties satisfied by the m^x as stated in Theorem 6.18 imply by the analysis in Chapter I that left translation L_u which maps $G^{s(u)}$ to $G^{r(u)}$ must transform $\mathrm{Tr}(m^{s(u)})$ into $\mathrm{Tr}(m^{r(u)})$ for almost all $u \in G$. Thus for almost all pairs x, y with $x \sim y$, $\mathrm{Tr}(m^x)$ on G^x is the same as $\mathrm{Tr}(m^y)$ on G^y after identifying G^x and G^y. Moreover the countable group G^x_x acts by left translation on G^x and hence on $L^2(G^x, \lambda^x_{G(X)})$ and m^x commutes with these translations. Again by Chapter I, $\mathrm{Tr}(m^x)$ is invariant under G^x_x and hence $\mathrm{Tr}(m^x)$ uniquely determines a measure $\mathrm{Tr}'(m^x)$ on $G^x_x \backslash G^x$. But this quotient space is just the equivalence class $\ell(x)$ of x. Hence for each leaf ℓ, and each

$x \in \ell$ we obtain a positive measure $\mathrm{Tr}'(m^x)$ on ℓ. The invariance properties cited above tell us that this measure does not depend on which x we choose and depends only on the leaf ℓ; we denote it by $\lambda_m(\ell)$.

This description is simpler if there is no holonomy so that G is an equivalence relation. Then G^x is the equivalence class or leaf of x, and the local trace of m^x gives a measure $\mathrm{Tr}(m^x)$ on G^x; invariance properties say that $\mathrm{Tr}(m^x) = \mathrm{Tr}(m^y)$ and so there is a measure $\lambda_m(\ell)$ depending only on the leaf ℓ; this can be thought of as the local trace of $m(\ell)$ for all or almost all ℓ. But now $\lambda_m(\ell)$ is what we called a tangential measure and it is the sort of object that can be integrated against a transverse measure to give a real number.

Proposition 6.23. *For every $m \in W^*(G, \tilde{\mu})^+$, the above prescription yields a tangential measure $\lambda_m(\ell)$ (perhaps not σ-finite). The integral in the sense of Chapter IV*

$$\phi_\nu(m) = \int \lambda_m(\ell)\, d\nu(\ell)$$

(finite or not) defines a semifinite normal weight on $W^*(G, \tilde{\mu})$.

Proof. For the assignment of a measure $\lambda_m(\ell)$ to each leaf to be a tangential measure, it must satisfy some smoothness conditions transversally. From Chapter IV we see that these amount to the requirement that the field of measures $\lambda_m^x = \mathrm{Tr}(m^x)$ on G^x should be Borel viewed as measures on G in that

$$\int f(u)\, d\lambda^x$$

should be a Borel function of x for any nonnegative Borel function f on G. This is clearly satisfied by the local traces of the Borel field of operators m^x. We note once more that m^x is not assumed to be locally traceable in the sense that $\lambda^x_{G(X)}$ is a σ-finite measure. The integral we write down in the statement still always makes sense as everything is nonnegative. It is clear that ϕ_ν as defined is additive and positively homogeneous. That it is normal is clear from the properties of the local trace and the integration process of Chapter IV. Equivalently it is not hard to produce a family of vectors ξ_i in the Hilbert space $\tilde{H}$ such that

$$\phi_\nu(m) = \sum (m\xi_i, \xi_i),$$

which is an equivalent definition of normality. Finally the dense subalgebra used in [Hahn 1978] to define the algebra $W^*(G, \tilde{\mu})$ synthetically contains a weakly dense set of operators where ϕ_ν is evidently finite so that ϕ_ν is semifinite. □

One of the features of this definition is that it is clear for which positive operators ϕ_ν is finite.

Corollary 6.24. *Let $m \in W^*(G, \tilde{\mu})^+$. Then $\phi_\nu(m) < \infty$ if and only if m^x is locally traceable on almost all G^x in the sense that*

$$\lambda_m^x = \mathrm{Tr}(m^x)$$

is a σ-finite measure; if so, then the integral

$$\int \lambda_m(\ell)\, d\nu(\ell)$$

is finite.

If an operator $a \in W^*(G, \tilde{\mu})$ is given by a kernel function f so that $a = \pi(f)$ and

$$(\pi(f)\psi)(u) = \int f(u^{-1}v)\psi(v)\, d\lambda_{G(X)}^x(v) \quad u \in G^x, \psi \in L^2(G^x, \lambda_{G(X)}^x)$$

with f integrable in the sense of Chapter IV, then we can give an alternate formula for $\phi_\nu(a)$. If $b = a^*a$ then b is given as $\pi(g)$, where

$$g(u) = f^*f(u) = \int \bar{f}(v^{-1}) f(v^{-1}u)\, d\lambda^{r(u)}(v)$$

according to formula 6.1 If $x \in X$, the unit space of G, then x can be thought of as an element of G and to keep matters straight let us call this element $e(x)$. (In case G is an equivalence relation on X, $e(x) = (x, x)$ is a diagonal element.) Now although f and g above are measurable functions on G defined only almost everywhere and as the units $e(x)$ form a null set in G, the restriction of g to $e(X)$ appears to have no sense. However if $u = e(x)$ is a unit, then

$$g(e(x)) = \int |f(v^{-1})|^2\, d\lambda_{G(X)}^x(v)$$

has a well defined meaning for almost all x. When we write $g(e(x))$ for a g of the form f^*f, it is this function that we shall understand. The following shows that as one expects, traces of integral operators are obtained by integrating the kernel on the diagonal.

Proposition 6.25. *For a transverse measure ν, let $\mu = \int \lambda^\ell\, d\nu$ be the integral of the tangential measure λ with respect to ν, the result viewed as a measure on the unit space X. For an operator*

$$b = \pi(g) \in W^*(G, \tilde{\mu})$$

with $g = f^*f$, then

$$\phi_\nu(b) = \int g(e(x))\, d\mu(x),$$

where $g(e(x))$ is as defined above. Equivalently $g(e(x)) \cdot \lambda$ defines a new tangential measure λ' whose derivative with respect to λ is $g(e(x))$. Then

$$\phi_\nu(b) = \int_X \lambda' \, d\nu$$

(the integral of λ' with respect to ν).

Proof. This is simply a matter of identifying the tangential measure λ' (or rather $(\lambda')^x$ as a measure on B^x for each x) as the local trace of the operator $\pi_x(f^*f)$ on $L^2(G^x, \lambda^x_{G(X)})$; this is self evident as $\pi_x(f^*f) = \pi_x(f)^*\pi_x(f)$, where $\pi_x(f)$ is given by a kernel defined by the function f. Then the result follows. □

By the general Tomita–Takesaki theory [Takesaki 1983], any semifinite normal faithful weight ϕ on a von Neumann algebra has associated to it a one parameter group of automorphisms of the algebra, the so called *modular automorphism group*, $\sigma_\phi(t)$. The standard construction of this group via unbounded operators can be exploited easily to construct this group explicitly for the weights ϕ_ν above. (These weights will always be normal, faithful and semifinite as the transverse measure ν was restricted to lie in the same equivalence class that defines the von Neumann algebra itself.) This is worked out in [Feldman and Moore 1977; Hahn 1978; Connes and Takesaki 1977].

Proposition 6.26. *Let Δ be the modular function of the transverse measure ν* (Definition 4.9). *Then the modular automorphism group σ_ν associated to the weight ϕ_ν of $W^*(G, \tilde{\mu})$ is spatially implemented by the one parameter group of unitary operators $U_\nu(t)$ on $L^2(G, \tilde{\mu})$ defined by multiplication by the functions Δ^{it} on G. Thus*

$$\sigma_\nu(t)m = U_\nu(t)mU_\nu(-t) \quad \textit{for } m \in W^*(G, \tilde{\mu}).$$

Moreover for operators of the form $\pi(f)$ in $W^*(G, \tilde{\mu})$ (see definition on page 142) *we have*

$$\sigma_\nu(t)\pi(f) = \pi(f\Delta^{it}),$$

where $f\Delta^{it}$ is pointwise multiplication of f and Δ^{it}.

Proof. The operators $\pi(f)$ form a Hilbert algebra with the $*$ operator given very concretely by $f^*(u) = \overline{f(u^{-1})}$. One then easily computes the polar decomposition of the unbounded conjugate linear operator $f \to f^*$ and following the standard recipe in [Takesaki 1983], one finds the result. The final formula is a simple calculation. □

Recall that the centralizer of a weight ϕ on a von Neumann algebra R is equivalently the von Neumann algebra generated by those unitaries u in the algebra such that $\phi(uxu^*) = \phi(x)$, or equivalently it is the fixed point algebra of the modular automorphism group [Pedersen 1979, Lemma 8.14.6]. A weight is a trace if and only if its centralizer is the entire algebra. As the modular automorphism group σ_ν of the weight ϕ_ν on $W^*(G, \tilde{\mu})$ is given explicitly and clearly fixes the diagonal subalgebra D_s of $W^*(G, \tilde{\mu})$ (Proposition 6.22), the first half of the following is immediate.

Proposition 6.27. *The centralizer of ϕ_ν contains the diagonal subalgebra D_s. Conversely if almost all of the holonomy groups are i.c.c.* (see Proposition 6.22) *then any faithful normal semifinite weight whose centralizer contains D_s is of the form ϕ_ω for some transverse measure ω.*

Proof. For the second part we fix a weight ϕ_ν and let ψ be any other faithful normal semifinite weight with centralizer containing D_s. Then compute the Radon–Nikodým derivative $(\psi : \phi_\nu)_t$ ([Connes 1973], or see [Takesaki 1983, p. 23]). This is a one parameter family of unitary operators in $W^*(G, \tilde{\mu})$ satisfying a certain cocycle condition. Since D_s centralizes both ψ and ϕ_ν, it follows that $(\psi : \phi_\nu)_t$ must commute with D_s for each t. But under the condition on G_x^x, the relation commutant of D_s is by Proposition 6.22 the abelian subalgebra A_s. Because of commutation properties, the derivative $(\psi : \phi_\nu)_t$ is actually a one parameter unitary group in A_s and so has the form $\exp(ith(x))$, where h is a measurable function on X, which by positivity properties of ψ and ϕ_ν is positive. Then $w = h\nu$ is another transverse measure, and it is evident that $\psi = \phi_{h\nu}$. □

The argument just given provides an answer in general to the question of finding all weights whose centralizer contains D_s, but one has to introduce an extended class of weights. As we will not need this, we sketch this only briefly. Suppose that in addition to a transverse measure ν on X one is given for each $x \in X$, a semifinite normal faithful trace τ^x on R^x, the group von Neumann algebra of G_x^x. Then one can construct in an obvious way a trace τ on the diagonal algebra D_s because D_s is given as a direct integral of the algebras R^x. The transverse measure ν itself also defines a weight τ_ν on D_s. The Radon–Nikodým derivative $(\tau : \tau_\nu)$ computed in D_s can then be used to define a weight ϕ on $W^*(G, \tilde{\mu})$ by the condition $(\tau : \tau_\nu) = (\phi : \phi_\nu)$ (computed in $W^*(G, \tilde{\mu})$).

The weights ϕ constructed in this fashion are, we claim, the most general weights on $W^*(G, \tilde{\mu})$ with centralizer containing D_s. The data entering into ϕ, namely a transverse measure ν and a family of traces τ^x on R^x are not independent for we can multiply each τ^x by a positive scalar $c(x)$, replace ν by the transverse measure ν' with

$$\frac{d\nu'}{d\nu} = c(x)^{-1},$$

and the resulting weight will be the same. When the traces τ^x are finite, then they can be normalized so $\tau^x(1) = 1$ and then the transverse measure ν is determined. Of course when τ^x is taken to be the Plancherel trace, then the resulting weight is ϕ_ν that we constructed previously. It is evident that values of the more general weights discussed in this paragraph can be given by integral formulas analogous to those in Properties 6.23 and 6.25. In addition it is not difficult to compute the modular automorphism group of these weights because there is a simple formula for the Radon–Nikodým derivative of these with respect to a ϕ_ν, where we already know the modular automorphism group.

Returning to the ϕ_ν, we see that we have determined when ϕ_ν is a trace because this is true if and only if the modular automorphism group is trivial.

Corollary 6.28. *The weight ϕ_ν is a trace if and only if ν is an invariant transverse measure, that is, its modular function Δ is identically one almost everywhere.*

It is not so easy to tell when the more general weights defined by fields of traces τ^x together with a ν are traces because in general it is hard to determine what the center of $W^*(G, \tilde{\mu})$ is.

To conclude this chapter let us return to the topological and geometric context of a locally compact topological groupoid G, or in particular the holonomy groupoid of a foliated space. As before G is assumed to come equipped with a fixed continuous tangential measure. Then for any transverse measure ν, the reduced C^* algebra $C_r^*(G)$ has a natural representation into $W^*(G, \tilde{\mu})$ as described in Proposition 6.19. The weight ϕ_ν may be restricted then to the image $C_r^*(G)$ to produce a weight on this C^*-algebra, which we denote by the same symbol. If the transverse measure ν is *finite* relative to the tangential measure λ in the sense that $\mu = \int \lambda \, d\nu$ is a finite measure on the unit space X of G (and in particular if it is a Radon transverse measure on the groupoid of a foliated space in the sense of 4.17) then the restriction of ϕ_ν to $C_r^*(G)$ enjoys finiteness properties. In particular for any g in $C_c(G)$, the norm dense subalgebra of compactly supported functions on G used in the definition of $C_r^*(G)$, the positive element $f = g^* g$ satisfies $\phi_\nu(f) < \infty$ in view of Proposition 6.25 or Corollary 6.24. This finiteness property plus the known continuity properties of ϕ_ν on $W^*(G, \tilde{\mu})$ assure that ϕ_ν as a weight on $C_r^*(G)$ is densely defined and lower semicontinuous [Pedersen 1979, 5.6.7]. Quite evidently we can recapture the von Neumann algebra $W^*(G, \tilde{\mu})$ from $C_r^*(G)$ and ϕ_ν via the GNS construction as the image of $C_r^*(G)$ is dense in $W^*(G, \tilde{\mu})$ by Proposition 6.19.

If ν is an invariant transverse measure, then ϕ_ν is of course a trace on $C_r^*(G)$, and as $C_r^*(G)$ is dense in $W^*(G, \mu)$, the converse is true. Thus Corollary 6.28 and Corollary 4.25 combine to yield the following Theorem in the setting of foliated spaces.

Theorem 6.29. *For a Radon transverse measure ν on a compact foliated space X with continuous tangentially smooth modular function Δ, the following are equivalent*:

(1) *The Ruelle–Sullivan current C_ν is closed and so defines a homology class*

$$[C_\nu] \in H_p^\tau(X;\mathbb{R}).$$

(2) *The 1-form $\sigma = 0$.*

(3) *The modular function $\Delta \equiv 1$.*

(4) *The transverse measure ν is an invariant transverse measure.*

(5) *The weight ϕ_ν on $W^*(G(X), \tilde{\mu})$ is a trace.*

In general $C_r^*(G)$ will have traces other than ϕ_ν; for instance if G is the holonomy groupoid of the Reeb foliation, the closed leaf and its holonomy produces a quotient isomorphic to $C^*(\mathbb{Z}^2) \otimes \mathcal{K}$, where $C^*(\mathbb{Z}^2)$ is the group C^*-algebra of $\mathbb{Z}^2$ and $\mathcal{K}$ is the compact operators. The only ϕ_ν which factors through this quotient comes by taking ν to be the transverse measure corresponding to the closed leaf: then ϕ_ν is $P \otimes \mathrm{Tr}$, where P is the Plancherel trace on $C^*(\mathbb{Z}^2)$.

However in the absence of holonomy, traces are always given, as one suspects, by transverse measures.

Theorem 6.30. *Let G be the groupoid of a compact foliated space X and assume there is no holonomy (so that G is the equivalence relation). If ϕ is any densely defined lower semicontinuous trace on the C^* algebra $C_r^*(G)$, then there is a unique invariant transverse Radon measure ν on X with $\phi = \phi_\nu$.*

Proof. We pick a complete transversal N and an open neighborhood U of it as in the discussion preceding Theorem 6.14. We make use of the structural fact that $C_r^*(G) \cong C_r^*(G_N^N) \otimes \mathcal{K}$, and we recall that any densely defined lower semicontinuous trace is finite on the Pedersen ideal — the unique minimal dense two-sided ideal [Pedersen 1979, Theorems 5.6.1, 5.6.7]. As this ideal intersects any subalgebra in a dense ideal, it follows that ϕ is densely defined on the subalgebra $C_r^*(G_N^N) \otimes e \simeq C_r^*(G_N^N)$, where e is a minimal projection in $\mathcal{K}$. Finally since the equivalence relation when restricted to N is discrete, $C_r^*(G_N^N)$ contains a Cartan subalgebra $C_0(N)$ by the remarks following Definition 6.10. For the same reasons as above, ϕ is densely defined on $C_0(N)$ and so is given by a Radon measure ν on N. Moreover by the construction of N, there is a larger transversal N' containing N with the closure $\overline{N}$ of N in N' compact. As the measure ν is by the same reasoning the restriction of a Radon measure ν' on N' it follows that ν is a finite measure on N. Since $C_0(N)$ contains an approximate identity for $C_r^*(G_N^N)$ and ϕ remains bounded on this approximate identity, it follows that ϕ is a finite trace on $C_r^*(G_N^N)$.

Since there is no holonomy, G_N^N is an equivalence relation on N. We know by Proposition 6.8 that G_N^N has a covering by open sets of the form $U(f, O) = \{(x, f(x)), x \in O\}$, where O is an open set in N and f is a homeomorphism of O onto an open subset of N with $f(x) \sim x$, where $\sim$ is the equivalence relation on N. As the diagonal ΔN of N in G_N^N is open and closed, its complement may be covered by sets of the form $U(f, O)$, where f has no fixed points. If a is any compactly supported function on $U(f, O)$ and b any compactly supported function on $\Delta N = U(\mathrm{id}, N)$, then viewed as elements in $C_r^*(G_N^N)$ their convolution products in both orders are again compactly supported on open sets $U(f, O)$ and

$$(a * b - b * a)(x, f(x)) = a(x, f(x))\big(b(f(x), f(x)) - b(x, x)\big).$$

Since $\phi(c)$ for c compactly supported in $U(f, O)$ can be expressed as

$$\phi(c) = \int c\, d\lambda$$

for a (signed) Radon measure on $U(f, O)$, the equality

$$\phi(a * b - b * a) = 0$$

plus the fact that f has no fixed points tells us that λ is zero. As any compactly supported function on $G_N^N - \Delta N$ can be written as a finite sum of functions supported on open sets $U(f, O)$, it follows that

$$\phi(a) = \int a(x, x)\, d\nu(x)$$

for every compactly supported function on G_N^N, where ν is the measure on N constructed above.

An argument similar to the one above shows that ν as a measure on N is invariant under the equivalence relation; that is, its modular function on N is trivial. Then, as in Chapter IV, ν can be extended to all Borel transversals to give an invariant Radon transverse measure, which we denote by ν. Then clearly $\phi = \phi_\nu$ on $C_r^*(G_N^N)$ and hence on $C_r^*(G)$. □

We have seen in Chapter IV that von Neumann factors of type II_∞ and of type III_λ for all λ occur as the von Neumann algebras of foliated spaces. Proposition 6.20 shows that with minimal assumptions on tangential measures, the von Neumann algebra has the form $\widetilde{W} \otimes B(H)$ for an infinite-dimensional Hilbert space H. We also have seen that the von Neumann algebra comes equipped with a family of semifinite normal faithful weights, with corresponding modular automorphism groups. Given this much structure, it is natural to wonder just which von Neumann algebras can occur as von Neumann algebras of foliated spaces. Here is an answer.

Theorem 6.31. *Any purely infinite approximately finite von Neumann algebra A is isomorphic to $W^*(X, \mu)$ for some compact foliated space X and transverse measure μ.*

Proof. According to the classification of such algebras [Connes 1973; Haagerup 1987; Krieger 1976], one may find a Borel space Y, an automorphism ϕ of Y (so that there is an associated action of $\mathbb{Z}$ on Y), and a transverse measure μ_0 so that the group measure construction associated to these data produces a von Neumann algebra A_0 so that

$$A \cong A_0 \otimes B(H).$$

Equivalently, if G is the measure groupoid generated by (Y, ϕ, μ), then A_0 is the von Neumann algebra of this measure groupoid as defined in Chapter VI.

Now according to [Varadarajan 1963, Theorem 3.2] we may assume without loss of generality that Y is a compact metric space and that the map ϕ is a homeomorphism. Form the associated compact foliated space X obtained by suspending (Y, ϕ), and let μ be the associated transverse measure on X constructed from μ_0 as in Chapter IV. Then the von Neumann algebra of (X, μ) is A as desired. □

We note that we have proved more than we stated, for the foliated space produced is always of leaf dimension 1. There are obvious questions which arise in this connection. May Y be chosen to be zero-dimensional? May Y be chosen to be a smooth manifold and ϕ a diffeomorphism, so that X is a smooth manifold? We do not know the answers to these questions.

If we are in the situation of a compact foliated space X with foliated space groupoid $G(X)$ and a tangentially smooth Hermitian vector bundle E on X, we may make the same modification to the construction of the W^*-algebra of G to include the vector bundle. Since a vector bundle is always trivial measure theoretically, the end result is that the original von Neumann algebra is tensored with $\mathcal{B}(V)$, where V is a Hilbert space of dimension equal to the dimension of E.

We conclude this chapter with a brief discussion of some aspects of the K-theory of operator algebras in the context of the C^*-algebras of groupoids. In the following chapter, K-theory will enter in a more extended fashion. We assume that the reader is familiar with the basics of the K-theory of operator algebras (see [Karoubi 1978], [Atiyah and Singer 1968a] and especially [Blackadar 1998]). Given a unital C^*-algebra A, let $M_n(A)$ denote the $n \times n$ matrices over A) Regard $M_n(A) \subset M_{n+1}(A)$ via the map sending an $n \times n$ matrix M to the upper left corner of an $(n+1) \times (n+1)$ matrix, with zeros inserted in the remaining slots. Let

$$M_\infty(A) = \bigcup_n M_n(A).$$

One looks at all projections in $M_\infty(A)$ and subjects them to the natural equivalence relation that $e \sim f$ if there are $u, v \in \bigcup_n M_n(A)$ with

$$uv = e \quad \text{and} \quad vu = f.$$

These classes form a semigroup, and one forms the associated Grothendieck group which is denoted $K_0(A)$. One may thnk of it as classes of formal differences of projections. If A does not have a unit, append one to obtain A^+, compute $K_0(A^+)$ as above, and note that the natural homomorphism $e : A^+ \to \mathbb{C}$ induces a homomorphism $e_* : K_0(A^+) \to K_0(\mathbb{C})$, where the latter group is easily seen to be isomorphic to the integers. Then define $K_0(A)$ to be the kernel of e_*. For a compact space X, $K_0(C(X))$ is the usual topological K-theory of compact spaces $K^0(X)$. For X locally compact, $K_0(C_0(X))$ is the usual K-theory of the space X with compact supports (see [Atiyah and Singer 1968a; Karoubi 1978]).

We define

$$K_j(A) = K_0(S^j A),$$

where $S^k A = C_0((0,1)^k, A)$. Then Bott periodicity asserts that

$$K_j(A) \cong K_j(S^2 A).$$

We recall three further properties of K-theory. First, $K_*(A)$ is homotopy-invariant; that is, if $f^t : A \to A'$ is a 1-parameter family of $*$-homomorphisms (continuous in the sense that the associated map $A \to C([0,1], A')$ is a $*$-homomorphism) then

$$f^0_* = f^1_* : K_*(A) \to K_*(A').$$

Second, if J is a closed ideal of A then there is a natural long exact sequence

$$\begin{array}{ccccc} K_0(J) & \longrightarrow & K_0(A) & \longrightarrow & K_0(A/J) \\ \uparrow & & & & \downarrow \\ K_1(A/J) & \longleftarrow & K_1(A) & \longleftarrow & K_1(J). \end{array}$$

Third, K-theory is invariant under stable isomorphism: if $A \otimes \mathcal{K} \cong B \otimes \mathcal{K}$ then $K_j(A) \cong K_j(B)$.

The group $K_0(C_r^*(G))$ is going to be a central player in index theory and will be the group where the abstract index lives. If G is the groupoid of a compact manifold foliated by a single leaf, $C_r^*(G) = \mathcal{K}$ is the compact operators and it is well known and easily seen that $K_0(\mathcal{K}) = \mathbb{Z}$, and the usual index of an elliptic operator is interpreted as an element of this group.

Recall that an invariant transverse measure ν on a foliation groupoid $G(X)$ corresponds to a trace ϕ_ν on $C_r^*(G(X))$. More generally, if E is some tangentially smooth vector bundle on X, the measure ν gives rise to a trace ϕ_ν^E on $C_r^*(G(X), \mathrm{End}_\tau(E))$. If E_1 and E_2 are two different bundles, we constructed in Theorem 6.15 a stable isomorphism

$$C_r^*\big(G(X), \mathrm{End}_\tau(E_1)\big) \cong C_r^*\big(G(X), \mathrm{End}_\tau(E_2)\big)$$

and hence we have an isomorphism of abelian groups

$$K_0\big(C_r^*(G(X), \operatorname{End}_\tau(E_1))\big) \cong K_0\big(C_r^*(G(X), \operatorname{End}_\tau(E_2))\big).$$

The traces above induce homomorphisms

$$\operatorname{Tr}_\nu^{E_i} : K_0\big(C_r^*(G(X), \operatorname{End}_\tau(E_i))\big) \longrightarrow \mathbb{R}$$

and it is reasonable to ask how these traces are related. Here is the answer.

Theorem 6.32. *Suppose that X is a compact foliated space and that E_1, E_2 are tangentially smooth Hermitian vector bundles over X. Let ν be an invariant tranverse measure on X and let*

$$\operatorname{Tr}_\tau^{E_i} : C_r^*\big(G(X), \operatorname{End}_\tau(E_{i,\infty})\big) \longrightarrow \mathbb{R}$$

be the associated traces. Suppose that

$$f^i : C_r^*\big(G(X), \operatorname{End}_\tau(E_{i,\infty})\big) \otimes \mathcal{K}(H_\infty) \longrightarrow C_r^*(G(X)) \otimes \mathcal{K}(H_\infty)$$

are stable isomorphisms of the sort constructed in Theorem 6.15. Then there is a natural commutative diagram

$$\begin{array}{ccc} K_0\big(C_r^*(G(X), \operatorname{End}_\tau(E_{1,\infty}))\big) & \xrightarrow{(f^2)^{-1} f^1} & K_0\big(C_r^*(G(X), \operatorname{End}_\tau(E_{2,\infty}))\big) \\ & {\scriptstyle \operatorname{Tr}_\nu^{E_1}} \searrow \quad \swarrow {\scriptstyle \operatorname{Tr}_\nu^{E_2}} & \\ & \mathbb{R} & \end{array}$$

Proof. Let

$$h = (f^2)^{-1} \circ f^1 : C_r^*\big(G(X), \operatorname{End}_\tau(E_{1,\infty})\big) \longrightarrow C_r^*\big(G(X), \operatorname{End}_\tau(E_{1,\infty})\big)$$

be the associated automorphism. It suffices to show that the trace is invariant under this automorphism. The automorphism is not inner, and hence this is not automatic. However, h is really conjugation by a continuous field of unitary operators $\{U_x\}$ operating on $C_r^*\big(G(X), \operatorname{End}_\tau(E_{1,\infty})\big)$ by conjugating in the range, and it is obvious that the trace respects the action of this type of automorphism. □

K-theory is intimately related to index theory. We briefly recall what happens in the classical situation, as a way of motivating our interest in the pseudodifferential operator extension. We will revisit this connection in detail in the following chapter.

Let $\mathcal{P}$ denote the C^*-algebra of norm limits of pseudodifferential operators of order ≤ 0 (say, with matrix coefficients) on a compact manifold M. There is a natural sequence of C^*-algebras

$$0 \longrightarrow \mathcal{K} \longrightarrow \mathcal{P} \xrightarrow{\pi} C(S^*M) \otimes M_n \longrightarrow 0,$$

where S^*M is the cosphere bundle. If $P \in \mathcal{P}$ is elliptic with principal symbol σ, then $\pi(P) = \sigma$ and

$$[\sigma] \in K_1(C(S^*M) \otimes M_n) \cong K^{-1}(S^*M).$$

The boundary map

$$\partial : K_1(C(S^*M) \otimes M_n) \longrightarrow K_0(\mathcal{K}) \cong \mathbb{Z}$$

corresponds to the Fredholm index map

$$\partial[\sigma] = \text{ index } (P)$$

as may be seen easily by a naturality argument involving the commuting diagram

$$\begin{array}{ccccccccc} 0 & \longrightarrow & \mathcal{K} & \longrightarrow & \mathcal{P} & \longrightarrow & C(S^*M) \otimes M_n & \longrightarrow & 0 \\ & & \| & & \downarrow & & \downarrow & & \\ 0 & \longrightarrow & \mathcal{K} & \longrightarrow & \mathcal{B}(H) & \longrightarrow & \mathcal{B}(H)/\mathcal{K} & \longrightarrow & 0. \end{array}$$

If G is the groupoid of a foliated space coming from a fibration with base B, $C_r^*(G)$ is, as we have seen, isomorphic to $C(B) \otimes \mathcal{K}$, and so by stability,

$$K_0(C_r^*(G)) \cong K_0(C(B)) \cong K^0(B).$$

Recall that the Atiyah–Singer index for families of elliptic operators [1971] with a parameter space B is an element of $K^0(B)$.

What we will describe here is a kind of Chern character on $K_0(C_r^*(G(X)))$, $G(X)$ the groupoid of a foliated space, or more properly a *partial* Chern character. This Chern character will take values in the reduced tangential cohomology group $\overline{H}_\tau^p(X)$ in top degree p (the leaf dimension) as defined in Chapter III. We shall assume without further notice that the foliated space is tangentially oriented and that the groupoid of the foliated space is Hausdorff. This partial Chern character sees only part of the structure of $K_0(C_r^*(G(X)))$, specifically the part that transverse measures can see. The "full" Chern character is conjecturally a homomorphism from $K_0(C_r^*(G))$ into the cyclic homology $H_*^\lambda(A^0)$ of a suitable dense subalgebra A^0 of $C_r^*(G)$, (see [Connes and Skandalis 1984] and, for cyclic theory, [Connes 1985a; 1985b]. While the outline of this is clear and specific cases are known, there do remain some details. The "partial" Chern character that we will define directly would be obtained in general by composing the full Chern character with a natural homomorphism from $H_*^\lambda(A^0)$ to $\overline{H}_\tau^p(X)$.

For the definition of our Chern character, we start with a typical element of K-theory, $u = [e]-[f]$, where e and f are projections in $M_n(C_r^*(G)^+)$ with the same images in $K_0(\mathbb{C})$, where $G = G(X)$. Then we can assume without loss of generality that the images of e and f in $M_n(\mathbb{C})$ are exactly the same. Let ν be a positive Radon invariant transverse measure on X and form the corresponding trace ϕ_ν on $C_r^*(G)$. Extend ϕ_ν to $\phi_\nu^n = \phi_\nu \otimes \mathrm{Tr}$ on $M_n(C_r^*(G))$.

Theorem 6.33. (a) *The element* $e - f$ *may be chosen to be in the ideal of definition of* ϕ_ν^n.

(b) *The map* $\nu \to \phi_\nu(e-f)$ *extends to a linear functional on the set of all Radon signed transverse measures* $MT(X)$ *which depends only on the* K*-theory class* $u = [e]-[f] \in K_0(C_r^*(G))$. *Denote it by* $c'(u)$.

(c) *The map* c' *takes values in the space of weak-$*$ continuous functionals on* $MT(X)$ *(viewed as the dual space of* $\overline{H}_\tau^p(X)$ *as in* (4.27), (4.29)) *and hence yields uniquely a map*

$$c : K_0(C_r^*(G(X))) \longrightarrow \overline{H}_\tau^p(X)$$

which we call the partial Chern character $c(u)$ *of* u.

(d) *If* E *is a tangentially smooth Hermitian vector bundle over* X *then the partial Chern character extends uniquely to*

$$c : K_0\big(C_r^*(G(X), \mathrm{End}_\tau(E))\big) \longrightarrow \overline{H}_\tau^p(X).$$

Before turning to the proof, we offer some observations. Note that the partial Chern character is given very explicitly as follows. If $[u] \in K_0(C_r^*(G))$ is represented by $[e]-[f]$, where $e, f \in M_n(C_r^*(G)^+)$ with common images in $M_n(\mathbb{C})$ and if e and f are in the domain of ϕ_ν^n, then $c[u]$ is the cohomology class of the tangentially smooth p-form ω_u which (after identifying p-currents with Radon invariant transverse measures) is given by

$$\omega_u(\nu) = \phi_\nu^n(e-f),$$

where ϕ_ν^n is the trace $\phi_\nu \otimes \mathrm{Tr}$ on $C_r^*(G) \otimes M_n$ associated to the invariant transverse measure ν.

Suppose that $[u]$ is the index class of a tangential, tangentially elliptic operator D on X as defined in the following chapter. One might try to construct ω_u as follows. The restriction of D to a leaf ℓ is locally traceable and has an associated p-form $(\rho_u)_\ell \in \Omega^p(\ell)$. One is tempted, then, to try to amalgamate the p-forms $(\rho_u)_\ell$ to a p-form $\rho_u \in \Omega_\tau^p(X)$. Unfortunately the forms $(\rho_u)_\ell$ do not vary continuously in the transverse direction and it is not at all clear that it is possible to alter the $(\rho_u)_\ell$ in some direct fashion to obtain a global class. We avoid this difficulty by regularizing at the C^*-algebra level with respect to $MT(X)$.

Proof of Theorem 6.33. In view of the Hilsum–Skandalis result, Theorem 6.14, and the fact that $K_0(A \otimes \mathcal{K}) \cong K_0(A)$, we may assume that $u \in K_0(C_r^*(G_N^N))$ for a transversal N of the type described in Theorem 6.14 and consequently that e and f are in $M_n(C_r^*(G_N^N)^+)$.

We need to look more carefully at how $C_r^*(G_N^N)$ sits inside $C_r^*(G)$. As before we may arrange matters so that there is larger transversal N' containing N and the closure $\overline{N}$, which we may assume is compact. Moreover we may arrange that a neighborhood U' of N' has the form $U' = N' \times \mathbb{R}^p$, p the leaf dimension, so that the second coordinates describe the leaves locally. Then

$$G_U^U = G_{N'}^{N'} \times \mathbb{R}^p \times \mathbb{R}^p.$$

Suppose that the graph is Hausdorff. Then elements of $G_{N'}^{N'}$ and G_N^N can be represented by Proposition 6.9 as continuous functions vanishing at ∞ on these spaces. We then pick a fixed compactly supported C^∞ function ϕ on $\mathbb{R}^p$ and extend a function ψ on $G_{N'}^{N'}$ to one on G_U^U by the formula $\psi_U(g,x,y) = \psi(g)\phi(x)\phi(y)$ and one extends ψ_U to ψ_G on all of G by making it zero on the complement of G_U^U. In particular if ψ is supported on G_N^N and represents an element of $C_r^*(G_N^N)$, then ψ_U and ψ_G have compact support and ψ_G represents an element of the dense subalgebra A of functions used to define $C_r^*(G)$. It may be checked that this map $\psi \longrightarrow \psi_G$ gives an embedding i of $C_r^*(G_N^N)$ into $C_r^*(G)$. In the non-Hausdorff case the same argument works after localizing to open Hausdorff subsets. It follows from the discussion here and in Theorem 6.14 that the isomorphism θ of $C_r^*(G_N^N) \otimes \mathcal{K}$ with $C_r^*(G)$ can be arranged so that $\theta(x \otimes e_1) = i(x)$, where e_1 is a one-dimensional projection.

In particular any finite matrix of elements in $C_r^*(G_N^N)$ is always represented in $C_r^*(G_N^N)$ by a kernel operator where the kernel is continuous and has compact support. Further, the kernel, when extended to G, is tangentially smooth (Chapter III) for the natural foliated space structure of G. Finally as every element of $C_r^*(G_N^N)$ can be written as a linear combination of elements of the form a^*a, it follows by Proposition 6.25 that any element b of $C_r^*(G)$ represented as a finite matrix of elements of $C_r^*(G_N^N)$ via the isomorphism θ is in the ideal of definition of any weight ϕ_ν for any (positive) Radon transverse measure, and that $\phi_\nu(b)$ is given by integrating the kernel of b on the unit space. Specifically if ν is a Radon transverse measure, and λ is the fixed smooth tangential measure, then the integral of λ with respect to ν

$$\mu = \int \lambda \, d\nu$$

is a measure on X. If k_b is the kernel function on G for b, then

$$\phi_\nu(b) = \int k_b(e(x)) \, d\mu(x),$$

where e is the function embedding X as the set of units in G. As k_b is tangentially smooth on G, $k_b(e(x))$ is tangentially smooth on X. Finally as the foliated space is oriented, we may view the tangential measure λ as a tangentially smooth p-form, and then $\omega_b = k_b(e(\cdot))\lambda$ is also a tangentially smooth p-form. Recasting the formula above, we see that

$$\phi_\nu(b) = \int \omega_b \, d\nu$$

is given by integrating the tangentially smooth p-form ω_b against the transverse measure ν.

The proposition is now obvious for we can arrange the two projections e and f defining the K-theory element $u = [e]-[f]$ to be in $M_n(C_r^*(G_N^N)^+)$ and their difference $e-f$ to be a finite matrix over $C_r^*(G_N^N)$ to which the above analysis applies. For an invariant (positive) Radon transverse measure, $\phi_\nu(e-f)$ can be given by integrating a fixed tangentially smooth p-form ω_{e-f} against ν. This in fact constructs the value of the partial Chern character $c(u)$ in $\overline{H}_\tau^p(X)$; namely it is the class of the form ω_{e-f}. That it is well defined and independent of the choice of e and f results from the fact that ϕ_ν is a trace and the duality result, Proposition 4.29.

Finally, the presence of the bundle E is easily accommodated with the assistance of Theorem 6.32. □

As we will be working with projections that often do not lie in the C^*-algebras under consideration, but rather in a von Neumann algebra containing the C^*-algebra of interest, we shall add a few words about K-theory for von Neumann algebras. As any von Neumann algebra W is a C^*-algebra one could just define $K_0(W)$ using the C^* definition. However, the presence of infinite projections leads to bad behavior; for instance, $K_0(\mathcal{B}(H)) = 0$ for an infinite-dimensional Hilbert space H. We want to stick to finite projections. Recall the definition, which is reminiscent of Dedekind's definition of a finite set.

Definition 6.34. A projection e in a von Neumann algebra W is *finite* if e is not equivalent in the sense above to a proper projection of itself.

Equivalently, one may first define a von Neumann algebra W to be finite if given $w \in W^+$ there is a finite normal trace ϕ on W^+ with $\phi(w) \neq 0$; then define $e \in W$ to be a finite projection if eWe is a finite von Neumann algebra. For this approach, see [Dixmier 1969a].

One then forms the semigroup of classes of finite projections in $\bigcup_n M_n(W)$ and then the corresponding Grothendieck group, thus obtain a group that we denote by $K_0^f(W)$. Evidently

$$K_0^f(\mathcal{B}(H)) = \mathbb{Z},$$

while

$$K_0^f(W) = \begin{cases} \mathbb{R} & \text{if } W \text{ is a factor of type II,} \\ 0 & \text{if } W \text{ is a factor of type III.} \end{cases}$$

From this one can readily compute $K_0^f(W)$ for any W.

Now if we start with a C^*-algebra A and a representation π of A into a von Neumann algebra W, we would like to define, at least under some conditions, a homomorphism

$$\pi_* : K_0(A) \longrightarrow K_0^f(W).$$

At the very least we would want this map to exist when $A = C_r^*(G(X))$ and $W = W^*(G(X), \tilde{\mu})$ with $\tilde{\mu}$ arising from a Radon invariant transverse measure for the foliated space.

Proposition 6.35. *Let A be a C^*-algebra of the form $A = B \otimes \mathcal{K}$ with a representation π into a von Neumann algebra W, such that $\pi(A)$ is dense and when we write $\pi(B)'' = eWe$ for a projection e in W, then e is a finite projection. Then there is a well defined homomorphism*

$$\pi_* : K_0(A) \longrightarrow K_0^f(W).$$

We omit the obvious proof that is based on the equality

$$K_0(B) \cong K_0(A)$$

and observe that the conditions are satisfied in the case at hand since

$$A = C_r^*(G(X)) = C_r^*(G_N^N) \otimes \mathcal{K}$$

and since the trace ϕ_ν has been shown to be finite on $C_r^*(G_N^N)$ in Theorem 6.31 it follows that $\phi_\nu(e)$ is finite, where e is the projection in the statement of the proposition. Finally since ϕ_ν is a faithful trace on $W^*(G, \tilde{\mu})$ it follows that e is a finite projection. □

Corollary 6.36. *For any finite Radon invariant transverse measure ν there is a natural homomorphism*

$$\pi_\nu : K_0(C_r^*(G)) \longrightarrow K_0^f(W^*(G, \tilde{\mu}))$$

and the associated trace ϕ_ν on $C_r^*(G)$ and on $W^*(G, \tilde{\mu})$ extends to yield a commuting diagram

$$\begin{array}{ccc} K_0(C_r^*(G)) & \xrightarrow{\pi_\nu} & K_0^f(W^*(G, \tilde{\mu})) \\ & {\scriptstyle \mathrm{Tr}_\nu} \searrow \quad \swarrow {\scriptstyle \mathrm{Tr}_\nu} & \\ & \mathbb{R} & \end{array}$$

We note that if $W^*(G, \tilde{\mu})$ is a factor then it is of Type II_∞ and

$$\mathrm{Tr}_\nu : K_0^f(W^*(G, \tilde{\mu})) \longrightarrow \mathbb{R}$$

is an isomorphism.

Looking ahead more explicitly to the next chapter, we consider the following situation: we have an exact sequence

$$0 \longrightarrow A \longrightarrow P \longrightarrow C \longrightarrow 0$$

of C^*-algebras. We assume that P has a representation π into a von Neumann algebra W such that $\pi(A)$ is weakly dense. As above we assume that $A = B \otimes \mathcal{K}$, where $\pi(B)'' = eWe$ with e a finite projection. We suppose that P and hence C are unital. Now let $d \in P$ and suppose that $\dot{d}$, its image in C is invertible (that is, to adumbrate the following chapter, d is elliptic). We regard $\dot{d}$ as an element of $K_1(C)$ and then according to the exact sequence of K-theory, the index of $\dot{d}$ is a well defined element $\mathrm{ind}(\dot{d})$ in $K_0(A)$.

On the other hand, we can view $\pi(d)$ as an element of the von Neumann algebra W and then its kernel $\operatorname{Ker}\pi(d)$, and also $\operatorname{Ker}\pi(d^*)$, are projections in W. What one hopes, using the map of Proposition 6.35 is indeed the case, as follows from Breuer's theory [1968] of Fredholm operators in von Neumann algebras. The following summarizes the result and will play a crucial role in Chapter VII.

Proposition 6.37. *Under the assumptions above,* $\operatorname{Ker}\pi(d)$ *and* $\operatorname{Ker}\pi(d^*)$ *are finite projections in* W. *Moreover the difference*

$$[\operatorname{Ker}\pi(d)] - [\operatorname{Ker}\pi(d^*)]$$

(the analytic index of d*) is an element of* $K_0^f(W)$, *and if* π_* *is the map from* $K_0(A)$ *to* $K_0^f(W)$ *of Proposition 6.35, then*

$$\pi_*(\mathrm{ind}(\dot{d})) = [\operatorname{Ker}\pi(d)] - [\operatorname{Ker}\pi(d^*)].$$

Proof. If m is the smallest norm closed ideal in W containing the finite projections, then evidently $m \supset \pi(B)$ by hypothesis, and hence $m \supset \pi(B \otimes \mathcal{K}) = \pi(A)$. Since $\dot{d}$ is invertible in C, it follows that the image of $\pi(d)$ in W/m is invertible and hence that $\pi(d)$ is Fredholm by [Breuer 1968, Theorem 1]. It follows from Breuer that $\operatorname{Ker}\pi(d)$ and $\operatorname{Ker}\pi(d^*)$ are finite projections in W. Finally a close examination of the definition of the index map $K_1(C) \to K_0(A)$ as for instance given in [Blackadar 1998, Definition 8.7] shows directly that

$$\pi_*(\mathrm{ind}(\dot{d}) = [\operatorname{Ker}\pi(d)] - [\operatorname{Ker}\pi(d^*)]. \qquad \square$$

The point here is that the naively defined "spatial" analytic index

$$[\operatorname{Ker}\pi(d)] - [\operatorname{Ker}\pi(d^*)]$$

of d in the von Neumann algebra W, a very measure theoretic type of object, is always the image via π_* of an element in $K_0(A)$, an element which in turn has important topological invariance properties. This will be applied to the extension

$$0 \longrightarrow C_r^*(G(X), \mathrm{End}_\tau(E)) \longrightarrow \bar{\mathcal{P}}^0 \longrightarrow \Gamma(S^*F, \mathrm{End}_\tau(E)) \longrightarrow 0$$

of tangential pseudodifferential operators defined on a bundle over a foliated space. The von Neumann algebra W will be $W^*(G, \tilde{\mu})$ constructed from a Radon invariant transverse measure ν.

□ □□□□□ □□□□

The class of C^*-algebras of foliated spaces has turned out to be a premier source of examples of C^*-algebras in the last fifteen years. It is a very interesting proving ground for general conjectures. A prime example is the Baum–Connes conjecture. There is a huge literature on this subject; we limit ourselves to mentioning the classic paper [Baum and Connes 2000], written in 1982, and the recent book [Valette 2002] for a thorough discussion. The version of the Conjecture for foliations goes roughly as follows. Given a foliated space X (the authors consider only foliated manifolds but presumably the conjecture would be the same), let $BG(X)$ denote the classifying space of the associated holonomy groupoid. There is an appropriate sort of topological K-theory denoted K_*^τ to apply to this space and a natural map

$$\mu : K_*^\tau(BG(X)) \to K_*(C_r^*(G(X)))$$

and the Baum–Connes Conjecture is that this map μ is an isomorphism. They show in [Baum and Connes 2000, Proposition 8] that μ is rationally injective and that if $G(X)$ is torsion-free (in the sense that the holonomy groups are all torsion-free), then μ is an isomorphism. Since then the conjecture has been established for various classes of foliations. For instance, J. L. Tu [1999] showed that the conjecture holds when X is an amenable foliation. On the other hand, Higson, Lafforgue, and Skandalis [Higson et al. 2002] have given some examples to show that sometimes the conjecture is false. (These examples involve non-Hausdorff foliation groupoids.) So the situation is really complicated.

The C^*-algebras of groupoids have played an important role in the theory of graph C^*-algebras, as in the work of Kumjian, Pask, Raeburn, and Renault [Kumjian et al. 1997; 1998; Kumjian and Pask 1999]. For a fine general treatment, see [Paterson 1999].

We also note the very recent results of Tu [2004], who introduces a notion of properness for G that is invariant under Morita equivalence of groupoids. (See [Muhly et al. 1987] for definitions.) He shows that any generalized morphism between two locally compact groupoids which satisfies some properness conditions induces a C^*-correspondence from $C_r^*(G_1)$ to $C_r^*(G_2)$, and thus two Morita-equivalent groupoids have Morita-equivalent C^*-algebras.

CHAPTER VII

Pseudodifferential Operators

This chapter is devoted to the study of tangential pseudodifferential operators and their index theory. The chapter has four topics, treated in turn:

- the general theory of pseudodifferential operators on foliated spaces (VII-A on page 169);
- differential operators and finite propagation (VII-B on page 190);
- Dirac operators and the McKean–Singer formula (VII-C on page 197);
- superoperators and the asymptotic expansion of the heat kernel (VII-D on page 202).

We discuss each of them briefly before revisiting them in their respective sections.

We are deeply grateful to Steve Hurder, Peter Gilkey, Jerome Kaminker, John Roe, and Michael Taylor for their enormously helpful assistance in the preparation of this chapter. We especially recommend Roe's papers [1988a; 1988b], his CBMS booklet [1996], and his book [1998] for further early thought on core areas of interest.

Pseudodifferential operators. We begin the chapter by introducing the machinery of tangential differential operators, smoothing operators, and pseudodifferential operators, first in a local setting and then globally. We demonstrate that a tangentially elliptic pseudodifferential operator has an inverse modulo compactly smoothing operators. Letting $\overline{\mathcal{P}}(G(X), E, E)$ denote the closure of the $*$-algebra of pseudodifferential operators of order ≤ 0 on a bundle E over a foliated space X, there is a short exact sequence

$$0 \longrightarrow C_r^*(G(X), \mathrm{End}_\tau(E)) \longrightarrow \overline{\mathcal{P}}(G(X), E, E) \longrightarrow \Gamma(S^*F, \mathrm{End}_\tau(E)) \longrightarrow 0,$$

where S^*F is the cotangent sphere bundle of the foliated space. This leads to formulas which relate the abstract index class

$$\mathrm{ind}(P) \in K_0(C_r^*(G(X))),$$

the Connes index $\mathrm{ind}_\nu(P)$, and the Type II von Neumann index. In general, the index of a tangential, tangentially elliptic operator may be regarded as a class

$K_0(C_r^*(G(X)))$ or in $K_0^f(W^*(G(X), \tilde{\mu}))$. The natural map

$$\beta_* : K_0(C_r^*(G(X))) \longrightarrow K_0^f(W^*(G(X), \tilde{\mu}))$$

commutes with the homomorphisms from these groups to $\mathbb{R}$ induced by an invariant transverse measure ν, so

$$\operatorname{ind}_\nu(P) = \phi_\nu\big(\operatorname{Ker}[\beta P] - \operatorname{Ker}[\beta P^*]\big) \in \mathbb{R},$$

where ϕ_ν is the trace associated to the invariant transverse measure ν. These results imply that the index of the operator depends only upon the homotopy class of the tangential principal symbol of the operator.

Differential operators and finite propogation. Turning next to tangential differential operators, we introduce bounded geometry and finite propagation conditions. We show that a tangential differential operator D on a compact foliated space has a unique (leafwise) closure, so that the Hilbert fields $\operatorname{Ker} D$ and $\operatorname{Ker} D^*$ are well-defined. It makes sense to form the index measure ι_D and then to define the $\mathbb{R}$-valued index by

$$\operatorname{ind}_\nu(D) = \int \iota_D \, d\nu.$$

This is formally the same as the definition for operators of order zero, of course, but some further work is required to make the connection between the two more concrete and transparent.

Dirac operators and the McKean–Singer formula. The key differential operators for the purposes of index theory are the tangential Dirac operators. Having introduced these operators in an abstract context and having verified that the general machinery of Section VII-B applies to these operators, we establish the McKean–Singer formula: for $t > 0$,

$$\operatorname{ind}_\nu(D) = \phi_\nu\big([e^{-tD^*D}] - [e^{-tDD^*}]\big).$$

Superoperators and the asymptotic expansion. We introduce superoperators and restate the McKean–Singer formula in the form

$$\operatorname{ind}_\nu(D) = \phi_\nu^s(e^{-t\widehat{D}}),$$

where $\widehat{D}$ is the superoperator

$$\widehat{D} = \begin{bmatrix} 0 & D^* \\ D & 0 \end{bmatrix}^2 = \begin{bmatrix} D^*D & 0 \\ 0 & DD^* \end{bmatrix}$$

and ϕ_ν^s is the supertrace. Next we introduce complex symbols and prove that as $t \to 0$ there is an asymptotic expansion

$$\phi_\nu^s(e^{-t\widehat{D}}) \sim \sum_{j \geq -p} t^{j/2p} \int_X \lambda_j(\widehat{D}) \, d\nu,$$

where each $\lambda_j(\widehat{D})$ is a signed tangential measure independent of t. As $\mathrm{ind}_\nu(D)$ is independent of t, an easy argument shows that

$$\mathrm{ind}_\nu(D) = \int \omega_D(g,E)\,d\nu = \langle [\omega_D(g,E)], [C_\nu] \rangle,$$

where

$$\omega_D(g,E) = \lambda_0(\widehat{D})|d\lambda| = (\lambda_0(D) - \lambda_0(D^*))\,|d\lambda|$$

is the associated tangentially smooth p-form and $[C_\nu]$ is the homology class of the Ruelle–Sullivan current associated to ν. The identification of ω_D for twisted signature operators and the completion of the proof are left to Chapter VIII.

VII-A. Pseudodifferential Operators

Fix a tangential Riemannian metric on X and corresponding tangential Riemannian metric on $G(X)$. This determines a volume form on each leaf of X and on each leaf of $G(X)$. There is a corresponding tangential measure λ_X on X and a tangential measure $\lambda_{G(X)}$ on $G(X)$. Recall that

$$\lambda_{G(X)} = \{\lambda^x_{G(X)}\},$$

where $\lambda^x_{G(X)}$ is a measure on G^x. The measure $\lambda_{G(X)}$ is invariant under the left action of the holonomy groupoid. Precisely, if $u \in G^y_x$ and if f is a nonnegative Borel function on G, then

$$\int f(uu')\,d\lambda^x_{G(X)}(u') = \int f(u')\,d\lambda^y_{G(X)}(u').$$

We fix once and for all a transverse measure $d\nu$. Note that in view of the results of Chapter IV, $d\nu$ may be regarded as a measure on the transversals of $G(X)$ or equivalently as a measure on the transversals of X. (For most of this chapter there would be no harm in letting ν have a nontrivial modular function, but our applications require that ν be an *invariant* transverse measure, so we assume that as needed.) This determines measures $\mu = \lambda_X\,d\nu$ on X and $\lambda_{G(X)}\,d\nu$ on $G(X)$ by the procedure of Chapter IV.

Let U be an open subset of $\mathbb{R}^p \times N$ with the induced foliated structure. Define

$$d^\alpha_x = \left(\frac{\partial}{\partial x_1}\right)^{\alpha_1} \cdots \left(\frac{\partial}{\partial x_p}\right)^{\alpha_p}$$

and

$$D^\alpha_x = (-i)^{|\alpha|} d^\alpha_x.$$

Recall that $C^\infty_\tau(U)$ denotes the continuous, tangentially smooth functions on U, and $C^\infty_{\tau c}(U)$ denotes those which are compactly supported. We topologize these by insisting that convergence means convergence on compact subsets of a function and its tangential derivatives.

Definition 7.1. Let X be a foliated space with foliation bundle F. The *bundle of densities of order α on X* (a complex line bundle) is defined by

$$|F|_{\alpha,x} = \{\phi : \Lambda^p F_x - \{0\} \to \mathbb{C} \mid \phi(\lambda w) = |\lambda|^\alpha \phi(w) \text{ for all } \lambda \in \mathbb{R} - \{0\} \text{ and } w \in \Lambda^p F_x - \{0\}\}.$$

Define $|F| = |F|_1$. Densities of order 1 on a leaf are measures on that leaf, so it makes sense to define

$$C_0^\infty(|\ell|) = \Gamma_0(\ell, |T\ell|)$$

and then *distributions* on the leaf ℓ by

$$\mathcal{D}'(\ell) = (C_0^\infty(|\ell|))^*.$$

Similarly, *compactly supported distributions* $\mathcal{E}'(\ell)$ are defined on the leaf ℓ as dual to $\Gamma(\ell, |T\ell|)$.

These are examples of an assignment to each leaf ℓ of a topological vector space $E(\ell)$, and we shall informally speak of such an assignment as a field of topological vector spaces, leaving undefined what kind of transverse measurability is required. Further examples include

$$\mathcal{B}_\tau^\infty(X) = \{C^\infty(\ell)\} \quad \text{and} \quad \mathcal{B}_{\tau c}^\infty(X) = \{C_c^\infty(\ell)\}.$$

One particular case of importance is when these spaces are Hilbert spaces.

Definition 7.2. A *Borel field of Hilbert spaces* E over a foliated space X consists of

(a) an assignment of a (separable) Hilbert space E_x to each x in X which is Borel in the sense of direct integral theory (see Chapter VI, page 142, and [Takesaki 1979, IV, §8]), and

(b) a map $u \to u_*$ from $G(X)$ into unitary operators from $E_{s(u)}$ to $E_{r(u)}$ in the language of Chapter IV,

such that:

1. $(uv)_* = u_* v_*$,
2. $(u^{-1})_* = (u_*)^{-1}$,
3. each u_* is a Borel function of u.

In this case we say that u defines a representation of $G(X)$ on the field E. A *bounded operator*

$$P : E \to E'$$

of Borel fields of Hilbert spaces is a Borel family of operators

$$P_x : E_x \to E'_x$$

with uniformly bounded norms which is invariant under the left action of each G_x^x.

If one has a tangential measure λ^x on X, one may form

$$E_x = L^2(\ell^x, \lambda^x)$$

as in Chapter IV, and this determines a field $\{E_x\}$ of Hilbert spaces. In fact it is clearly a Borel field of Hilbert spaces where u_* for any u is defined as the identity map from $E_{s(u)}$ to $E_{r(u)}$. This is called the *regular representation* of the groupoid $G(X)$ with the tangential measure λ.

Let E and E' be finite-dimensional tangentially smooth complex bundles over X. A *tangential operator* from E to E' is a family $P = \{P_x : x \in X\}$, where, for each x, P_x is a linear map

$$P_x : C_c^\infty(G^x, s^*(E)) \to C^\infty(G^x, s^*(E')) \tag{7.3}$$

which is invariant under the left action of each G_x^x.

Left invariance implies that there exists a vector-valued distribution on G such that for each $x \in X$ the distributional kernel associated to P_x (on G^x) is $K(\gamma, \gamma') = K(\gamma^{-1}\gamma')$ so that

$$(P_x\xi)(\gamma) = \int K(\gamma^{-1}\gamma')\xi(\gamma')\, d\lambda^x_{G(X)}(\gamma') \tag{7.4}$$

for all $\xi \in C_c^\infty(G^x, s^*(E))$ and $\gamma \in G^x$. Note that in this generality, the operators $\{P_x\}$ vary measurably but not necessarily continuously in the transverse direction. To obtain continuous control transversely one must assume that the distribution kernel varies continuously transversely.

If we assume that $G(X)$ is Hausdorff, the distributions

$$K_x = K(\gamma, \cdot), \qquad x = r(\gamma) \in X$$

corresponding to the operator P_x fit together to form a distribution K corresponding to the operator P on $G(X)$ because $G(X)$ is a fibre space over X with G^x as the fibre over x. This goes as follows. One defines

$$K(\varphi) = \int K_x(\varphi_x)\, d\mu(x),$$

where φ_x is the restriction of a compactly supported test function φ on $G(X)$ to G^x and $\mu = \lambda d\nu$ is the measure on X obtained by integrating the tangential measure λ with respect to the fixed transverse measure ν as in Chapter IV. The distribution K is called the *distribution kernel* of P.

The usual constructions for operators on manifolds may be conducted leaf by leaf. For instance, if T is a tangential operator then a *formal adjoint* T^t on C_c^∞ is defined leafwise by

$$\langle \psi, T^t\phi\rangle = \langle T\psi, \phi\rangle.$$

Definition. A *tangential differential operator*

$$D : \Gamma_\tau(E) \to \Gamma_\tau(E')$$

is a continuous linear operator which, locally, is given by a linear combination of partial differential operators along the leaves.

We extend D to tangential distributional sections ψ by

$$\langle D\psi, \phi \rangle = \int \psi(x) D^t \phi(x)\, dx,$$

where D^t is the formal adjoint of D.

A tangential differential operator D has a local expansion on a coordinate patch of the form

$$D = \sum_{|\alpha| \le m} a_\alpha(x) D^\alpha,$$

where the a_α vary continuously in x and vary smoothly on each leaf. The maximal global value for m is the *order* of D. A tangential differential operator from E to E' induces an operator

$$D : \mathcal{B}_\tau^\infty(E) \to \mathcal{B}_\tau^\infty(E')$$

by restriction. This operator varies continuously as one moves transversely. More generally, one sometimes wishes to consider operators $D = \{D_\ell\}$ where the transverse variation is only measurable.

The *Hodge–Laplace operator* provides a key example of a tangential differential operator. Suppose given a foliated space X with leaves of dimension p and with a tangential Riemannian connection. Recall that the de Rham operator is a map $d = \{d_x\}$, where, for $x \in \ell$,

$$d_x : \Omega^k(\ell) \to \Omega^{k+1}(\ell).$$

The orientation on F determines the Hodge $*$-operator

$$* : \Omega^j(\ell) \to \Omega^{p-j}(\ell).$$

Define

$$\delta = (-1)^{pk+p-1} * d * : \Omega^{k+1}(\ell) \to \Omega^k(\ell)$$

and

$$\Delta_k = d\delta + \delta d : \Omega^k(\ell) \to \Omega^k(\ell).$$

This determines the tangential Hodge–Laplace operator

$$\Delta_k : \Omega_\tau^k(X) \to \Omega_\tau^k(X)$$

on forms over X and similarly on forms over $G(X)$. Each Δ_k is a second order tangential differential operator. In flat space,

$$\Delta_0 = -\sum \frac{\partial^2}{\partial x_i^2}$$

is the classical Laplacian.

Given a tangential differential operator

$$D : \Gamma_\tau(E) \to \Gamma_\tau(E'),$$

define the *tangential* (*total*) *symbol* of D locally by

$$\sigma(x,\xi) = \sum_{|\alpha|\le m} a_\alpha(x)\xi^\alpha.$$

and define the *tangential principal symbol* of D by

$$\sigma_m(x,\xi) = \sum_{|\alpha|=m} a_\alpha(x)\xi^\alpha.$$

The tangential total symbol is a purely local notion; it depends on the choice of a coordinate system. In contrast, the local tangential principal symbols patch together to yield the global tangential principal symbol

$$\sigma_m(D) : S^*F \longrightarrow \mathrm{Hom}(\pi^*E, \pi^*E')$$

on the cosphere bundle S^*F of F, where $\pi : S^*F \to X$ denotes the obvious projection. If $\sigma_m(D)$ is invertible, so that

$$\sigma_m(D) : S^*F \longrightarrow \mathrm{Isom}(\pi^*E, \pi^*E')$$

then D is said to be *tangentially elliptic*. For example, the principal symbol of the tangential Hodge–Laplace operator is given by

$$\sigma_2(\Delta_\ell) = -\sum \xi_i^2$$

and is invertible on unit vectors, so the tangential Hodge–Laplace operator Δ is a tangentially elliptic operator.

Next recall a bit of the classical theory of pseudodifferential operators; see [Atiyah and Segal 1968; Taylor 1981; Gilkey 1984], for more detail. Suppose first that U is an open subset of $\mathbb{R}^p$. If

$$P(x,D) = \sum_{|\alpha|\le m} a_\alpha(x) D^\alpha$$

is a differential operator with smooth coefficients one can write for $u \in C_c^\infty(U)$, extended to $\mathbb{R}^p$, ($\hat{u}$ the Fourier transform),

$$P(x,D)u(x) = \sum_{|\alpha|\le m} a_\alpha(x) \int \xi^\alpha e^{2i\pi\langle x,\xi\rangle}\,\hat{u}(\xi)\,d\xi$$

so that, with the total symbol of P given by

$$\sigma(x,\xi) = p(x,\xi) = \sum_{|\alpha|\leq m} a_\alpha(x)\xi^\alpha \in C^\infty(U \times \mathbb{R}^p),$$

one has

$$P(x,D)u(x) = \int p(x,\xi)e^{2i\pi\langle x,\xi\rangle}\hat{u}(\xi)\,d\xi. \tag{7.5}$$

Sometimes one writes

$$P(x,D) = OP(p(x,\xi)).$$

The class of differential operators is not large enough to include, for instance, the parametrix of a differential operator of positive order, since such an operator would have negative order. The general idea then is to admit a larger class of symbols and use (7.5) to define a larger class of operators. We define two such classes, $S^m(U)$ and $S_0^m(U)$, as follows.

For any integer m, let $S^m(u)$ be the set of all smooth functions $p(x,\xi)$ on $U\times\mathbb{R}^p$ which satisfy the following condition: for each compact subset K of U and for all multi-indices α,β,

$$|D_x^\beta D_\xi^\alpha p(x,\xi)| \leq C_{\alpha,\beta,K}(1+|\xi|)^{m-|\alpha|} \qquad \text{for } x\in K, \text{ for } \xi\in\mathbb{R}^p.$$

For instance, polynomials in ξ of degree m with smooth coefficients lie in $S^m(U)$. More general, if ϕ is some smooth function, let

$$p(x,\xi) = \phi(x)(1+|\xi|^2)^{m/2}I.$$

This is an elliptic symbol of order m whenever $\phi\neq 0$. For $p\in S^m(U)$, define

$$P = OP(p) : C_c^\infty(U)\to C^\infty(U)$$

by

$$Pu(x) = (2\pi)^{-p}\int p(x,\xi)e^{i\langle x,\xi\rangle}\hat{u}(\xi)\,d\xi.$$

The class $S_0^m(U)$ consists of those symbols $p\in S^m(U)$ which satisfy the following additional condition: for each nonzero value of ξ, the limit

$$\sigma_m(p)(x,\xi) \;=\; \lim_{\eta\to\infty}\frac{p(x,\eta\xi)}{\eta^m}$$

exists. Then $\sigma_m(p)$ is a C^∞ function on $U\times(\mathbb{R}^p - 0)$ and it is homogeneous of degree m in ξ.

Finally, a *pseudodifferential operator* is an operator

$$P : C_c^\infty(U)\to C^\infty(U)$$

such that for each $f\in C_c^\infty(U)$ the associated operator Pf is a pseudodifferential operator in local coordinates; i.e., it is of the form $OP(p_f)$ for some $p_f\in S_0^m$.

The set of such operators is denoted $\mathcal{P}^m(U)$. There is an obvious extension to matrix-valued functions.

Lemma 7.6. *Let $r(x,\xi,y)$ be a matrix-valued system which is smooth in each variable. We suppose that r has compact x-support inside U (an open set in $\mathbb{R}^p$ with compact closure) and that there are estimates*

$$|D_x^\alpha D_\xi^\beta D_y^\gamma r| \le C_{\alpha,\beta,\gamma}(1+|\xi|)^{m-|\beta|}$$

for all multiindices (α,β,γ), where $m<-p-k$, so that the associated operator

$$OP(r)f(x) = \iint e^{i(x-y)\xi} r(x,\xi,y) f(y)\, dy d\xi$$

is a pseudodifferential operator of order m. The distribution kernel $K(x,y)$ is given by

$$K(x,y) = \int e^{i(x-y)\xi} r(x,\xi,y)\, d\xi.$$

Then K is C^k in (x,y) and

$$OP(r)f(x) = \int K(x,y) f(y) dy.$$

Proof. See [Gilkey 1984, Lemma 1.2.5, p. 19]. □

Lemma 7.7. *Let $K(x,y)$ be a smooth kernel with compact x, y support in U (an open set in $\mathbb{R}^p$ with compact closure). Let P be the operator defined by K. If k is a nonnegative integer, then*

$$|K|_{\infty,k} \le C(k)|P|_{-k,k}.$$

Proof. See [Gilkey 1984, Lemma 1.2.9, p. 21]. □

The *principal symbol* $\sigma_m(P)$ of a pseudodifferential operator P is defined by

$$\sigma_m(P)(x,\xi) = \sigma_m(p_f)(x,\xi),$$

where f is any function equal to 1 near x. The algebra $\mathcal{P}^m(U)$ is invariant under diffeomorphisms of U and hence determines uniquely a corresponding class of operators $\mathcal{P}^m(M)$ for a (paracompact) manifold M, and, more generally, for $\mathcal{P}^m(M,E,E')$, where E and E' are smooth bundles over M. The principal symbol yields a map

$$\sigma_m(P) : S^*M \to \mathrm{Hom}(\pi^*(E), \pi^*(E')),$$

where π is the canonical projection of the cotangent sphere bundle of M to M. Give $\mathcal{P}^m(M,E,E')$ the natural Fréchet topology using coordinate neighborhoods. Then

$$\sigma_m : \mathcal{P}^m(M,E,E') \to \Gamma\big(S^*M, \mathrm{Hom}(\pi^*(E), \pi^*(E'))\big).$$

If M is compact then

$$\mathcal{P}^m(M) \to \mathcal{B}(W^s(E), W^{s-m}(E'))$$

is continuous for each m and s, where $W^s(E)$ denotes the (classical) Sobolev space associated to the smooth sections over the (compact) manifold M, so bounded families of symbols yield bounded families of operators.

A pseudodifferential operator P from E to E' on a compact manifold M is *smoothing* if for all s, t, P induces bounded maps on Sobolev spaces

$$P : W^s(E) \to W^{s+t}(E').$$

Equivalently, P is smoothing if

$$P : \mathcal{E}'(E) \to C^\infty(E').$$

The conditions are equivalent since

$$\bigcup_s W^s(E) = \mathcal{E}'(E) \quad \text{and} \quad \bigcap_s W^s(E) = C^\infty(E)$$

by the Sobolev lemma. A smoothing operator has a smooth distributional kernel.

Let us return to the realm of foliated spaces. Let X be a compact foliated space with leaves of dimension p equipped with a tangential Riemannian metric and let $G = G(X)$ be its holonomy groupoid, which we assume to be Hausdorff. Let E and E' be finite-dimensional tangentially smooth complex bundles over X.

Definition 7.8. Fix a real number s. The *tangential Sobolev field*

$$W_\tau^s(G(X)) \equiv W_\tau^s = \{W_x^s\}$$

is defined as follows: the Hilbert space W_x^s is the completion of

$$\mathrm{Dom}(1+\Delta_x)^{s/2}$$

with respect to the norm

$$\|\xi\|_{s,x} = \|(1+\Delta_x)^{s/2}\xi\|_{L^2(G^x)}.$$

The representation of $G(X)$ on the Hilbert field $W_\tau^s(G(X))$ by left translation is by construction equivalent to the regular representation of $G(X)$ (compare Definition 7.2). Note that up to equivalence the field $W_\tau^s(G(X))$ is independent of choice of tangential Riemannian metric.

Definition. A tangential operator P is *smoothing* if P induces a bounded operator

$$P : W_\tau^s(G(X)) \to W_\tau^{s+t}(G(X))$$

for all s, t. The distribution kernel which determines P is in fact a smooth function on each leaf, though it may be only measurable transversely. The kernel dies off in a complicated way on each leaf; it is not necessarily compactly supported on $G(X)$. A tangential operator P is *compactly smoothing* if P is smoothing and if the distribution kernel of P is compactly supported on $G(X)$.

If C is a compact subset of $G(X)$ then the *support* of P is in C if the distribution vanishes off C. A tangential operator P is *pseudolocal* if for all neighborhoods S of G^0 there is a compactly smoothing operator R with $\mathrm{Supp}(P+R) \subset S$. Say $P_1 \sim P_2$ if $P_1 - P_2$ is compactly smoothing.

Suppose that if $\Omega \cong L \times N$ is a distinguished coordinate patch of the holonomy groupoid $G(X)$ with L open and connected in $\mathbb{R}^{2p}$. A tangential operator P from E to E' over Ω corresponds by invariance to a measurable family $P = \{P_n : n \in N\}$, where

$$P_n : C^\infty(L \times \{n\}, E) \to C^\infty(L \times \{n\}, E').$$

To make P a tangential pseudodifferential operator one naturally requires that each P_n be a classical pseudodifferential operator and that these operators vary continuously in n. The invariance condition on the family of operators translates into the condition that the distribution kernel $K(\gamma, \gamma', n)$ is really a function of $\gamma^{-1}\gamma'$, so write

$$K(\gamma, \gamma', n) = K(\gamma^{-1}\gamma', n).$$

Thus K may be regarded as being defined on an open set of $G(X)$ itself.

On the question of what support for K should be allowed, one has some choice. We insist that K has compact support on $G(X)$. The set of such P of order $\leq m$ is denoted $\mathcal{P}^m_c(\Omega, E, E')$. Each element of $C^\infty_\tau(G(\Omega))$ determines a compactly smoothing operator.

If $P \in \mathcal{P}^m_c(\Omega, E, E')$ with distribution kernel K, then K extends naturally to all of $G(X)$ by setting it equal to zero outside of Ω. It is then the distribution kernel for a unique tangential operator on G, denoted P'. This operator decomposes as $P' = \{P'_x\}$, where P'_x has support contained in $G^x \cap s^{-1}(\Omega)$. Finally:

Definition. A *tangential pseudodifferential operator on* X is a finite linear combination of compactly smoothing operators with transversely continuous distribution kernels and operators of the form P' above.

By construction, each tangential pseudodifferential operator is pseudolocal and has a continuous compactly supported distribution kernel. Transverse continuity implies that the tangential principal symbol of such an operator is continuous.

Let $\mathcal{P}^m(G(X), E, E')$ be the linear space of tangential pseudodifferential operators of order $\leq m$ from E to E'; that is, finite linear combinations of operators arising on the various $\mathcal{P}^m(\Omega, E, E')$ and compactly smoothing operators. When the context is appropriate we abbreviate to $\mathcal{P}(E, E')$ or to $\mathcal{P}$. The linear space

$$\mathcal{P}^{-\infty}(E, E') = \bigcap_m \mathcal{P}^m(E, E')$$

consists of the compactly smoothing operators with transversely continuous tangentially smooth kernels.

Note that one can compose two elements of $\mathcal{P}^{-\infty}(E, E')$ when $E = E'$ (and the proposition below implies that the set is closed under composition in an appropriate sense.)

All of this has been for $G(X)$ Hausdorff. If $G(X)$ is only locally Hausdorff then we modify as in the construction of $C_r^*(G(X))$. Cover the space $G(X)$ by open Hausdorff sets Ω, for which $\mathcal{P}^m(E, E')$ does make sense, and then define $\mathcal{P}^m(G(X), E, E')$ to be the vector space of linear combinations of these local pseudodifferential operators and compactly smoothing operators.

Proposition 7.9 [Connes 1979, page 126]. (a) *$\mathcal{P}^m \circ \mathcal{P}^n \subset \mathcal{P}^{m+n}$ for all m, n.*

(b) *If $P \in \mathcal{P}^0(E, E')$, then the family $\{P_x : x \in X\}$ extends to a bounded intertwining operator*

$$L^2(G(X), \lambda_{G(X)}, E_s) \to L^2(G(X), \lambda_{G(X)}, E'_s).$$

(c) *If $P \in \mathcal{P}^m(\mathbb{C}, \mathbb{C})$, $m < 0$, then $P \in C_r^*(G(X))$.*

(d) *If $P \in \mathcal{P}^m(E, E')$ with $m < -p/2$, then its associated distribution kernel K is measurable on $G(X)$ with*

$$\sup_y \int \|K(\gamma^{-1})\|_{HS}^2 \, d\nu^y(\gamma) < \infty.$$

Proof (Connes). (a) Suppose first that $n = -\infty$. One may assume that $P' \in \mathcal{P}^m$ corresponds to a continuous family $P \in \mathcal{P}_c^m(\Omega, E, E')$ with $\Omega \cong L \times N$. A partition of unity argument shows that we may study functions f (with associated multiplication operators M_f) supported on

$$W' \cong L \times L' \times N,$$

where $\Omega' \cong L' \times N$ compatibly with $\Omega \cong L \times N$. The kernel associated to PM_f is of the form

$$K_1(t, t'', n) = \int K(t, t', n) f(t', t'', d)\alpha\, |dt'|$$

and is tangentially smooth. Thus PM_f is smoothing, and this implies that $\mathcal{P}^m \mathcal{P}^{-\infty} \subset \mathcal{P}^{-\infty}$. For the general case assume that $P' \in \mathcal{P}^m$, $Q' \in \mathcal{P}^n$ arise from $\mathcal{P}_c(\Omega, E, E')$, where $\Omega \cong L \times N$, and then invoke the classical argument. In particular, this shows that $\mathcal{P}^0(G(X), E, E)$ is an algebra.

(b) Assume that the operator is of the form P' for $P \in \mathcal{P}_c^0(\Omega, E, E')$. The assertion follows from the inequality

$$\|P'_x\| \le \sup \|P_n\|.$$

(c) This follows from the natural inclusion

$$C_r^*(\Omega) \to C_r^*(G(X))$$

and the continuity of the map given by $n \mapsto P_n$.

(d) It suffices to prove the assertion for P', with $P \in \mathcal{P}_c^m(\Omega, E, E')$. One has

$$K(t, t', n) = \int e^{i\langle t-t', \xi\rangle} a(t, \xi, n)\, d\xi,$$

where

$$\|a_{t,n}\|_2^2 = \int |a(t, \xi, n)|^2\, |d\xi|$$

is uniformly bounded; i.e.,

$$|a(t, \xi, n)| \le c(1 + |\xi|)^m.$$

Then the Parseval equality shows that

$$\int |K(t, t', n)|^2\, dt' = \|a_{t,n}\|_2^2$$

is uniformly bounded. □

Let $P \in \mathcal{P}^m(G(X), E, E')$ be a tangential pseudodifferential operator from E to E'. We define its *principal symbol* $\sigma_m(P)$ to be that of the operator $s(P)$ (which acts on bundles over X, rather than on bundles over G.) If P is a smoothing operator with associated kernel K, then $s(P)$ is the operator associated with the kernel function

$$K'(y, x) = \sum K(\gamma) \in E_x^* \otimes E_y \qquad \text{(sum over all } \gamma : x \to y\text{)}.$$

This is indeed a smoothing operator and its principal symbol $\sigma_m(P)$ is zero for all m. It follows that σ_m induces a homomorphism

$$\sigma_m : \mathcal{P}^m(G(X), E, E') \to \Gamma_\tau(S^*F, \mathrm{Hom}(E, E')).$$

One defines ellipticity of P by the invertibility of $\sigma_m(P)$ which is the same as the ellipticity of $s(P)$, namely, we must have

$$\sigma_m : \mathcal{P}^m(G(X), E, E') \to \Gamma_\tau(S^*F, \mathrm{Isom}(E, E'))$$

and if this is the case then we say that P is *tangentially elliptic*.

Proposition 7.10 [Connes 1979, page 128]. *Suppose that $P \in \mathcal{P}^m(E, E')$ is a tangentially elliptic pseudodifferential operator. Then there exists a tangential parametrix, that is, a tangentially elliptic pseudodifferential operator $Q \in \mathcal{P}^{-m}(E', E)$ such that $PQ - \mathrm{id}_{E'}$ and $QP - \mathrm{id}_E$ are compactly smoothing.*

Proof (Connes). Let $\{\Omega_i\}$ be a finite open cover of X by coordinate charts of the form $\Omega_i \cong L_i \times N_i$. Let $\{\phi_i\}$ be a tangentially smooth partition of unity subordinate to this cover. Let C be a compact neighborhood of $G^0 \subset G(X)$ such that for each i,

$$\{\gamma \in C : s(\gamma) \subset \operatorname{Supp} \phi_i'\} \subset W_i = L_i \times L_i \times N_i,$$

where $\phi_i' \in C_{\tau c}^\infty(\Omega_i)$ has value 1 on the support of ϕ_i and s is the source map. We may suppose that $\operatorname{Supp} P \subset C$.

For each i, define M_i to be the tangential operator from E to E' given by multiplication by $\phi_i' \circ s$. The distribution K_i associated to PM_i is supported in W_i, so there exists $P_i \in \mathcal{P}_c^m(\Omega_i, E, E')$ such that $P_i' = \mathrm{PM}_i$. The usual multiplicative property of principal symbols implies that

$$\sigma_m(P_i') = \sigma_m(P)\phi_i'$$

so that P_i is tangentially elliptic on the support of ϕ_i. We must show that there exists $Q_i \in \mathcal{P}_c^{-m}(\Omega_i, E', E)$ such that $P_i Q_i - \phi_i$ is compactly smoothing.

Since P_i is elliptic on the support of ϕ_i with total symbol p and principal symbol $p_m \in S^m$ there exists some $q \in S^{-m}$ with $p_m q - \phi_i$ smoothing. Define q_k inductively by $q_0 = q$ and

$$q_k = -q \cdot \sum \frac{1}{\alpha!} d_\xi^\alpha p \cdot D_\xi^\alpha q_j \in S^{-m-k},$$

where the sum is taken over all α, j, k with $j < k$ and $|\alpha| + j = k$. Let $\tilde{Q}_i \in \mathcal{P}^{-m}$ with total symbol $q_0\phi_i' + q_1\phi_i' + \cdots$. This defines $\tilde{Q}_i \in \mathcal{P}^{-m}$ so that $\sigma(P_i\tilde{Q}_i - \phi_i) \sim 0$ on $\operatorname{Supp}(\phi_i)$. Similarly we could solve $\sigma(\hat{Q}_i P_i - \phi_i) \sim 0$ for $\hat{Q}_i \in \mathcal{P}^{-m}$. We compute

$$\begin{aligned}\sigma(\phi_i\tilde{Q}_i - \phi_i\hat{Q}_i) &= \sigma(\phi_i\tilde{Q}_i - \hat{Q}_i P_i \tilde{Q}_i) + \sigma(\hat{Q}_i P_i \tilde{Q}_i - \phi_i \tilde{Q}_i)\\ &= \sigma((\phi_i - \hat{Q}_i P_i)\tilde{Q}_i) + \sigma((\hat{Q}_i P_i - \phi_i)\tilde{Q}_i),\end{aligned}$$

so $\phi_i(\tilde{Q}_i - \hat{Q}_i) \sim 0$ modulo smoothing operators on the support of ϕ_i, which implies that $\tilde{Q}_i$ and $\hat{Q}_i$ agree modulo smoothing operators. Their distributional kernels are compactly supported since ϕ_i' is compactly supported. Set $Q_i = \tilde{Q}_i\phi_i$; then $P_i Q_i - \phi_i$ is compactly smoothing. Set $Q = \sum M_i Q_i'$. Then $PQ - I_{E'}$, is compactly smoothing, which implies the result. □

Corollary 7.11 [Connes 1979, page 128]. *Suppose that*

$$P_1, P_2 \in \mathcal{P}_m(G(X), E, E')$$

with P_2 elliptic. Then there is a constant $c < \infty$ such that

$$\|P_{1,x}\xi\| \le c\big(\|P_{2,x}\xi\| + \|\xi\|\big)$$

for all $x \in X$ and for all $\xi \in C_c^\infty(G^x)$.

Proof (Connes). Let $Q_2 \in \mathcal{P}^{-m}(G(X), E', E)$ with $Q_2 P_2 - \mathrm{id}_E$ smoothing. Because $P_1 Q_2 \in \mathcal{P}^0$ by Proposition 7.9(d), there is a constant $c_1 < \infty$ with

$$\|P_1 Q_2(P_2\xi)\| \le c_1 \|P_2\xi\|$$

for each $\xi \in C_c^\infty(G^x)$. As $P_1(Q_2P_2 - \mathrm{id}_E)$ is smoothing, one has

$$\|P_1Q_2P_2\xi - P_1\xi\| \le c_2\|\xi\|$$

for each $\xi \in C_c^\infty(G^x)$, which implies the result. □

Remark 7.12 (Connes). We note two special cases of this corollary. First, suppose that P_2 is the identity. Then

$$\|P_{1,x}\xi\| \le c(2\|\xi\|)$$

so that P_1 is a bounded operator. Second, suppose that $P_2 = (1+\Delta)^m$, some power of the identity plus the tangential Laplacian. Then the corollary implies that

$$\|P_{1,x}\xi\| \le \|(1+\Delta)^m\xi\| + \|\xi\|.$$

In particular,

$$\|(1+\Delta)^k\xi\|_s \le \|\xi\|_{s+2} + \|\xi\|_s$$

for any k.

Corollary 7.11 implies that if $P \in \mathcal{P}^s(E, E')$ is tangentially elliptic, then P defines a bounded invertible $G(X)$-operator

$$P : W_\tau^s \to \operatorname{Dom} P,$$

where Dom P has norm $\|\xi\| + \|P\xi\|$. This implies that each $Q \in \mathcal{P}^m(E, E')$ extends for each s to a bounded $G(X)$-invariant operator

$$Q : W_\tau^{s+m}(E) \to W_\tau^s(E').$$

Proposition 7.13 [Connes 1979]. (a) *Let $U = L \times N$ be a distinguished coordinate patch, let $P \in \mathcal{P}_c^m(U, E, E')$, and let*

$$P' : W_\tau^{s+m}(E) \to W_\tau^s(E')$$

be the canonical extension. Then there is a constant $b > 0$ (independent of P) such that

$$\|P'\|_{W_\tau^{s+m}, W_\tau^s} \le b \ \sup_n \|P_n\|_{W^{s+m}, W^s}.$$

(b) *Let ν be an invariant transverse measure with associated trace ϕ_ν on*

$$W^*(G(X), \tilde{\mu}).$$

Then each $T \in W^*(G(X), \tilde{\mu})$ having a continuous extension to

$$W_\tau^{-s}(E) \to W_\tau^s(E')$$

for some $s > p$ (the dimension of the leaves) is in the domain of ϕ_ν and there is a constant c, independent of T, such that

$$|\phi_\nu(T)| \le c\|T\|_{W^{-s}, W^s}.$$

Proof. (a) If $m = 0$ then this estimate follows as in the proof of Proposition 7.9(b). In general, fix some s' and consider the tangential operator

$$Q = (1+\Delta)^{-s'/2m} P(1+\Delta)^{-s/2m},$$

where Δ is the tangential Hodge–Laplace operator $\Delta = \{\Delta_n\}$, Δ_n defined over $L \times \{n\}$, formed from the underlying tangential Riemannian connection. Then

$$\|Q\| = c\|P\|_{W^s,W^{s'}}.$$

If Q were in $\mathcal{P}^0$ the argument would be complete, but this is not so in general. However, we may uniformly approximate the distributional kernel of Q by kernels K_j supported on compact neighborhoods of the diagonal $\{(x,x)\} \times N$. Let T_j be the associated operator to K_j. Then $T_j \in \mathcal{P}^0$, so that

$$\|T_j\| \leq \sup \|T_{j,n}\|$$

by the earlier estimate and the T_j uniformly approximate Q, which completes the argument.

(b) There is some $S \in W^*(G(X), \tilde{\mu})$ such that

$$T = (1+\Delta)^{-s/2m} S(1+\Delta)^{-s/2m}$$

with $\|S\| = \|T\|_{-s,s}$. Proposition 7.9 implies that S has finite trace. So it suffices to show that $(1+\Delta)^{-s/m}$ is in the domain of ϕ_ν. Corollary 7.10 implies that there is a tangential pseudodifferential operator P of order $-s$ with

$$(1+\Delta)^{-s/m} \leq P^* P.$$

So it suffices to show that $\phi_\nu(P^* P)$ is finite. Let K_P denote the distributional kernel of P. Restrict to a leaf ℓ. Proposition 1.12 implies that $(P^* P)_\ell$ is a locally traceable operator with local trace given by

$$\mu_{(P^*P)_\ell} = \int_y |K_P(y,x,n)|^2 \, d\lambda(y)\lambda(x).$$

Thus

$$\phi_\nu(P^* P) = \int_X \mu_{(P^*P)_\ell} \, d\nu = \int_X \int_y |K_P(y,x,n)|^2 \, d\lambda(y)\lambda(x) \, d\nu,$$

which is finite by Proposition 7.9(d) and the fact that

$$\int \|K_P\|_{HS}^2 \, d\nu < \infty. \qquad \square$$

Recall from Proposition 7.9(b) that each pseudodifferential operator

$$P \in \mathcal{P}^0(G(X), E, E')$$

extends to a bounded intertwining operator

$$L^2(G(X), \lambda_{G(X)}, E_s) \to L^2(G(X), \lambda_{G(X)}, E'_s),$$

which we denote in Hilbert field notation as

$$P : L^2_\tau(G(X), E) \to L^2_\tau(G(X), E')$$

We norm these as usual by

$$\|P\| = \sup_{x \in X} \|P^x\|,$$

where

$$P^x : L^2_\tau(G^x, E|_{G^x}) \to L^2_\tau(G^x, E'|_{G^x})$$

and denote the associated normed space of pseudodifferential operators of order $\leq m$ by $\mathcal{P}^m(G(X), E, E')$ We note that for any m this space contains the space of tangentially smooth compactly supported sections $\Gamma_{\tau c}(G(X), \mathrm{Hom}(E, E'))$.

The most important case of interest to us is $\mathcal{P}^0(G(X), E, E)$. This is obviously a $*$-algebra containing $\Gamma_{\tau c}(G(X), \mathrm{End}_\tau(E))$ as a two-sided ideal. Taking closures we obtain a C^*-algebra $\overline{\mathcal{P}}(G(X), E, E)$ called the (closed) *pseudodifferential operator algebra* with closed two-sided ideal $C^*_r(G(X), \mathrm{End}_\tau(E))$.

Given some foliated space X with canonical bundle $F \to X$, fix some tangential Riemannian metric. This fixes an isomorphism $F \cong F^*$ of F with its dual cotangent bundle. We denote the vectors of length at most one in the total space by D^*F and the vectors of length exactly one by S^*F. (To be precise, we should write D^*F^* and S^*F^* but this gets to be an awkward burden, and in any event unnecessary since the spaces are canonically homeomorphic.) The bundle $\pi : S^*F \to X$ is called the *cosphere* bundle of X. It is elementary that the zero section $X \to D^*F$ is a homotopy equivalence, since sending a vector v to tv $0 \leq t \leq 1$ is a deformation retraction of D^*F to X.

We regard the tangential principal symbol map as a map taking values in

$$\Gamma_\tau(S^*F, \mathrm{End}_\tau(E)).$$

Proposition 7.14 [Connes 1979, p. 138]. *The tangential principal symbol map*

$$\sigma : \mathcal{P}^0(G(X), E, E) \to \Gamma_\tau(S^*F, \mathrm{End}_\tau(E))$$

is a $*$-homomorphism with dense image. It extends to a surjection of C^*-algebras and induces a canonical short exact sequence of C^*-algebras

$$0 \longrightarrow C^*_r(G(X), \mathrm{End}_\tau(E)) \longrightarrow \overline{\mathcal{P}}^0(G(X), E, E) \xrightarrow{\sigma} \Gamma(S^*F, \mathrm{End}_\tau(E)) \longrightarrow 0.$$

Proof. That σ is surjective is proved in the classical setting in [Palais 1965, pp. 269, 246] by the construction of a continuous linear section. The general idea is to use partition of unity arguments to reduce down to the case of trivial vector bundles over open balls in Euclidean space, and then to explicitly write down the section. All this generalizes in an obvious way to our setting. It suffices, then, to compute $\mathrm{Ker}\,\sigma$. It is clear that $\mathrm{Ker}\,\sigma$ contains $C^*_r(G(X))$, so it suffices to prove the opposite inclusion. Note that since σ has a continuous linear section, any $T \in \mathcal{P}^0$ with $\|\sigma(T)\|$ small has small spectral radius in $\overline{\mathcal{P}}^0/C_r^*(G(X))$. The proposition then follows from the next Lemma (with $A = C_r^*(G(X))$ and $B = \operatorname{Ker}\sigma$). □

Lemma 7.15. *Let $\mathcal{P}$ be a dense $*$-subalgebra of a C^*-algebra $\overline{\mathcal{P}}$ and let $A \subseteq B \subset \overline{\mathcal{P}}$ be ideals. Suppose that the following condition holds:*

If $x \in \mathcal{P}$ with $|x|$ small in $\overline{\mathcal{P}}/B$ then the spectral radius $\rho(x)$ is small in $\overline{\mathcal{P}}/A$.

Then $A = B$.

Proof. Let $\mathcal{P}_A \subset \overline{\mathcal{P}}/A$ be the (dense) image of $\mathcal{P}$ and similarly for $\mathcal{P}_B \subset \overline{\mathcal{P}}/B$. Let

$$\psi : \mathcal{P}_A \to \mathcal{P}_B$$

be the obvious surjection. If $x \in \mathcal{P}_A$ with $\psi(x) = 0$ then $|\psi x| = 0$ in $\overline{\mathcal{P}}/B$ by the condition in the lemma. Then $\rho(x) = 0$ in $\overline{\mathcal{P}}/A$ and $x = 0$; thus ψ is injective and so an isomorphism. Let

$$\phi = \psi^{-1} : \mathcal{P}_B \to \mathcal{P}_A.$$

Then ϕ is a bounded map, again by the condition in the lemma, and it extends to

$$\bar{\phi} : \overline{\mathcal{P}}/B \to \overline{\mathcal{P}}/A.$$

It is easy to see that $\bar{\phi}$ is the inverse to the natural projection

$$\bar{\psi} : \overline{\mathcal{P}}/A \to \overline{\mathcal{P}}/B,$$

so $\bar{\psi}$ is an isomorphism, and $A = B$. □

Note that if P is a smoothing operator of order 0 which is not compactly smoothing then it might not be in $\overline{\mathcal{P}}$ and in particular not in $C_r^*(G(X))$. Such operators are, however, in the Breuer ideal of compact operators (cf. the proof of Proposition 6.37) in $W^*(G(X), \tilde{\mu})$, as we shall see in Proposition 7.37. Similarly, if P is (say) compactly smoothing with distribution kernel which is measurable but not continuous then the same conclusion holds.

The previous proposition enables us to extend the definition of tangential ellipticity to any P in the closure of $\mathcal{P}^0$ by declaring P to be *tangentially elliptic* if $\sigma(P)$ is invertible.

For $P \in \overline{\mathcal{P}}^0(G(X), E_1, E_2)$ the principal symbol restricts to a map

$$\sigma(P) : S^*F \longrightarrow \operatorname{Hom}_\tau(\pi^* E_1, \pi^* E_2),$$

so that $\sigma(P)$ induces for each $x \in S^*(F)$ a linear map

$$\sigma(P)_x : (\pi^* E_1)_x \longrightarrow (\pi^* E_2)_x,$$

and to say that P is tangentially elliptic simply says that each $\sigma(P)_x$ is an isomorphism of vector spaces.

In order to finish this section, two tasks remain:

(1) We must define the abstract analytic index of a tangential, tangentially elliptic pseudodifferential operator, as the class

$$\operatorname{ind}(P) \in K_0(C^*(G(X)))$$

and relate this index class with families of projections and the associated von Neumann algebra projections.

(2) We must find a topological home for $\sigma(P)$ in order to be able to form $\operatorname{ch}_\tau(P)$ and hence complete the definition of the topological index of P.

Both tasks involve some subtleties; we take each one in turn.

Suppose that $P \in \overline{\mathcal{P}}^0(G(X), E_1, E_2)$ is a tangential, tangentially elliptic pseudodifferential operator of order zero, and suppose first that $E_1 \cong E_2$. Then

$$\Gamma_\tau(S^*F, \operatorname{End}_\tau(\pi^* E_1))$$

is a C^*-algebra and $\sigma(P)$ is an invertible element in it. So

$$[\sigma(P)] \in K_1(\Gamma(S^*F, \operatorname{End}(\pi^* E_1))).$$

The short exact sequence (7.14) induces a long exact sequence in K-theory and, in particular, there is a natural connecting homomorphism

$$\partial : K_1\big(\Gamma(S^*F, \operatorname{End}_\tau(E_1))\big) \to K_0\big(C_r^*(G(X), \operatorname{End}_\tau(E_1))\big).$$

Then the idea is to define

$$\operatorname{ind}(P) = \partial[\sigma(P)] \in K_0(C_r^*(G(X), \operatorname{End}_\tau(E))).$$

Let us examine this construction of $\operatorname{ind}(P)$ very explicitly, keeping track of the bundles. Let $Q \in \overline{\mathcal{P}}^0(E_2, E_1)$ be a parametrix for P. Then

$$QP - I \in C_r^*(G(X), \operatorname{End}_\tau(E_1)) \quad \text{and} \quad PQ - I \in C_r^*(G(X), \operatorname{End}_\tau(E_2)).$$

Define a matrix

$$T : L^2(G(X), E_1) \oplus L^2(G(X), E_2) \longrightarrow L^2(G(X), E_2) \oplus L^2(G(X), E_1)$$

by

$$T = \begin{pmatrix} P+(I-PQ)P & PQ-I \\ I-QP & Q \end{pmatrix}$$

Then T is invertible with

$$T^{-1} = \begin{pmatrix} Q & I-QP \\ PQ-I & P+P(I-QP) \end{pmatrix}.$$

Letting $e_0 = \left(\begin{smallmatrix} 1 & 0 \\ 0 & 0 \end{smallmatrix}\right)$, we have

(7.16) $$\operatorname{ind}(P) = [Te_0T^{-1}] - [e_0] \in K_0\big(C_r^*(G(X), \operatorname{End}_\tau(E_1 \oplus E_2))\big).$$

It may seem problematic that $\operatorname{ind}(P)$ does not take values in $K_0(C_r^*(G(X)))$, but in fact there is no difficulty, for Theorem 6.15 demonstrates that

$$C_r^*(G(X), \operatorname{End}_\tau(E_1 \oplus E_2))$$

is stably isomorphic to $C_r^*(G(X))$, so the two K_0-groups are isomorphic, and these particular stable isomorphisms preserve the natural traces that arise from invariant transverse measures, by Theorem 6.32, so that the partial Chern character (Theorem 6.33) of the index class

$$c(\operatorname{ind}(P)) \in \overline{H}_\tau^p(X)$$

is well-defined.

In fact formula (7.16) is even better than it seems at first glance. For suppose given a pseudodifferential operator

$$P \in \overline{\mathcal{P}}^0(E_1, E_2),$$

where E_1 and E_2 are *not necessarily* isomorphic. Then $\overline{\mathcal{P}}^0(E_1, E_2)$ is no longer a ring and so formally the long exact K-theory sequence is not available. This turns out not to be an obstacle. Let $Q \in \overline{\mathcal{P}}^0(E_2, E_1)$. be a parametrix for P. The operator T is still an isomorphism, and the resulting classes $[Te_0T^{-1}]$ and $[e_0]$ still lie in the group $K_0(C_r^*(G(X), \operatorname{End}_\tau(E_1 \oplus E_2)))$. Thus there is still an abstract index class $\operatorname{ind}(P)$ given by formula (7.16), and there is a well-defined partial Chern character to apply to obtain $c(\operatorname{ind}(P)) \in \overline{H}_\tau^p(X)$.

So, given a tangential, tangentially elliptic operator, we have constructed an abstract analytic index class $\operatorname{ind}(P)$. Next, we relate the index class $\operatorname{ind}(P)$ to the families of kernels $\operatorname{Ker} P_L$ and $\operatorname{Ker} P_L^*$, to the associated families of local traces, and to the associated von Neumann algebra projections. In this measure theory context we need not keep track of the bundles, since measurably they are all stably equivalent.

Fix an invariant transverse measure ν and form the associated von Neumann algebra $W^*(G(X), \tilde{\mu})$ with trace ϕ_ν. It is clear from the construction that there is a natural map

$$\beta : \overline{\mathcal{P}} \to W^*(G(X), \tilde{\mu})$$

whose image is weakly dense. Let $\pi : C_r^*(G(X)) \to W^*(G(X), \tilde{\mu})$ be the canonical map and let

$$\pi_* : K_0(C_r^*(G(X))) \to K_0^f(W^*(G(X)), \tilde{\mu})$$

be the induced homomorphism. Recall that $\iota_P = \{\iota_P^x\}$ is the index measure of P and that $\operatorname{ind}(P) \in K_0(C_r^*(G(X)))$ is the image of the tangential principal symbol of P.

Theorem 7.17. *Let $P \in \overline{\mathcal{P}}^0$ be a tangentially elliptic operator. Then*

(a) $\operatorname{Ker}(\beta P)$ *and* $\operatorname{Ker}(\beta P^*)$ *are finite projections in* $W^*(G(X), \tilde{\mu})$ *such that*

$$[\operatorname{Ker}(\beta P)] - [\operatorname{Ker}(\beta P^*)] \in K_0^f(W^*(G(X), \tilde{\mu})).$$

(b) $\pi_*(\operatorname{ind}(P)) = [\operatorname{Ker}(\beta P)] - [\operatorname{Ker}(\beta P^*)]$.

(c) $c(\operatorname{ind}(P)) = [\iota_P] \in \bar{H}_\tau^p(X)$.

(d) $\operatorname{ind}_\nu(P) \equiv \int \iota_P \, d\nu = \phi_\nu\big([\operatorname{Ker}(\beta P)] - [\operatorname{Ker}(\beta P^*)]\big)$.

Proof. This is immediate from Proposition 6.37. □

Corollary 7.18. *Let* $P \in \overline{\mathfrak{P}}^0$ *be a tangentially elliptic operator. Then*

$$\operatorname{ind}_\nu(P) = \phi_\nu\big([\operatorname{Ker}(\beta P)] - [\operatorname{Ker}(\beta P^*)]\big)$$

depends only upon the homotopy class of the principal symbol of P in the group $K_0(C_r^*(G(X)))$.

Proof. Immediate from Theorem 7.17 and the fact that $\operatorname{ind}(P) \in K_0(C_r^*(G(X)))$ depends only upon the homotopy class of the tangential principal symbol $\sigma_0(P)$ of P. □

This completes our discussion of the analytic index. We turn now to the second task — that of preparing the way for the topological index. Suppose given a tangential, tangentially elliptic pseudodifferential operator P with principal symbol $\sigma(P)$. Where does this symbol *really* live? It lives in $K^0(F^*)$, as we now explain.

Given some foliated space X with canonical bundle $F \to X$, fix some tangential Riemannian metric. This fixes an isomorphism $F \cong F^*$ of F with its dual bundle, and hence the spaces D^*F and S^*F as introduced earlier. The natural inclusion $D^*F \subseteq F^*$ induces a homeomorphism

$$D^*F/S^*F \longrightarrow F^+,$$

called the *Thom–Pontryagin map*. Identify the quotient space D^*F/S^*F, which is the *Thom space* of the bundle F^*, with the one-point compactification of F^*.

Proposition 7.19. *Let X be a compact foliated space with canonical bundle F and tangential Riemannian metric. Then*

(1) *For* $j = 1, 2$ *there are natural identifications*

$$K^j(D^*F/S^*F) \cong \tilde{K}^j((F^*)^+) \cong K^j(F^*).$$

(2) *There is a natural long exact cohomology sequence*

$$\cdots \longrightarrow K^0(D^*F) \longrightarrow K^0(S^*F) \xrightarrow{\partial} K^1(F^*)$$
$$\longrightarrow K^1(D^*F) \longrightarrow K^1(S^*F) \xrightarrow{\partial} K^0(F^*) \longrightarrow K^0(D^*F) \longrightarrow \cdots$$

Proof. Part (1) is immediate from definitions and the Thom–Pontryagin homeomorphism. Part (2) follows from the long exact K-theory sequence of the pair (D^*F, S^*F) together with (1). □

Coming back to

$$[\sigma(P)] \in K^1(S^*F),$$

apply $\partial : K^1(S^*F) \to K^0(F^*)$ to obtain a class

$$\partial[\sigma(P)] \in K^0(F^*).$$

Normally the map ∂ is suppressed and the class is simply written

$$[\sigma(P)] \in K^0(F^*).$$

and referred to as the class of the principal symbol of P.

This entire construction has been under the assumption that $E_1 \cong E_2$. However, what if E_1 is not isomorphic to E_2? Then it is necessary to proceed differently—and to proceed in a way that generalizes the construction above. We need a new description of the group $K^0(F^*)$.

If X is a locally compact space then we have previously defined the K-theory of X with compact supports as

$$K^0(X) = \widetilde{K}^0(X^+).$$

There is another approach to this group which is essential to our purposes. Here is how it is described in [Atiyah and Singer 1968a, p. 489], where it is introduced for essentially the same reason.

An *elliptic complex of vector bundles* over X is a sequence of Hermitian bundles and bundle maps

$$0 \to E^0 \xrightarrow{\alpha} E^1 \xrightarrow{\alpha} E^2 \xrightarrow{\alpha} \cdots \to E^n \longrightarrow 0$$

with $\alpha^2 = 0$. The *support* of the complex is the set of points $x \in X$ such that the sequence of vector spaces

$$0 \longrightarrow E^0_x \xrightarrow{\alpha} E^1_x \xrightarrow{\alpha} E^2_x \xrightarrow{\alpha} \ldots \longrightarrow E^n_x \longrightarrow 0$$

is *not* exact. The prototype example is obtained, of course, by taking a tangential, tangentially elliptic operator P and forming the elliptic complex

$$0 \longrightarrow \pi^* E_0 \xrightarrow{\sigma(P)} \pi^*(E_1) \longrightarrow 0.$$

Consider only complexes of compact support. Homotopy classes of these complexes form an abelian semigroup under $\oplus$ and there is a sub-semigroup consisting of those complexes with empty support. The quotient of these two turns out to be a group, and in fact it is $K^0(X)$, as demonstrated in [Segal 1968].[1]

[1] The map from elliptic complexes to $K^0(X)$ is given roughly as follows. Starting with an elliptic complex, we take alternating sums to reduce to complexes of the form

$$0 \longrightarrow E^0 \xrightarrow{\alpha} E^1 \longrightarrow 0.$$

The ring structure in K-theory corresponds to splicing complexes. In the case of $K^0(F^*)$ more can be said. Let $\pi : F^* \to X$ be the natural projection. Then it is the case that every element of $K^0(F^*)$ may be represented as a complex

$$0 \longrightarrow \pi^*(E^0) \xrightarrow{\alpha} \pi^*(E^1) \longrightarrow 0,$$

where E^0 and E^1 are Hermitian bundles over X itself.

Now, let

$$P : \Gamma_\tau(E_1) \longrightarrow \Gamma_\tau(E_2)$$

be a tangential, tangentially elliptic pseudodifferential operator. Pulling the bundles back along $\pi : F^* \to X$ and taking tangential principal symbols, we obtain a complex

$$0 \to \pi^*(E_1) \xrightarrow{\sigma(P)} \pi^*(E_2) \to 0.$$

This is indeed an elliptic complex, and its homotopy class gives naturally

$$[\sigma(P)] \in K^0(F^*)$$

If in fact $E_1 = E_2$ so that our previous construction yields

$$[\sigma(P)] \in K^1(S^*F)$$

then it is evident from the definition of ∂ that this class maps correctly to $K^0(F^*)$ under ∂. So now it makes sense to define $\mathrm{ch}_\tau(P)$ via the composite

$$[\sigma(P)] \in K^0(F^*) \xrightarrow{\mathrm{ch}_\tau} H^*_{\tau c}(F^*) \xrightarrow{\Phi_\tau^{-1}} H^*_\tau(X)$$

and, adding a sign (the peculiar choice of which is explained in [Atiyah and Singer 1968b, p. 557]):

$$\mathrm{ch}_\tau(P) = (-1)^{p(p+1)/2} \Phi_\tau^{-1}\, \mathrm{ch}_\tau(\sigma(P)).$$

This completes our introduction to abstract tangential pseudodifferential operators.

VII-B. Differential Operators and Finite Propagation

The most natural operators on foliated spaces are parametrized versions of the classical differential operators. These operators are unbounded, and it is necessary to exercise some care in promoting them to bounded operators in defining an index. There are at least two possible technical approaches. Connes prefers to use methods from geometric asymptotics. We have chosen to use finite propagation techniques, in part because of their lovely simplicity, and in

---

We alter α by adding on a trivial bundle if necessary and then deforming α by a homotopy so that $\operatorname{Ker}\alpha$ and $\operatorname{Cok}\alpha$ are vector bundles over X. Then the corresponding class in $K^0(X)$ is $[\operatorname{Ker}\alpha] - [\operatorname{Cok}\alpha]$.

part because we have been impressed by their efficacy as demonstrated, e.g., in [Taylor 1979; Cheeger et al. 1982; Roe 1987].

Definition 7.20. Let D be a first order differential operator over a noncompact complete manifold with self-adjoint principal symbol $\sigma_1(D)$. The *propagation speed* of D is defined by

$$c(x) = \sup\{\|\sigma_1(x,\xi)\| \mid \|\xi\| = 1\}.$$

If $c(x) \leq c$ then D is said to have *finite propagation speed* [Cheeger et al. 1982; Taylor 1979; Chernoff 1973; Roe 1987]. In that case, solutions to the hyperbolic system

$$\left(\frac{\partial}{\partial t} + iD\right)u = 0.$$

exist [Friedrichs 1954] and propagate at speeds bounded by c.

Recall that if D is a densely defined operator then the *formal adjoint* D^t of D is defined by $(D^t u, v) = (u, Dv)$. If $D = D^t$ then D is *formally self-adjoint.* In general, the closure $\bar{D}$ of D satisfies $\bar{D} \subset D^t$. A symmetric operator T is *essentially self-adjoint* provided that $\bar{U}$ is self-adjoint, or equivalently, T^t is symmetric, in which case $\bar{U} = T^t$.

Theorem 7.21 [Chernoff 1973, Lemma 2.1]. *Suppose that*

$$D : \Gamma(E) \to \Gamma(E)$$

is a first-order, not necessarily elliptic, differential operator over a noncompact complete manifold and suppose that D is formally self-adjoint and has finite propagation speed with a uniform bound

$$c(x) \leq c < +\infty.$$

Then D is essentially self-adjoint and, more generally, D^k is essentially self-adjoint for all k. Thus for any bounded Borel function on $\mathbb{R}$, $f(D)$ is defined as a bounded operator on $L^2(E)$.

Proof. We repeat Chernoff's proof. Fix a positive integer k and let $A = D^k$. It suffices to show that there is no nontrivial solution to the eigenvalue equation $A^t u = \pm iu$; that is, there is no nonzero choice for u such that

$$\langle u, v\rangle \pm \langle u, Av\rangle = 0$$

for all $v \in \operatorname{Dom} A$.

Suppose that $A^t u = iu$. We want to show that $u = 0$. Let $v \in C_c^\infty(M)$. Then $U_t = e^{itA}$ extends to a unitary operator on L^2. Define $F(t)$ by

$$F(t) = \langle U_t v, u\rangle.$$

The function F is bounded on $\mathbb{R}$ since U_t is unitary. The k-th derivative $F^{(k)}$ of $F(t)$ is given by

$$F^{(k)}(t) = \langle i^k D^k U_t v, u\rangle = \langle i^k A U_t v, u\rangle = \langle i^k U_t, A^t u\rangle = -i^{k+1} F(t).$$

Hence $F(t)$ is a linear combination of exponential functions $e^{\alpha t}$, where α runs through the solutions of the equation $\alpha^k = -i^{k+1}$. So none of the α's is pure imaginary. As F is bounded, this implies that F is identically zero, so that $\langle U_t v, u\rangle = 0$. Finite propagation implies that U_t restricts to an isomorphism $C_c^\infty(M) \to C_c^\infty(M)$. Thus $\langle C_c^\infty(M), u\rangle = 0$ and so $u = 0$ as required. A similar argument applies to the solutions of $A^t u = -iu$. This establishes the theorem. □

Pick some point $x \in X$. The map

$$\mathbb{R}^p \cong F_x \xrightarrow{\exp_x} X$$

maps some open p-ball B about the origin to a chart of ℓ_x, the leaf which contains x. Choose an orthonormal base for F_x and extend thé map to

$$F_x \times N \xrightarrow{\exp_x} X$$

to obtain a "tangential normal coordinate system" at x. It is determined uniquely up to an element of $C(N, O(p))$, where $O(p)$ is the orthogonal group. Choose an orthonormal basis for S_x, the fibre of the bundle S at x. For

$$y \in \exp(B \times N) \cap \ell$$

there is a well-defined isomorphism $S_x \to S_y$ given by parallel transport. Thus a basis is determined for the sections of S over the patch. So fix a choice of basis at S_x; the resulting system is called a *canonical coordinate system*. Letting $\{e_i\}$ denote the basis vector-fields on $\exp(B \times N)$ corresponding to the canonical coordinate system on S, the tangential Levi-Civita connection acts by

$$\nabla_i(e_j) = \sum \Gamma_{ij}^k e_k \qquad \text{and} \qquad \nabla_i(s_\alpha) = \sum \Gamma_{i\alpha}^\beta s_\beta.$$

Definition 7.22. (X, S) has *bounded geometry* if

(1) X has positive tangential injectivity radius; that is, there is a nonempty open ball $B \subset \mathbb{R}^p$ which is injected by the exponential map at very point of X,

(2) For each leaf, the Christoffel symbols of the tangential connection on X lie in a bounded set of the Fréchet space $C^\infty(B)$, and

(3) For each leaf, the Christoffel symbols of the tangential connection of the bundle S lie in a bounded set of $C^\infty(B)$.

Proposition 7.23. *Let M be a smooth Riemannian manifold with a C^∞ bounded geometry covered by open sets $\{U_j\}$ with exponential coordinate charts on each U_j of fixed radius c. Let D be an elliptic differential operator of positive order whose coefficients are bounded in C^∞ with a uniform ellipticity estimate. Then D and its formal adjoint D^t act as unbounded operators on $L^2(M)$ with domain $C_0^\infty(M)$, and the closure of D^t is the Hilbert space adjoint D^* of D.*

Proof. (This proof was kindly supplied to us by Michael Taylor.) We define D and D^t as unbounded operators on $L^2(M)$ with domain

$$\text{Dom } D = \text{Dom } D^t = C_0^\infty(M).$$

We aim to prove that the closure of D^t is D^*. Suppose first that the order of D is even. Recall from 7.21 that all powers of the Laplace operator Δ are essentially self-adjoint since M is complete. Since, by definition,

$$u \in \text{Dom } D^* \iff |(u, Dv)| \le C_u \|v\|_{L^2} \text{ for all } v \in C_0^\infty(M),$$

using local elliptic regularity of D^t, we can state

$$u \in \text{Dom } D^* \iff u \in L^2(M),\ u \in W^{2m}_{\text{loc}}(M), \text{ and } D^t u \in L^2(M),$$

where D^t is a priori applied to u in the distributional sense. Since the weak and strong extensions of Δ^m coincide, we can say both that

$$u \in \text{Dom } \Delta^m \iff u \in L^2(M),\ u \in W^{2m}_{\text{loc}}(M), \text{ and } \Delta^m u \in L^2(M)$$

and that

$$u \in \text{Dom } \Delta^m \iff u \in L^2(M) \text{ and there exists a sequence } v_j \in C_0^\infty(M),$$
$$\big(v_j \to u \text{ in } L^2(M) \Rightarrow \Delta^m(v_j - v_k) \to 0 \text{ in } L^2(M) \text{ as } j,k \to \infty\big).$$

Now elliptic estimates bound L^2 norms of $D^t u$ over a ball $V_j \subset M$, where $V_j \subset U_j$, say of radius $c_0/2$, in terms of L^2 norms of $\Delta^m u$ and of u over U_j (with bounds independent of j) and conversely, one has a bound on L^2 norms of $\Delta^m u$ over V_j in terms of L^2 norms of $D^t u$ and u over U_j. One can suppose the V_j cover M and that the U_j do not have too many overlaps, so we deduce

$$\text{Dom } D^* = \text{Dom } \Delta^m.$$

From here it is easy to complete the proof. Indeed, given $u \in \text{Dom } D^* = \text{Dom } \Delta^m$, we know by the last characterization that there exist $v_j \in C_0^\infty(M)$ such that $v_j \to u$ in $L^2(M)$ and $\Delta^m(v_j - v_k) \to 0$ in $L^2(M)$, as $j,k \to \infty$. The boundedness hypotheses on the coefficients of D^t, together with elliptic estimates, imply

$$\|D^t w\|_{L^2(M)} \le C\|\Delta^m w\|_{L^2(M)} + C\|w\|_{L^2(M)} \quad \text{for } w \in C_0^\infty(M).$$

Thus

$$\|D^t(v_j - v_k)\|_{L^2} \le C\|\Delta^m(v_j - v_k)\|_{L^2} + C\|v_j - v_k\|_{L^2} \to 0 \quad \text{as } j,k \to \infty,$$

and the theorem is established for D of even order.

It remains to consider the case when D is of odd order. Let P_0 be the closure of D^t, the minimal extension of D^t, and let $P_1 = D^*$, the Hilbert space adjoint, which is the maximal extension of D^t. Clearly $P_0 \subset P_1$. Let $A = P_0^* P_0$ and $B = P_1^* P_1$. By von Neumann's theorem, A and B are self-adjoint and

$$\text{Dom}\, A^{1/2} = \text{Dom}\, P_0, \qquad \text{Dom}\, B^{1/2} = \text{Dom}\, P_1.$$

However A and B are extensions of the even order elliptic operator $D^t D$. The previous case implies that $A = B$. Thus Dom $P_0 =$ Dom P_1 and we are through. □

If D is a tangential differential operator then Ker $D = \{\text{Ker}\, D_\ell\}$ forms a measurable field of Hilbert spaces. If D is tangentially elliptic then by (4.11) there is also associated a tangential measure

$$\mu_{\text{Ker}\, D} = \{\mu_{\text{Ker}\, D_\ell}\},$$

where $\mu_{\text{Ker}\, D_\ell}$ is the local dimension of the orthogonal projection onto the subspace Ker D_ℓ. Similarly there is a natural tangential measure $\mu_{\text{Ker}\, D^*}$. These measures would appear to depend upon the choice of closure of D. This problem is disposed of by the following Corollary.

Corollary 7.24. *Let X be a compact foliated space with some fixed tangential Riemannian metric and let D be a tangentially elliptic differential operator. Then the (leafwise) closure of the (leafwise) formal adjoint of D is the (leafwise) Hilbert space adjoint of D. Thus D has a unique closure. Hence* Ker D *and* Ker D^* *are uniquely defined Hilbert fields, and $\mu_{\text{Ker}\, D}$ and $\mu_{\text{Ker}\, D^*}$ are uniquely defined tangential measures.*

Proof. This follows immediately from the preceeding proposition and the observation that if ℓ is a leaf in X then ℓ is a Riemannian manifold with bounded geometry as required. □

It still remains to define the index of a tangential differential operator of positive order. The most natural definition at this point is to form an index measure

$$\iota_D = \mu_{\text{Ker}\, D} - \mu_{\text{Ker}\, D^*}$$

which is unique, by 7.24, and let the index be the total mass of this measure:

$$\text{ind}_\nu(D) = \int \iota_D \, d\nu.$$

As this stands it is not at all clear how this corresponds to the index of order zero operators and the canonical pseudodifferential operator extension, nor is it clear how to compute. We turn to these matters next.

Let D be a tangential, tangentially elliptic differential operator of positive order m from sections of E to sections of E' over a compact foliated space X. Then D extends to a densely defined unbounded operator $D = \{D_{\tilde{\ell}}\}$ of Hilbert fields

$$L^2_\tau(\widetilde{E}) \to L^2_\tau(\widetilde{E}'),$$

where $\tilde{\ell}$ is the holonomy covering of the leaf ℓ, the bundles $\widetilde{E}, \widetilde{E}'$ are the pull-backs of the bundles E, E' respectively to the holonomy groupoid $G = G(X)$ and L^2 denotes the corresponding Hilbert fields obtained by pulling the bundles back to $G(X)$, lifting the action of D, and then restricting. The operator D has a unique leafwise closure, by Corollary 7.24, which for convenience we also denote by D. By standard functional analysis, $(1 + D^*D)$ is a positive operator which is bounded below and hence has an inverse $(1 + D^*D)^{-1}$ which is a *bounded* operator

$$(1 + D^*D)^{-1}\colon L^2_\tau(\widetilde{E}_\ell) \longrightarrow L^2_\tau(\widetilde{E}_\ell)$$

for each leaf ℓ.

Recall that

$$\text{Dom}\, D^*D = \{\phi : \phi \in \text{Dom}\, D,\ D\phi \in \text{Dom}\, D^*\}.$$

Then $(1+D^*D)$ has a square root $(1+D^*D)^{1/2}$ by standard functional analysis. The spectral theorem implies that

$$\text{Dom}\ (1 + D^*D)^{1/2} = \text{Dom}\ (D^*D)^{1/2}.$$

As $A = (D^*D)^{1/2}$ is the positive part of the polar decomposition $D = UA$ (U partial isometry), Dom A = Dom D and so

$$\text{Dom}\ (1 + D^*D)^{1/2} = \text{Dom}\ D.$$

This implies that the operator $(1 + D^*D)^{-1/2}$ has range equal to Dom D. Since the operator $(1 + D^*D)^\alpha$ is onto for each $\alpha > 0$, the operator $(1 + D^*D)^{-1/2}$ is defined on all of $L^2(\widetilde{E})$. Thus

$$L = D(1 + D^*D)^{-1/2}$$

makes sense and is bounded by direct composition. In polar form, $L = UB$. That is, L has the same polar part U as $D = UA$; D has been replaced by $D(1 + D^*D)^{-1/2}$, a bounded version of D, and

$$B = A^2(1 + A^2)^{1/2} = \left(D^*D(1 + D^*D)^{-1}\right)^{1/2}.$$

Note that $L = UB$ and $D = UA$ have the same kernel. The closure of the ranges is likewise the same. Hence

$$\text{Ker}\, L = \text{Ker}\, D \quad \text{and} \quad \text{Ker}\, L^* = \text{Ker}\, D^*$$

in the von Neumann algebra $W^*(G(X), \tilde{\mu})$. If we knew that L were in $\mathcal{P}^0$ or even in $\overline{\mathcal{P}}^0$ then we would know that these projections were ν-finite and that the ν-index of D was just the ν-index of L. One can establish this in greater generality using methods of Connes, but we specialize to first order operators.

Theorem 7.25 [Taylor 1981, Chapter XII; Roe 1987]. *Let $D = \{D_\ell\}$ be a tangential, tangentially elliptic and tangentially formally self-adjoint operator. Lift each D_ℓ to its holonomy covering $D_{\tilde{\ell}}$. Let f be a bounded Borel function, so that $f(D_{\tilde{\ell}})$ is defined by the spectral theorem. Let $f(D) \equiv \{f(D_{\tilde{\ell}})\}$ act on the canonical Hilbert field*

$$f(D) : L^2_\tau(G(X), E) \longrightarrow L^2_\tau(G(X), E)$$

of $C^*_r(G(X))$. Then:

(1) *If f is a Schwartz function with Fourier transform $\hat{f}$, then*

$$f(D) = \frac{1}{2\pi} \int \hat{f}(t) e^{itD}\, dt,$$

where the integral is understood to be in the weak sense along the leaves.

(2) *If D is of first order wth finite propagation speed on each leaf and $f \in C_0(\mathbb{R})$ with Fourier transform $\hat{f} \in C_c^\infty(\mathbb{R})$ then*

$$f(D) \in C^\infty_{\tau c}(G(X), \mathrm{End}_\tau(E)).$$

(3) *If D is of first order with finite propagation speed on each leaf, $f \in C_0(\mathbb{R})$, then*

$$f(D) \in C^*_r(G(X), \mathrm{End}_\tau(E)).$$

Proof. Part (1) is proved in [Taylor 1981, Chapter XII]. For parts (2) and (3) see [Roe 1987, Theorem 2.1 and Corollary 2.2]. □

Corollary 7.26 (Roe). *Let D be a first order tangential tangentially elliptic and tangentially formally self-adjoint differential operator from sections of E to sections E' with uniformly bounded propagation speed on all leaves. Define*

$$L = D(1 + D^2)^{-1/2}.$$

Then L is a bounded operator on L^2, and $L \in \overline{\mathcal{P}}^0$.

Proof. It suffices to prove that $L \in \overline{\mathcal{P}}^0$. Let

$$f(x) = x(1 + x^2)^{-1/2}.$$

Then $f'(x) = (1 + x^2)^{-3/2}$ and $f''(x) = O(|x|)^{-3}$ at ∞.

Regard f as a tempered distribution (i.e., as a functional on the Schwartz space) and let $g(\xi)$ be the Fourier transform of f. Then g is itself a tempered distribution, and

$$(f')\hat{} = i\xi g(\xi), \qquad (f'')\hat{} = -\xi^2 g(\xi).$$

Thus $\xi g(\xi)$ is a function and f'' is in L^2, which implies that

$$(f'')\hat{} = -\xi^2 g(\xi)$$

is bounded, so that $g(\xi) = O(\xi^{-2})$ at ∞. Write $g = g_1 + g_2$, where g_1 has support very near 0 and $g_2 \in L^1(\hat{\mathbb{R}})$. Then

$$f(D) = \int g_1(\xi)e^{i\xi D}\,d\xi + \int g_2(\xi)e^{i\xi D}\,d\xi.$$

The inverse Fourier transform of g_2 belongs to $C_0(\mathbb{R})$ by the Riemann–Lebesgue lemma, so the second term is in $C_r^*(G(X))$. The first term is properly supported, by the finite propagation speed condition, and it is a pseudodifferential operator by the argument of [Taylor 1981, Theorem 1.3, p. 296]; thus it belongs to $\mathcal{P}_0$, and hence $f(D) \in \overline{\mathcal{P}}^0$. □

The preceeding corollary shows us how to fit classical first order tangentially elliptic operators into the general framework of tangential pseudodifferential operators presented in Section VII-A. For arbitrary higher order differential operators we adopt an alternate strategy: we work directly at the von Neumann algebra level.

Proposition 7.27. *Let X be a compact foliated space with invariant transverse measure ν. Let T be a tangential, tangentially elliptic pseudodifferential operator of order $m > 0$, and let Δ be the tangential Hodge–Laplace operator associated to the bundle of T. Define*

$$P = (1+\Delta)^{-m/2}T.$$

Then $P \in \overline{\mathcal{P}}^0$, $\sigma_0(P)$ is homotopic to $\sigma_m(T)$, and

$$\phi_\nu(\operatorname{Ker} P) = \phi_\nu(\operatorname{Ker} T)$$

and

$$\phi_\nu(\operatorname{Ker} P^*) = \phi_\nu(\operatorname{Ker} T^*)$$

in $W^*(G(X)), \tilde{\mu})$.

Proof. Since $P =$ (invertible)T, $\sigma_0(P)$ is homotopic to $\sigma_m(T)$. It suffices to prove that $P \in \overline{\mathcal{P}}^0$ and $\phi_\nu(\operatorname{Ker} P^*) = \phi_\nu(\operatorname{Ker} T^*)$. For the first, note that Δ is the 0-form component of $D = d + d^*$ extended to the bundle via the connection. Use the leafwise finite propagation speed property of the operator D to write

$$(1+\Delta)^{-m/2}T = \int \hat{g}_1(\xi)e^{i\xi D}T\,d\xi + \int \hat{g}_2(\xi)e^{i\xi D}T\,d\xi = g_1(D)T + g_2(D)T.$$

Then $g_1(D)T \in \mathcal{P}^0$ as in 7.26. The operator $g_2(D)$ is smoothing and tends to 0 if we make g_1 have large support. Thus $\|g_2(D)T\|_{L^2} \to 0$ and thus $P \in \overline{\mathcal{P}}^0$.

It remains to prove that $\phi_\nu(\operatorname{Ker} P^*) = \phi_\nu(\operatorname{Ker} T^*)$ in W^*. If π is the orthogonal projection onto $\operatorname{Ker} T^*$ then the orthogonal projection onto $\operatorname{Ker} P^*$ is given by

$$\pi' = (1+\Delta)^{-m/2}\pi(1+\Delta)^{m/2}.$$

We should like to say that π and π' have the same trace. This is not immediate, since $(1+\Delta)^{m/2}$ is an unbounded operator. The ellipticity estimate in general takes the form

$$|(1+\Delta)^{m/2}\zeta| \le |T^*\zeta| + c|\zeta|.$$

If $\zeta \in \operatorname{Ker} T^*$ then

$$|(1+\Delta)^{m/2}\zeta| \le c|\zeta|$$

and thus $(1+\Delta)^{m/2}$ is bounded on $\operatorname{Ker} T^*$, and $\pi(1+\Delta)^{m/2}$ *is* bounded. Thus

$$\begin{aligned}\phi_\nu(\pi') &= \phi_\nu((1+\Delta)^{-m/2}\pi(1+\Delta)^{m/2})\\ &= \phi_\nu((1+\Delta)^{-m/2}\pi\pi(1+\Delta)^{m/2})\\ &= \phi_\nu(\pi(1+\Delta)^{m/2}(1+\Delta)^{-m/2}\pi) = \phi_\nu(\pi),\end{aligned}$$

as desired. □

This completes our general study of tangential differential operators with finite propagation speed. These results will be used in Section VII-C, which deals with a special class of tangential differential operators which are closely tied to the geometry of foliated spaces.

VII-C. Dirac Operators and the McKean–Singer Formula

We turn now to the study of generalized Dirac operators and asymptotics. The goal of this section is the McKean–Singer formula (7.39) which is the bridge to the asymptotic development of the index $\operatorname{ind}_\nu(D)$. References [Gilkey 1974] and [Roe 1998] serve as valuable general background for this section and the next.

Assume for the rest of the chapter that X is a compact foliated space with oriented foliation bundle F which is equipped with the Levi–Civita tangential connection 5.19 and associated tangential Riemannian metric. Each leaf of X is a complete Riemannian manifold with bounded geometry. Suppose that V is a real inner product space. We write $\operatorname{Cliff}(V)$ for its associated *Clifford algebra.* The Clifford algebra is universal with respect to linear maps $j : V \to A$, where A is a real unital algebra and

$$(v, v)1 + (jv)^2 = 0,$$

and this characterizes the algebra. More concretely, $\operatorname{Cliff}(V)$ may be regarded as the free associative unital algebra on the basis vectors $\{e_k\}$ of V modulo the relations

$$e_i e_j + e_j e_i = 0 \quad (i \neq j) \quad \text{and} \quad e_i^2 = -1 \quad \text{all } i, j.$$

Let

$$\text{Cliff}^c V = (\text{Cliff } V) \otimes_{\mathbb{R}} \mathbb{C}$$

be the complexified algebra. If $E \to X$ is any real Riemannian vector bundle, then $\text{Cliff}^c E$ is the associated bundle of Clifford algebras. In particular, if X is a foliated space with a tangential Riemannian metric then we may form

$$\text{Cliff}^c X \equiv \text{Cliff}^c F,$$

where F is the tangent bundle of the foliated space.

Definition 7.28. If S is a bundle of left modules over $\text{Cliff}^c X$, then S is a *tangential Clifford bundle* if it is equipped with a tangential Hermitian metric and compatible tangential connection such that

(a) if $e \in F_x$ then $e : S_x \to S_x$ is an isometry.

(b) if $\phi \in \Gamma_\tau(\text{Cliff}^c X)$ and $s \in S$, then

$$\Delta(\phi s) = \phi \Delta(s) + (\Delta \phi) s.$$

If S has an involution which anticommutes with the Clifford action of tangent vectors, then it is a *graded* Clifford bundle.

Associated to a tangential Clifford bundle S is a natural first order differential operator $D = D_S$ called the (*generalized*) *Dirac operator*. It is defined to be the composition

$$\Gamma_\tau(S) \to \Gamma_\tau(F^* \otimes S) \to \Gamma_\tau(F \otimes S) \to \Gamma_\tau(S),$$

where the first map is given by the tangential connection, the second by the tangential Riemannian metric, and the third by the Clifford module structure on S. In an orthonormal basis $\{e_1, \ldots, e_p\}$ for F_x one may write

$$(Ds)_x = \sum e_k (\nabla_k s)_x.$$

If S is graded then D is similarly graded; it interchanges sections of the positive and negative eigenbundles of the involution. In Chapter VIII we shall show that this definition encompasses the operators of primary interest in the proof (and in many applications) of the index theorem.

Lemma 7.29. *The Dirac operator is formally self-adjoint on each leaf and has finite propagation speed.*

Proof. Fix tangentially smooth sections r, s of S, one of which is compactly supported. Let α be the tangential 1-form

$$\alpha(v) = -(r, vs),$$

where vs is the module action of s on v. Let $e_1, \ldots, e_p$ be a normal basis of vector fields near x. Then

$$\begin{aligned}(Dr, s)_x &= \sum (e_i \nabla_i r, s)_x = -\sum (\nabla_i r, e_i s)_x \\ &= \sum \left(\nabla_i (r, e_i s) - (r, e_i \nabla_i s)\right) = (d^* \alpha)_x + (r, Ds)_x\end{aligned}$$

and hence $\langle Dr, s\rangle = \langle r, Ds\rangle$ by integration, as required. □

Form the Hilbert field $L^2_\tau(S)$ by completing the tangentially smooth sections of S along each leaf in the norm determined by the tangential Riemannian metric.

Proposition 7.30. *The Dirac operator is essentially self-adjoint regarded as an operator on the Hilbert field $L^2_\tau(S)$. Thus (by 7.21) if f is a bounded Borel function on $\mathbb{R}$ then $f(D)$ is defined as a bounded operator on $L^2_\tau(S)$.*

Proof. This follows immediately from 7.29 and 7.21. □

Let $R : \Lambda^2 F^* \to \mathrm{End}_\tau(S)$ be the tangential curvature operator associated to the tangential connection on S. Define $R' \in \mathrm{End}_\tau(S)$ by

$$R'(s) = \frac{1}{2} \sum e_i e_j R(e_i \wedge e_j) s$$

with respect to the orthonormal basis.

Proposition 7.31 (Weitzenbock formula). *For $s \in \Gamma_\tau(S)$,*

$$D^2 s = \nabla^* \nabla s + R' s.$$

Proof. Work in normal coordinates at a point. Then the result is formal:

$$\begin{aligned}D^2 s &= \sum e_i \nabla_i (e_j \nabla_j s) \\ &= -\sum \nabla_j \nabla_i s + \sum_{i<j} e_i e_j (\nabla_i \nabla_j - \nabla_j \nabla_i) s = \nabla^* \nabla s + R' s.\end{aligned}$$ □

This formula allows us to analyze the coefficients of the Dirac operator. Suppose that (X, S) has bounded geometry. Using tangential normal coordinates near a point of X, one may regard the operator D^2 as a partial differential operator along the leaves of $B \times N$ acting on matrix-valued functions. By the Weitzenbock formula, D^2 may be written as

$$-\sum_{i,j} g_{ij}(x) \frac{\partial}{\partial x^i} \frac{\partial}{\partial x^j} + \sum_j a_j \frac{\partial}{\partial x^j} + b, \tag{7.32}$$

where the a_j and b are matrix-valued tangentially smooth functions on $B \times N$ which are constant in n and which, by virtue of the bounded geometry, may be estimated independently of the particular point of X chosen. In particular one sees that D^2 is a tangentially elliptic operator with principal symbol $-\xi^2$. As the origin of the tangential normal coordinate system varies, the operators D^2

form a bounded family of tangentially elliptic operators with the same tangential principal symbol.

Suppose that f is a function on $\mathbb{R}^p$ supported within $B/2$. Then f may be regarded as defined on $B \times N$ and D^2 may be regarded as acting on f. The elliptic estimate 7.12 applied to D^2 gives

$$\|f\|_{k+2} \le C(\|f\|_k + \|D^2 f\|_k) \tag{7.33}$$

for some constant C and the usual Sobolev norms. Moreover, since $\det g$ is bounded away from zero locally and (by the compactness of X) globally with a global lower bound, the tangential principal symbol of D^2 is bounded away from zero with a global lower bound, so C may be chosen uniformly on X. This makes it possible to prove a Sobolev embedding theorem for X.

Definition 7.34. Suppose $r \ge 0$. The *uniform C^r space $UC^r_\tau(S)$* is the bundle obtained by taking over each leaf the Banach space of all C^r_τ sections s of S (restricted to the leaf) such that the norm

$$|||s|||_r = \sup\{|\nabla_{v_1} \dots \nabla_{v_q} s(x)|\},$$

is finite, where sup is over all $x \in X$ and over all choices $v_1, \dots, v_q$ $(0 \le q \le r)$ of unit tangent vectors at x.

Theorem 7.35 (Sobolev Embedding Theorem [Roe 1985, 5.20]). *If k is an even integer with $k > r + p/2$, then $W^k_\tau(S)$ is included continuously in $UC^r_\tau(S)$.*

Proof. We may immediately restrict attention to some leaf ℓ. (The constant involved in the elliptic estimate is continuous from leaf to leaf.) Choose some $s \in W^k(\ell)$. Then

$$|||s||| = \sup_{(B,f)} \|fs\|_{UC^r(\ell)},$$

where $B \subset \mathbb{R}^p$, $f : B \to [0, 1]$ is a smooth function supported on $B/2$ with $f \equiv 1$ on $B/4$, and fs is regarded as a function on $B/2$. Then

$$\|fs\|^2_{UC^r(\ell)} = \|fs\|^2_{C^r(\mathbb{R}^p)} \le \|R\| \|fs\|_{W^k(\mathbb{R}^p)}$$

by the classical Sobolev embedding; this is further bounded above by

$$c_1 \|s\|_{W^k(B/2)} \le c_2 \|s\|_{W^k(\ell)}$$

and so $|||s|||_r \le (\text{const})\|s\|_{W^k(\ell)}$ as required. □

Theorem 7.36 [Roe 1985, 5.21]. *Suppose that X is a compact foliated space and that P is a tangential, tangentially elliptic differential operator on the module S. Let f lie in $\mathcal{S}(\mathbb{R})$, the Schwartz space. Then the operator $f(P)$, which is defined (leafwise) by the spectral theorem, is a tangential smoothing operator and its distribution kernel*

$$K_f \in \Gamma_\tau(S^* \otimes \Lambda F^* \otimes S)$$

is uniformly bounded.

Proof. Since f is a Schwartz function, the functions $x \mapsto |x|^k f(x)$ are bounded on $\mathbb{R}$ for any k, implying by the spectral theorem that the operators $P^k f(P)$ are bounded on $L^2(\ell, S)$ for each leaf ℓ. Thus $f(P)$ maps $W^k(S)$ into $W^{k+n}(S)$ for any k and n. It follows in the usual way that $f(P)$ is a smoothing operator when restricted to each leaf. Thus $f(P)$ is tangentially smoothing. As for the uniform bound, let $x \in X$ and $v \in S_x^*$; let $\epsilon_{x,v}$ be the distributional section defined by

$$\epsilon_{x,v}(s) = \langle s_x, v \rangle$$

for $s \in \Gamma_\tau(S)$. Then $\epsilon_{x,v} \in UC^r(S)^* \subset W^{-k}(S)$ (by Theorem 7.35) and so

$$K_f(v, \cdot) = f(P)\epsilon_{x,v} \in W^k(S) \subset UC^r(S),$$

again by Theorem 7.35. This implies that K_f is uniformly bounded. □

Proposition 7.37. *Let P be a self-adjoint tangentially elliptic differential operator of any positive order on a module S with bounded geometry, and let $f \in C_0(\mathbb{R})$. Then $f(P)$ is in the Breuer ideal [1968] of compact operators in $W^*(G(X), \tilde{\mu})$. Similarly, if $P \geq 0$ then e^{-tP} is in the Breuer ideal.*

Proof. By a continuity and density argument we may assume that f is compactly supported and smooth. Then Theorem 7.36 gives a distribution kernel for $f(P)$ which is bounded on G, and similarly for $f(P)^2$. This implies that

$$\operatorname{Tr}(f(P)^2) = \int |K_{f(P)}(x, x)|^2 \, dv < \infty$$

so that $f(P)^2$ is trace class. Thus $f(P)$ is Hilbert–Schmidt, and so compact. The same argument applies to e^{-tP} for P positive since the function e^{-tz} may be replaced by a function which dies quickly off $\mathbb{R}^+$ and which agrees with e^{-tz} on $\mathbb{R}^+$. □

It is now possible to prove a generalization of the McKean–Singer formula, which provides a bridge to the asymptotic expansion.

Theorem 7.38. *Fix an invariant transverse measure ν on X and let*

$$D : \Gamma_\tau(E) \to \Gamma_\tau(E')$$

be a tangentially elliptic differential operator of order $m > 0$ on modules with vector bundles having Then for each $t > 0$, the operators e^{-tD^*D} and e^{-tDD^*} are tangential smoothing operators whose distribution kernels are functions which are uniformly bounded. The corresponding elements in $W^*(G(X), \tilde{\mu})$ have finite trace, and

$$\text{(7.39)} \qquad \operatorname{ind}_\nu(D) = \phi_\nu\big([e^{-tD^*D}] - [e^{-tDD^*}]\big).$$

Proof. The first part of the theorem is immediate from (7.37). To establish formula (7.39), we argue as follows. Write $D = UA$ in polar form, where $A = (D^*D)^{1/2}$ and U is a partial isometry. Then U^*U is the projection onto $(\operatorname{Ker} D)^\perp$, UU^* is the projection onto $(\operatorname{Ker} D^*)^\perp$, and

$$U^*(DD^*)U = U^*UAAU^*U = ID^*DI = D^*D,$$

so U is an equivalence between corresponding spectral projections of D^*D and DD^* for any Borel subset of $(0, +\infty)$. Thus

$$\phi_\nu\big([e^{-tD^*D}] - [e^{-tDD^*}]\big) = \phi_\nu\big([\beta \operatorname{Ker} D] - [\beta \operatorname{Ker} D^*]\big) = \operatorname{ind}_\nu(D),$$

where $\beta : C_r^*(G) \longrightarrow W^*(G, \tilde{\mu})$ is defined before Proposition 6.19 and ϕ_ν is the trace associated to the invariant transverse measure ν. □

The next step in our development is the reformulation of the McKean–Singer formula (7.39) in terms of superoperators, and the resulting asymptotic expansion of the heat kernel.

VII-D. Superoperators and the Asymptotic Expansion

In this section the McKean–Singer formula (7.39) is rephrased in terms of superoperators. Then symbols which depend upon a complex parameter introduced and the asymptotic expansion (Theorem 7.49) for $\operatorname{ind}_\nu(D)$ is developed. This leads to the formula (7.49), which expresses $\operatorname{ind}_\nu(D)$ as the total mass of the tangentially smooth p-form $\omega_D(g, E)$. More detailed study of this form for particular Dirac operators leads in Chapter VIII to the proof of the index theorem.

Definition 7.40. A *graded vector space* is a vector space of the form $V = V^+ \oplus V^-$ thought of as the eigenspace decomposition of an involution of V. A *superoperator* is an operator $T : V \to V$. A superoperator has an obvious 2 by 2 matrix decomposition and is said to be *grade-preserving* if $T_{ij} = 0$ for $i \neq j$. A trace φ on $\mathcal{L}(V^+)$ and $\mathcal{L}(V^-)$ extends to a *supertrace* φ^s on V by

$$\varphi^s(T) = \varphi(T_{11}) - \varphi(T_{22}).$$

If $D : V^+ \to V^-$ then define its *associated superoperator* $\widehat{D}$ by

$$\widehat{D} = \begin{pmatrix} 0 & D^* \\ D & 0 \end{pmatrix}^2 = \begin{pmatrix} D^*D & 0 \\ 0 & DD^* \end{pmatrix} : V \to V.$$

Then $\widehat{D}$ is a positive grade-preserving superoperator of order twice the order of D.

The utility of this construction is illustrated by the following corollary.

Corollary 7.41. *Fix an invariant transverse measure ν on X and let*

$$D : \Gamma_\tau(E^+) \to \Gamma_\tau(E^-)$$

be a tangentially elliptic differential operator on bundles having bounded geometry with associated superoperator $\widehat{D}$. Then

$$\operatorname{ind}_\nu(D) = \phi^s_\nu(e^{-t\widehat{D}}).$$

Proof. This is immediate from 7.39 and the definition of the supertrace. □

Next we develop the machinery of complex symbols in order to produce the asymptotic expansion of $\phi^s_\nu(e^{-t\widehat{D}})$. Let us assume given a tangentially elliptic differential operator D of order $m/2$ with positive definite principal symbol. Let $\widehat{D}$ be the associated superoperator of order m; say

$$\widehat{D} : \Gamma_\tau(E) \to \Gamma_\tau(E).$$

Let $\mathscr{C}$ be a fixed curve of distance ≥ 1 from the positive real axis as shown.

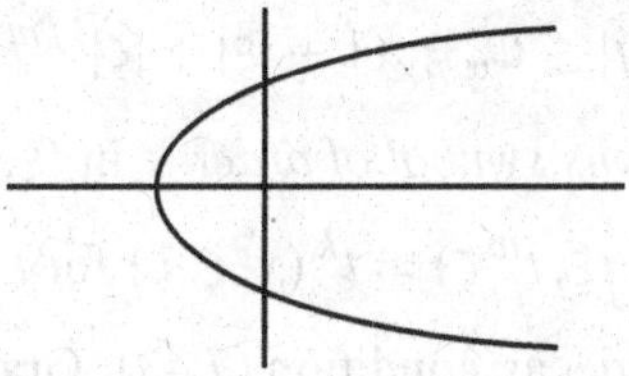

For $\zeta \in \mathscr{C}$, the operator $(\widehat{D} - \zeta)^{-1}$ is defined by the spectral theorem and has norm

$$|(\widehat{D} - \zeta)^{-1}| \leq 1.$$

The map

$$\zeta \to |(\widehat{D} - \zeta)^{-1}|$$

is continuous for $\zeta \in \mathscr{C}$, and hence we may write

$$e^{-t\widehat{D}} = (2\pi i)^{-1} \int_{\mathscr{C}} e^{-t\zeta} (\widehat{D} - \zeta)^{-1} \, d\zeta.$$

Extend $(\widehat{D} - \zeta)^{-1}$ to the graded tangential Sobolev spaces. Note that $|\zeta - x|^{-1} \leq 1$ for $\zeta \in \mathscr{C}$, $x \in \mathbb{R}^+$, so that

$$|(\widehat{D} - \zeta)^{-1} f|_0 \leq c|f|_0.$$

Then

$$|(\widehat{D} - \zeta)^{-1} f|_{km} \leq c\big(|\widehat{D}^k (\widehat{D} - \zeta)^{-1} f|_0 + |(\widehat{D} - \zeta)^{-1} f|_0\big)$$

by [Gilkey 1984, 1.3.5], which in turn is bounded above by

$$c\{|\widehat{D}^{k-1} f|_0 + |\zeta \widehat{D}^{k-1} (\widehat{D} - \zeta)^{-1} f|_0 + |f|_0\}$$
$$\leq c\{|f|_{km-m} + |\zeta|\,|(\widehat{D} - \zeta)^{-1} f|_{km-m}\}.$$

If $k = 1$, we obtain

$$|(\hat{D}-\zeta)^{-1} f|_m \leq c(1+|\zeta|)\,|f|_0$$

and then by induction,

$$|(\hat{D}-\zeta)^{-1} f|_{km} \leq c(1+|\zeta|)^{k-1}|f|_{km-m}.$$

By interpolation one obtains:

Proposition 7.42. *Let $\hat{D}$ be as above. Given s, there is a $k = k(s)$ and $c = c(s)$ so that*

$$|(\hat{D}-\zeta)^{-1} f|_s \leq c(1+|\zeta|)^{k-1}|f|_s$$

for all $\zeta \in \mathscr{C}$.

Definition. The function$q(x,\xi,\zeta,n) \in S^k(\zeta)(U \times N)$ is a *symbol of order k depending on ζ* if q is smooth in (x,ξ,ζ), continuous in n, has compact x-support in U, is holomorphic in ζ and if there are estimates

$$|D_x^\alpha D_\xi^\beta D_\zeta^\gamma q| \leq C_{\alpha,\beta\gamma}(1+|\xi|+|\zeta|^{1/m})^{k-|\beta|-m|\gamma|}. \tag{7.43}$$

Say that q is a *homogeneous symbol of order k* in (ξ,ζ) if

$$q(x,t\xi,t^m\zeta) = t^k(x,\xi,\zeta) \text{ for } t \geq 1.$$

Homogeneity implies the decay condition (7.43). Grading in this manner corresponds to regarding ζ as having order m. It follows that $(p_m-\zeta)^{-1} \in S^{-m}(\zeta)$. Further, the spaces $S^*(\zeta)$ are closed under multiplication and differentiation in the usual manner. In particular, given $n > 0$, there is some $k(n) > 0$ such that if Q has symbol in $S^k(\zeta)$ then it induces $Q(\zeta) : W^{-n} \to W^n$ and

$$|Q(\zeta)|_{-n,n} \leq C(1+|\zeta|)^{-n}. \tag{7.44}$$

Let $\mathcal{P}_\zeta^k(U \times N)$ denote those grade-preserving pseudodifferential superoperators

$$C_{\tau c}^\infty(U \times N) \to C_{\tau c}^\infty(U \times N)$$

with symbol in $S^k(\zeta)$ and x-support in U. For ζ fixed,

$$Q(\zeta) \in \mathcal{P}^k(U \times N).$$

A tangentially smooth homeomorphism

$$h : U \times N \to \tilde{U} \times \tilde{N}$$

induces a map

$$\mathcal{P}_\zeta^k(U \times N) \to \mathcal{P}_\zeta^k(\tilde{U} \times \tilde{N})$$

which respects principal symbols, so that it makes sense to speak of operators with complex symbol on $C_{\tau c}^\infty(X)$ or even of operators on bundles over X. Finally, define $\mathcal{P}_\zeta^k(G(X))$ as before, that is, as finite linear combinations of pseudodifferential operators from patches lifted from $\mathcal{P}^k_\zeta(U \times N)$ and compactly smoothing operators.

We wish to find an approximation for $(\widehat{D}-\zeta)^{-1}$, which is a pseudodifferential operator. Fix some finite open cover $\{V_i\}$ of X by distinguished coordinate patches and let η_i be a subordinate tangentially smooth partition of unity. On a coordinate patch, let $\widehat{D}$ have total symbol $p_0 + \cdots + p_m$. Let $p'_j = p_j$ for $j < m$ and $p'_m = p_m - \zeta$. Then

$$\sigma(\widehat{D} - \zeta) = \sum_{j=0}^{m} p'_j$$

so $\widehat{D} - \zeta$ is tangentially elliptic. Use the equation

$$\sigma\big(\eta_i R(\zeta)(\widehat{D} - \zeta)\big) - I \sim 0$$

to give a local solution for $R_i(\zeta)$, with symbol $\eta_i r_0 + \cdots + r_{n_0}$, n_0 large. Precisely, set

$$r_0 = \eta_i (p_m - \zeta)^{-1} \quad \text{and} \quad r_n = -r_0 \sum \frac{1}{\alpha!} d^\alpha_\xi r_j D^\alpha_x p'_k,$$

where we sum over all $j < n$ and $|\alpha| + j + m - k = n$. Define

$$R(\zeta) = \sum \eta_i R_i(\zeta).$$

The principal tangential symbol of $R(\zeta)$ is $(p_m - \zeta)^{-1}$, so $R(\zeta)$ is a parametrix of $\widehat{D}$. We have established the following proposition.

Proposition 7.45. *Let $\widehat{D} \in \mathcal{P}^m_\zeta(E, E)$ be a tangentially elliptic grade-preserving differential superoperator. Then n_0 may be selected sufficiently large so that $(\widehat{D} - \zeta)^{-1}$ is approximated arbitrarily well by the parametrix $R(\zeta)$ in the operator norm as $\zeta \to \infty$. That is,*

$$|\{(\widehat{D} - \zeta)^{-1} - R(\zeta)\} f|_k \le c_k (1 + |\zeta|)^{-k} |f|_{-k}$$

for $\zeta \in \mathcal{C}$, $f \in \Gamma_\tau(E)$. □

Proposition 7.45 implies that

$$\| R(\zeta)(\widehat{D} - \zeta) - \mathrm{id}_E \|_{-k,k} \le c_0 (1 + |\zeta|)^{-k-1}$$

and hence, for $t < 1$,

$$\| R(\zeta/t) - (\widehat{D} - \zeta/t)^{-1} \|_{-k,k} \le c_0 (1 + |\zeta/t|)^{-k-1}.$$

Define $E(t) \in \mathcal{P}$ by

$$E(t) = (2\pi i)^{-1} \int_{\mathcal{C}} R(\zeta) e^{-\zeta t}\, d\zeta = (2\pi i)^{-1} \int_{\mathcal{C}} R(\zeta/t) e^{-\zeta}\, d\zeta/t.$$

Then

$$\| e^{-t\widehat{D}} - E(t) \|_{-k,k} \le (2\pi)^{-1} \int_{\mathcal{C}} |e^{-\zeta}| (1 + |\zeta/t|)^{-k-1} \, |d\zeta/t|$$

by the analyticity in ζ. Thus

$$t^{-k}\|e(t) - e^{-t\hat{D}}\|_{-k,k} \leq (2\pi)^{-1} \int_{\mathscr{C}} |e^{-\zeta}|(t + |\zeta|)^{-k-1}\, |d\zeta|$$

is bounded at $t \to 0$. If $k > p/2$ then $\|\,.\,\|_{-k,k}$ bounds the uniform norm and hence

$$\phi_\nu(e^{-t\hat{D}}) - \phi_\nu(E(t)) = O(t^k).$$

So it suffices to find an asymptotic expansion for $\phi_\nu(E(t))$. Define

$$E^i(t) = (2\pi i)^{-1} \int_{\mathscr{C}} e^{-\zeta t} R_i(\zeta)\, d\zeta.$$

Then

$$\phi_\nu(E(t)) = \sum_i \phi_\nu(E^i(t)) \quad \text{(finite sum)}$$

so it suffices to expand $E^i(t)$.

Recall that the total symbol of $R(\zeta)$ is denoted by $\{r_j\}$. Define

$$e_{j,t}(x,\xi) = (2\pi i)^{-1} \int_{\mathscr{C}} e^{-t\zeta} r_j(x,\xi,\zeta)\, d\zeta.$$

Then $E^i(t)$ is a pseudodifferential operator with total symbol

$$e_{0,t} + \cdots + e_{n_0,t},$$

and $e_{j,t} \in S^{-\infty}$ for all t. Let $E^i_j(t)$ be the operator associated to $e_{j,t}$. Then $E^i_j(t)$ is represented by a distribution kernel $K_{j,t}$ defined by

$$K_{j,t}(x,y,n) = \int e^{i(x-y)\xi} e_{j,t}(x,\xi,n)\, d\xi.$$

Thus

$$K_{j,t}(x,x,n) = t^{(j-p)/m} e_j(x,n),$$

where

$$e_j(x,n) = (2\pi i)^{-1} \int\!\!\int_{\mathscr{C}} e^{-\zeta} r_j(x,\xi,\zeta,n)\, d\zeta d\xi.$$

Note that each $e_j(x,n)$ is tangentially smooth and is transversely bounded. If m is even then $e_j(x,n) = 0$ for j odd.

Define

$$\lambda_j(\hat{D})_{(x,n)} = \bar{e}_j(x,n)\,\mathrm{dvol}(x)$$

and

$$\lambda_j(\hat{D}) = \{\lambda_j(\hat{D})_{(x,n)}\}.$$

Then each $\lambda_j(\hat{D})$ is a signed tangential measure

$$\lambda_j(\hat{D}) = \lambda_j(D) - \lambda_j(D^*)$$

depending on the (X, F), D, and the tangential Riemannian metric g, but not on t.

Proposition 7.46. *Each signed tangential measure $\lambda_j(\widehat{D})$ is locally bounded.*

Proof. Note that $\lambda_j(\widehat{D})_\ell$ is given by

$$\lambda_j(\widehat{D})_\ell = e_j(x,n)\,\mathrm{dvol}(x) \quad \text{for } x \in \mathbb{R}^p,\ n \in N.$$

It is clear that $\lambda_j(\widehat{D})^x$ has a signed Borel density on $r^{-1}(x)$ for each x. So it suffices to show that the Radon–Nikodým derivative of $\lambda_j(\widehat{D})$ with respect to the standard tangential measure is bounded on any set $r^{-1}(C)$, C compact. This derivative is of course just the function $e_j(x,n)$. So the problem reduces to proving that $e_j(x,n)$ is locally bounded.

Recall that

$$e_j(x,n) = (2\pi i)^{-1} \iint e^{-\zeta} r_j(x,\xi,\zeta,n)\, d\zeta\, d\xi,$$

where the r_j are the homogeneous parts of the total symbol of $\widehat{D}_\xi$ given explicitly above, and $p_m + p_{m-1} + \cdots$ is the total symbol of $\widehat{D}$. Note further that

$$e_{j,t}(x,\xi,n) = (2\pi i)^{-1} t^{-k} \int_{\mathscr{C}} e^{-t\zeta} \frac{d^k}{d\zeta^k} r_j(x,\xi,\zeta,n)\, d\zeta.$$

Since $(d^k/d\zeta^k) r_j$ is homogeneous of degree $-m-j-km$ in (ξ,ζ), it follows that e_j is a smoothing operator on each leaf for any $t > 0$ (though not necessarily compactly supported) and hence $\phi_\nu(e_j)$ is finite, as required. □

This establishes the following theorem.

Theorem 7.47 (Asymptotic Expansion of the Trace [Connes 1979]). *Let X be a compact foliated space with foliation bundle F and fixed tangential Riemannian metric g. Fix an invariant transverse measure ν and a tangential, tangentially elliptic differential operator D from E^+ to E^-, where (X, E^+) and (X, E^-) have bounded geometry. Let $\widehat{D}$ be the associated superoperator, and let ϕ_ν^s be the associated supertrace on $W^*(G(X), E^+ \oplus E^-, \tilde{\mu})$. Then for $j \geq -p$ there is a family of signed tangential measures $\lambda_j(\widehat{D})$ on X (which depend on X, g, F, and D but not on t) and an asymptotic expansion*

$$\phi_\nu^s(e^{-t\widehat{D}}) \sim \sum_{j \geq -p} t^{j/2p} \int_X \lambda_j(\widehat{D})\, d\nu. \tag{7.48}$$

Corollary 7.49. *In the notation of Theorem 7.47,*

$$\mathrm{ind}_\nu(D) = \int \big(\lambda_0(D) - \lambda_0(D^*)\big)\, d\nu.$$

Proof of 7.49. Fix some $t > 0$. Then

$$\mathrm{ind}_\nu(D) = \phi_\nu^s(e^{-t\widehat{D}}) = \sum_{j \geq -p} t^{j/2p} \int_X (\lambda_j(D) - \lambda_j(D^*))\, d\nu.$$

As the left hand side is independent of t, each term in the summation which involves nontrivial powers of t must vanish. The remaining term (corresponding to $j = 0$) then gives the index. □

Corollary 7.50. *The tangential measure* λ_j *is homogeneous of weight* $j/2p$ *in the coefficients of* D. *That is,*

$$\lambda_j(\zeta D) = \zeta^{j/2p} \lambda_j(D).$$

Further, in the case $m = 1$, *then* $(\det a)^{1/2} \lambda_j(D)$ *is a polynomial in the coefficients of* D *relative to* x, *their derivatives relative to* x, *and* $\det^{-1} a$, *where* $\det a$ *is the leading term of the quadratic form.*

Write

$$\omega_D(g, E) = \big(\lambda_0(D) - \lambda_0(D^*)\big)\, |d\lambda| \tag{7.51}$$

for the tangentially smooth p-form which corresponds to D. Note that this form is measurable but not necessarily continuous transversely. In Chapter VIII this form will be identified for certain classical operators and this will enable us to complete the proof of the Index Theorem.

□ □□□□□ □□□□

The main development in this area related to index theory is the rise and domination of Fredholm triples, also known as spectral triples. This is discussed very nicely in [Connes 1994]. The idea originates, as does so much of our subject, with M. F. Atiyah [1970]. G. G. Kasparov built upon this idea in a very powerful way in order to form his KK-groups. (In fact one of the early goals of his work was to determine exactly the appropriate equivalence relation on Atiyah's $Ell(X)$, "elliptic operators" on the compact space X.) Baum and Douglas used the idea effectively in several of their papers on K-homology. Under Connes and his students the concept has become absolutely central; see [Connes 2002; 2000]. Dirac operators in concrete and abstract form remain vital to K-theory and especially to KK-theory, where the existence of "dual Dirac" is tied intimately to the Novikov conjecture.

CHAPTER VIII

The Index Theorem

In this chapter we put everything together to state and prove the Connes Index Theorem for compact foliated spaces.

Let X be a compact foliated space with leaves of dimension p and foliation bundle F which we assume oriented and equipped with a tangentially smooth oriented tangential Riemannian structure g. Let $G = G(X)$ denote the associated holonomy groupoid of the foliated space. Let D be a tangential, tangentially elliptic pseudodifferential operator on (bundles over) X. For each leaf ℓ the spaces Ker D_ℓ and Ker D_ℓ^* are well defined by Proposition 7.23 and are locally finite-dimensional with local index measure

$$\iota_{D_\ell} = \mu_{D_\ell} - \mu_{D_\ell^*}.$$

We define the analytic index of D to be the tangential measure

$$\iota_D = \{\iota_D^x\},$$

where $\iota_D^x = \iota_{D_\ell}$ for $x \in \ell$. If D is a differential operator of positive order m then Proposition 7.24 implies that the index measure ι_D is well-defined.

Given an invariant transverse measure ν, the analytic index ind_ν is the real number defined by

$$\mathrm{ind}_\nu(D) = \int \iota_D d\nu.$$

Alternatively, the operator $(1 + \Delta)^{-m/2} D$ is in the closure of the order-zero pseudodifferential operator algebra $\bar{\mathcal{P}}^0$ and has the same tangential principal symbol and same index class in the von Neumann algebra and thus may be used to replace D. The analytic index class $\mathrm{ind}(D)$ can be defined as in (7.16) as a K-theory class in $K_0(C^*(G(X)))$. Theorem 6.33 provides a map c, the partial Chern character, from this K-theory group to $H_\tau^*(X)$ and then $c[\mathrm{ind}(D)]$ as a cohomology class which we denote $[\mathrm{ind}(D)]$. Of course an invariant transverse measure ν defines a linear functional on $H_\tau^p(X)$, and it is clear from the definitions that

$$\nu(c(\mathrm{ind}(D))) = \mathrm{ind}_\nu(D).$$

The topological index of the operator D is defined by

$$\iota_D^{\mathrm{top}}(D) = \mathrm{ch}_\tau(D)\, Td_\tau(X),$$

with

$$\mathrm{ch}_\tau(D) = (-1)^{p(p+1)/2} \Phi_\tau^{-1}\, \mathrm{ch}_\tau(\sigma(D))$$

(see the end of Section VII-A). We can integrate this class with respect to an invariant transverse measure ν to get a real number

$$\mathrm{ind}_\nu^{\mathrm{top}}(D) = \int \iota_D^{\mathrm{top}}\, d\nu$$

which depends only on the component in dimension p of the class.

The Index Theorem asserts that $\mathrm{ind}_\nu(D)$ and $\mathrm{ind}_\nu^{\mathrm{top}}(D)$ coincide for every invariant transverse measure. Alternatively, we can interpret the analytic and topological indices as classes in $\overline{H}_\tau^p(X)$ and the Index Theorem can be restated as the equality of the two classes in $\overline{H}_\tau^p(X)$.

The Connes–Skandalis Index Theorem [1981; 1984], which is established for foliations, involves the analytic index, which just as above is defined as an element of $K_0(C^*(G(X)))$, and then a topological index is defined directly as an element of the same K-theory group, and their equality is proved directly without any intervening Chern maps.

With these preliminaries in hand, we may state the Connes Index Theorem (proved in [Connes 1979] for foliated manifolds and extended by us to foliated spaces).

Theorem 8.1 (Connes Index Theorem). *Let X be a compact foliated space with leaves of dimension p and foliation bundle F which we assume oriented and equipped with a tangentially smooth oriented tangential Riemannian structure g. Let D be a tangential, tangentially elliptic pseudodifferential operator on X and let ν be an invariant transverse measure. Then*

$$\mathrm{ind}_\nu(D) = \mathrm{ind}_\nu^{\mathrm{top}}(D).$$

That is,

$$\mathrm{ind}_\nu(D) = \int \mathrm{ch}_\tau(D) Td_\tau(X)\, d\nu.$$

Our study of invariant transverse measures and tangential cohomology enables us to reformulate Theorem 8.1 so as to avoid mention of transverse measures.

Theorem 8.2. *Let X be a compact foliated space with leaves of dimension p and foliation bundle F which we assume oriented and equipped with a tangentially smooth oriented tangential Riemannian structure g. Let D be a tangential, tangentially elliptic operator on X. Then*

$$[\iota_D] = [\mathrm{ch}_\tau(D) Td_\tau(X)]$$

as classes in $\overline{H}_\tau^p(X)$.

Theorem 8.2 implies Theorem 8.1 since an invariant transverse measure ν corresponds uniquely to a homomorphism $\bar{H}^p_\tau(X) \to \mathbb{C}$. If X has no invariant transverse measures then $\bar{H}^p_\tau(X) = 0$ and so the statement is simply

$$[\iota_D] = 0 \in \bar{H}^p(X).$$

Theorem 8.1 and the Riesz representation theorem (4.27) immediately imply Theorem 8.2.

The proof follows a well-known path: we establish Theorem 8.1 for twisted signature operators and then argue homotopy-theoretically that this suffices to prove the general case.

As an introduction to the techniques we first consider the de Rham and signature operators.

Define complex vector bundles E^k_X and E^k_G by

$$E^k_X = \Lambda^k(F^*_{\mathbb{C}}), \qquad E^k_G = \Lambda^k(s^* F^*_{\mathbb{C}}) = s^* E^k_X,$$

$$E_X = \bigoplus E^k_X, \qquad E_G = \bigoplus E^k_G.$$

The tangential de Rham operator d is defined in Chapter VII; we recall additional detail here. Let $f \wedge dx_I$ be a tangentially smooth k-form on $G(X)$ in local coordinates; i.e., a tangentially smooth section of the bundle E^k_G. Exterior differentiation

$$d(f \wedge dx_I) = \sum_{i=1}^{p} \frac{\partial f}{\partial x_i} dx_i \wedge dx_I$$

induces a natural map

$$\Gamma_\tau(E^k_G) \to \Gamma_\tau(E^{k+1}_G)$$

for each k and hence induces a natural map

$$d : \Gamma_\tau(E_G) \to \Gamma_\tau(E_G)$$

which agrees with the usual exterior derivative on each leaf G^x of $G(X)$. Thus d yields an unbounded operator on the Hilbert field

$$d : L^2(G(X), E_G) \to L^2(G(X), E_G).$$

If ξ is some vector then explicit computation yields

$$\xi \wedge dx_I = \sum \xi_j \wedge dx_I,$$

so that the principal symbol $\sigma(d)$ of d is given locally by

$$\sigma(d)(x,\xi)(v) = \xi \wedge v \quad \text{for } v \in F^*_{\mathbb{C}}. \tag{8.3}$$

The associated symbol sequence

$$\cdots \to E^k_G \xrightarrow{(\xi\wedge)_*} E^{k+1}_G \to \cdots$$

is an exact sequence for each $\xi \neq 0$ and hence d is a tangentially elliptic operator. To summarize:

Proposition 8.4. *The de Rham operator*

$$d : L^2(G(X), E_G) \to L^2(G(X), E_G)$$

is a densely defined unbounded tangential, tangentially elliptic operator with tangential principal symbol given by

$$\sigma(d)(x, \xi)(v) = \xi \wedge v.$$

The orientation of F induces a natural bundle isomorphism

$$* : E_G^k \to E_G^{p-k}$$

given locally in terms of an orthonormal basis $\{e_1, \ldots, e_s\}$ by $*(e_I) = \pm e_J$, where I and J are complementary multi-indices and the sign is determined by the parity of the permutation (I, J). This induces the Hodge inner product on sections $\Gamma_\tau(E_G)$:

$$\langle u, v \rangle = \int_{G(X)} u \wedge * \bar{v} \, d\mu.$$

With respect to this inner product the de Rham operator has a formal adjoint

$$\delta = \delta_{k+1} : \Gamma_\tau(E_G^{k+1}) \longrightarrow \Gamma_\tau(E_G^k)$$

given on $(k+1)$-forms by

$$\delta_{k+1} = (-1)^{pk+p+1} * d_k * ,$$

where d_k denotes the restriction of d to k-forms. As $*$ induces an isometry on forms, its symbol is invertible, so that $\sigma(\delta) = \pm\sigma(*)\sigma(d)\sigma(*)$ is also invertible. Hence δ is a tangentially elliptic operator.

The *tangential Hodge–Laplace operator* Δ is defined by

$$\Delta = d\delta + \delta d : \Gamma_\tau(E_G) \to \Gamma_\tau(E_G) \tag{8.5}$$

and its restriction to E_G^i is denoted by Δ_i.

We note that

$$\begin{aligned}(d+\delta)^2 &= d^2 + d\delta + \delta d + \delta^2 \\ &= \Delta \quad \text{since} \quad d^2 = \delta^2 = 0\end{aligned}$$

so that $(d+\delta)$ is a first order tangentially elliptic operator. Furthermore,

$$\operatorname{Ker} \Delta_i = \operatorname{Ker}((d+\delta)_i)$$

since

$$\langle \delta\omega, \omega \rangle = \langle (d+\delta)^2\omega, \omega \rangle = \langle (d+\delta)\omega, (d+\delta)\omega \rangle = |(d+\delta)\omega|^2.$$

Proposition 8.6. *The Hodge–Laplace operator is an essentially self-adjoint tangential, tangentially elliptic operator.*

Proof. This proposition follows from Theorem 7.21, but we prefer to give a more direct proof. Let ℓ be a leaf of $G(X)$. Restrict d to ℓ and consider the resulting commuting diagram

$$\begin{array}{ccc}
\Gamma_\tau(E_{G|\ell}) & \xrightarrow{\ d\ } & \Gamma_\tau(E_{G|\ell}) \\
\| & & \| \\
\Gamma(\Lambda^*((T\ell)^*_{\mathbb{C}})) & \xrightarrow{\ d\ } & \Gamma(\Lambda^*(T\ell^*_{\mathbb{C}})) \\
\downarrow & & \downarrow \\
L^2(\ell,(s^*,\alpha)^*) & \overset{T_\ell}{\dashrightarrow} & L^2(\ell,(s^*\alpha)^*)
\end{array}$$

where α is the density associated to (X,g) restricted to ℓ. Let T_ℓ be the closure of d. Then $\mathrm{Im}(T_\ell) \subseteq \mathrm{Ker}\, T_\ell$ and the operator

$$T_\ell^* T_\ell + T_\ell T_\ell^*$$

is a self-adjoint operator on $L^2(\ell,(s^*\alpha))$ which extends the operator $\Delta|_\ell$. This implies that the restriction of Δ to each leaf is a self-adjoint elliptic operator. □

The locally finite-dimensional space $(\mathrm{Ker}\,\Delta_i)_\ell$ is just the space of *square-integrable harmonic forms* of degree i on ℓ. The local dimension of this space is well-defined up to equivalence, since changing the metric g on F results in a change by similarity. Define the *Betti measure* β_i to be the tangential measure given by

$$\beta_i^x = \text{ local dimension of } (\mathrm{Ker}\,\Delta_i)_\ell = \mu_{(\mathrm{Ker}\,\Delta_i)_\ell},$$

where $x \in \ell$. The Betti numbers relative to some invariant transverse measure ν are given by $\int \beta_i d\nu$.

Note that the Hodge $*$-operator induces a natural isomorphism of Hilbert fields

$$\mathrm{Ker}\,\Delta_i \cong \mathrm{Ker}\,\Delta_{p-i}$$

and hence the Betti measures β_i and β_{p-i} coincide. Define the *tangential Euler characteristic* $\chi_\tau(X,F)$ to be the signed tangential measure

$$\chi_\tau(X,F) = \sum_{i=0}^{p} (-1)^i \beta_i.$$

If p is odd then

$$\chi_\tau(X,F) = \sum_{i=0}^{p} (-1)^i \beta_i = (\beta_0 - \beta_p) + (\beta_1 - \beta_{p-1}) + \cdots + (\beta_{\frac{p-1}{2}} - \beta_{\frac{p+1}{2}}) = 0$$

since $\beta_i = \beta_{p-i}$. Let us assume, then, that $p = 2q$ is even.

Let D be the restriction of $(d+\delta)$ to even forms, so that

$$D : \Gamma_\tau(\oplus E_G^{2i}) \to \Gamma_\tau(\oplus E_G^{2i+1}).$$

Then the local index of D_ℓ is just

$$\iota_{D_\ell} = (\Sigma(-1)^i \beta_i)^x \qquad \text{for} \quad x \in \ell.$$

Furthermore, D is a Dirac operator in the sense of Chapter VII, so that we may apply the heat equation argument as follows.

Define the *tangential Euler class* $e^\tau(X,F) \in H_\tau^p(X)$ by

$$e^\tau(X,F) = [Pf(K/2\pi)]$$

Theorem 8.7 (Chern–Gauss–Bonnet). *Let X be a compact foliated space with leaves of dimension p and foliation bundle F which we assume oriented and equipped with a tangentially smooth oriented tangential Riemannian structure g.*

(a) *For any invariant transverse measure ν,*

$$\int e_\tau(X,F)d\nu = \int \chi_\tau(X,F)d\nu.$$

(b)

$$[e_\tau(X,F)] = [\chi_\tau(X,F)] \in \overline{H}_\tau^p(X).$$

We emphasize the great difference between the two sides of the equation and hence the great depth of the result. The measure $\chi_\tau(X,F)$ is built from the various measures $\mu_{Ker \Delta_i \ell}$ which describes how the L^2-harmonic forms on the leaf ℓ are distributed on the leaf ℓ. On the other hand, the tangential Euler characteristic $e^\tau(X,F)$ is built out of the curvature of the various leaves, and thus is essentially a local property of the leaf. This difference is carried through to the general Index Theorem.

Proof. The index of the operator D may be expressed in two ways. On the one hand, the local index ι_{D_ℓ} is given by

$$\iota_{D_\ell} = \sum(-1)^i \beta_i^x$$

more or less by definition. On the other hand, D is a first order tangential tangentially elliptic operator and Theorem 7.47 implies that

$$\operatorname{ind}_\nu(D) = \int \omega_D(g,E)\, d\nu,$$

where ω_D is a tangentially smooth p-form which corresponds to D. Restrict $\omega_D(g,E)$ to a leaf ℓ. Then the local index theorem of Atiyah–Bott–Patodi [Atiyah et al. 1973] implies that

$$\omega_D(g,E)_\ell = Pf(K/2\pi)_\ell.$$

Thus

$$\int \Sigma(-1)^i \beta_i^x \, d\nu = \int Pf(K/2\pi)\, d\nu.$$

This holds for each invariant transverse measure ν, and hence

$$\sum(-1)^i \beta_i = Pf(K/2\pi) = e^\tau(X, F)$$

as classes in $\overline{H}^p(X)$. □

Corollary 8.8 ([Connes 1979]). *Let X be a foliated compact space with leaves of dimension 2. Let F be oriented and equipped with a tangentially smooth Riemannian metric. Fix some invariant transverse measure ν. Suppose that $\int K d\nu > 0$ (i.e., the ν-average curvature of X is strictly positive). Then X must have a closed leaf, and in fact, the set of closed leaves has positive ν measure.*

Proof. The Chern–Gauss–Bonnet theorem 8.7 and the curvature assumption imply that

$$\int (\beta_0 - \beta_1 + \beta_2)\, d\nu > 0.$$

Suppose that there is no generic closed leaf. Then

$$(\operatorname{Ker} \Delta_0)|_\ell = 0$$

for ν-almost every leaf, and hence $\int \beta_0 \, d\nu = 0$. By duality we have $\int \beta_2 \, d\nu = 0$. Thus $-\int \beta_1 \, d\nu > 0$ which is a contradiction since for any invariant transverse measure, $\int \beta_1 \, d\nu \geq 0$. □

We move next to the signature operator. Assume that $p = 2q$ is even. Then there is a natural involution $t : E_x \to E_x$ given by $t = (-1)^q * 1$. This decomposes E_G to

$$E_G = E_G^+ \oplus E_{G'}^-,$$

the $\pm$ eigenspaces. The elliptic operator

$$(d + \delta) : \Gamma_\tau(E_G) \to \Gamma_\tau(E_G)$$

anticommutes with t and hence restricts to an operator

$$A : \Gamma_\tau(E_G^+) \to \Gamma_\tau(E_G^-) \tag{8.9}$$

given by

$$A = (d + \delta)|_{\Gamma_\tau(E_G^+)}.$$

This is the *tangential signature operator*. The tangential principal symbol of A_ℓ is the restriction of the symbol of the elliptic operator $(d + \delta)_\ell$ to $\Gamma_\tau(E_G^+|_\ell)$ which is invertible, so A is tangentially elliptic. Graded as in (8.9), A is a Dirac operator in the sense of Chapter VII.

The involution t restricts to an involution of $\operatorname{Ker}(d+\delta) \cong \operatorname{Ker} \Delta$ since t anticommutes with $(d+\delta)$. The $\pm$ eigenspace decomposition is simply the decomposition of Hilbert fields

$$\operatorname{Ker} \Delta \cong \operatorname{Ker} A \oplus \operatorname{Ker} A^*.$$

Decompose $\operatorname{Ker} \Delta$ further as

$$\operatorname{Ker} \Delta = \bigoplus_{i=0}^{p} \operatorname{Ker} \Delta_i,$$

where Δ_i is the restriction of Δ to i-forms. The subspace

$$\operatorname{Ker} \Delta_k \oplus \operatorname{Ker} \Delta_{p-k}$$

is t-invariant for each k, $0 \leq k \leq q$, and there is a unitary equivalence

$$(\operatorname{Ker} \Delta_k \oplus \operatorname{Ker} \Delta_{p-k})_\ell^+ \to (\operatorname{Ker} \Delta_k \oplus \operatorname{Ker} \Delta_{p-k})_\ell^-$$

given by

$$x + t(x) \mapsto x - t(x).$$

Thus only the middle dimension $\operatorname{Ker} \Delta_q$ contributes to the index.

If $u, v \in \operatorname{Ker} \Delta_q \subset H_\tau^q(X)$ then $u \wedge v \, d\nu \in H_\tau^p(X)$ and for any invariant transverse measure ν, $\int u \wedge v \, d\nu \in \mathbb{R}$. This gives a natural bilinear form on $\operatorname{Ker} \Delta_q$ and it is reasonable to think of ι_A as the signature measure of this bilinear form, since

$$\int \iota_A \, d\nu = \int (+1 \text{ eigenspace of } t) \, d\nu - \int (-1 \text{ eigenspace of } t) \, d\nu \equiv \operatorname{Sign}(X, \nu).$$

If $X = M$ foliated as one leaf then $\operatorname{Ker} \Delta_i \cong H^i(M)$ and $\operatorname{Sign}(X, \nu)$ is exactly the usual signature of M.

Suppose that $p = 2q = 4r + 2$. Then $t = \pm i_*$ and so $** = -\operatorname{id}$. Thus $*$ is a real transformation on $\operatorname{Ker} \Delta_q$. The $\pm$ eigenspaces of $*$ (and hence of t) are conjugate via the map

$$a \otimes 1 - (*a) \otimes i \mapsto a \otimes 1 + (*a) \otimes i$$

and thus $(\operatorname{Ker} \Delta_q)^+$ is unitarily equivalent to $(\operatorname{Ker} \Delta_q)^-$ and ι_A is the zero measure. The topological index also vanishes. Thus the index theorem holds trivially. So we restrict attention to the case $p = 4r$.

Recall the Hirzebruch L-polynomials L_k are polynomials of degree $4k$ in the Pontryagin classes which are given by the splitting principle as

$$\sum_k L_k = \prod \frac{x_j}{\tanh x_j}.$$

The first few polynomials (in the tangential cohomology setting) are

$$L_0 = 1, \quad L_1 = \tfrac{1}{3} p_i^\tau, \quad L_2 = \tfrac{1}{45}(7p_2^\tau - (p_1^\tau)^2),$$
$$L_3 = \tfrac{1}{945}(62p_3^\tau - 13p_1^\tau p_2^\tau + 2(p_1^\tau)^3).$$

Lemma 8.10. *We have* $L_r(p_1^\tau, \dots, p_r^\tau) = \mathrm{ch}_\tau(A)\,\mathrm{Td}_\tau(F_\mathbb{C})|_p$, *where* $\omega|_p$ *is the component of* ω *in dimension* p.

We omit this calculation; a proof may be found in [Shanahan 1978, §6], and see also [Atiyah and Singer 1968b, p. 577].

Theorem 8.11 (Hirzebruch Signature Theorem). *Let* X *be a compact oriented foliated space with leaves of dimension* $4r$, *oriented foliation bundle* F, *and oriented tangential Riemannian structure* g, *assumed tangentially smooth. Let* $L_r(p_1^\tau, \dots, p_r^\tau)$ *denote the Hirzebruch L-polynomial in* $\Omega_\tau^p(X)$. *Then*

(a) *For any invariant transverse measure* ν,

$$\mathrm{Sign}(X, \nu) = \int L_r(p_1^\tau, \dots, p_r^\tau)\, d\nu.$$

(b) *The index class* ι_A *of the signature operator equals* $L_r(p_1^\tau, \dots, p_r^\tau)$ *in* $\overline{H}_\tau^p(X)$.

Proof. The index of the operator A may be expressed in two ways. On the one hand, the local trace ι_{D_ℓ} is given by

$$\iota_{D_\ell} = \mathrm{Sign}(X, \nu)_\ell$$

as explained above. On the other hand, D is a first order tangential tangentially elliptic operator and Theorem 7.47 implies that

$$\mathrm{ind}_\nu(A) = \int \omega_A(g, E)\, d\nu,$$

where ω_A is a tangentially smooth p-form which corresponds to A. Restrict $\omega_A(t, E)$ to a leaf ℓ. Then the local index theorem of Atiyah–Bott–Patodi [Atiyah et al. 1973] implies that

$$\omega_A(g, E)_\ell = L_r(p_1^\tau, \dots, p_r^\tau)_\ell.$$

Thus

$$\mathrm{Sign}(X, \nu) = \int L_r(p_1^\tau, \dots, p_r^\tau)\, d\nu.$$

This holds for each invariant transverse measure ν, and hence

$$\iota_D = L_r(p_1^\tau, \dots, p_r^\tau)$$

as classes in $\overline{H}_\tau^p(X)$. □

With this preparation in hand we consider the twisted signature operators. Let X be a compact foliated space with leaves of dimension $p = 2q$ and oriented foliation bundle F. Let V be a tangentially smooth complex vector bundle with a tangential Hermitian structure and tangential connection Δ_V. The bundle $E_X \otimes_{\mathbb{C}} V$ carries a twisted de Rham differential

$$d_V : \Gamma_\tau(E_X \otimes_{\mathbb{C}} V) \to \Gamma_\tau(E_x \otimes_{\mathbb{C}} V)$$

given by

$$d_V(u \otimes v) = du \otimes v + (-1)^i u \wedge \Delta_V v,$$

where $u \in \Gamma_\tau(\Lambda^i(F^*_{\mathbb{C}}))$, $v \in \Gamma_\tau(V)$, and $\wedge$ is the external pairing. The map $*$ acts as $*(u \otimes v) = (*u) \otimes v$. The involution $t : E_X \to E_X$ extends to a natural involution of $E_X \otimes V$ which fixes $1 \otimes V$. The twisted differential and the involution lift to $E_G \otimes V$, as usual.

Let δ_V denote the formal adjoint of d_V. Then $\delta_V = - * d_V *$ and

$$(d_V + \delta_V)t = -t(d_V + \delta_V).$$

Decompose $E_G \otimes V$ into $\pm$ eigenspaces with respect to t. Then the operator $d_V + \delta_V$ restricts to an operator

$$A_V : \Gamma_\tau((E_G \otimes V)^+) \to \Gamma_\tau((E_G \otimes V)^-) \tag{8.12}$$

called the *twisted signature operator*. This is a Dirac operator in the sense of Chapter VII. Define

$$\mathcal{L}(X) = \Sigma 2^{-2s} L_s(p_1^\tau, \ldots, p_1^\tau).$$

Lemma 8.13. $\operatorname{ch}(V) \cdot 2^q \mathcal{L}(X)|_p = \operatorname{ch}(A_V) \operatorname{Td}_\tau(X)|_p.$

This is a fairly involved purely topological calculation whose proof we omit; see [Shanahan 1978].

Let X be a compact oriented foliated space with leaves of dimension $4r$, oriented foliation bundle F, and tangentially smooth oriented tangential Riemannian structure g. Let $L_r(p_1^\tau, \ldots, p_r^\tau)$ denote the Hirzebruch L-polynomial in $\Omega_\tau^p(X)$.

Theorem 8.14 (Twisted Signature Theorem). *Let X be a compact and oriented foliated space with leaves of dimension $4r$, oriented foliation bundle F, and tangentially smooth oriented tangential Riemannian structure g. Let V be a complex vector bundle over X, and let A_V denote the associated twisted signature operator. Then:*

(a) *For every invariant transverse measure ν,*

$$\int \iota_{A_V}\, d\nu = \int \operatorname{ch}_\tau(V) \cdot 2^{2r} \mathcal{L}(X)\, d\nu.$$

(b) $[\iota_{A_V}] = \left[\operatorname{ch}_\tau(V) \cdot 2^{2r} \mathcal{L}(X)|_p\right] \in \overline{H}_\tau^p(X).$

(c) *The Index Theorem holds for twisted signature operators.*

Proof. The argument is virtually identical to the argument in Theorem 8.11. □

The remaining task before us is to demonstrate how knowledge of the index of twisted signature operators (that is to say, of certain natural differential operators) implies the index theorem for all tangential pseudodifferential operators. We begin with the following lemma.

Lemma 8.15. *Suppose that the index theorem holds for pseudodifferential operators of order zero. Then it holds for pseudodifferential operators of all orders.*

Proof. There is nothing to prove for operators of negative order, since such operators lie in the kernel of the tangential principal symbol map on $\bar{\mathcal{P}}^0$. Suppose that T is a tangential, tangentially elliptic pseudodifferential operator of positive order m. Let $\hat{T}$ be the associated superoperator of order $2m$. Then $\hat{T}$ is tangential, tangentially elliptic and formally self-adjoint of order $2m$, with

$$\operatorname{ind}_\nu(T) = \phi_\nu^s(\hat{T}) \quad \text{and} \quad \sigma_m(T) \simeq \sigma_{2m}(\hat{T}).$$

Let $P = (1+\Delta)^{-m}\hat{T}$. Then Proposition 7.27 implies that $P \in \bar{\mathcal{P}}^0$ with

$$\phi_\nu^s(\hat{T}) = \operatorname{ind}_\nu(P) \quad \text{and} \quad \sigma_{2m}(\hat{T}) \simeq \sigma_0(P).$$

The index theorem for P then implies the index theorem for T. □

We turn next to the case of a tangential, tangentially elliptic pseudodifferential operator of order zero on a compact foliated space X with leaves of dimension p and oriented foliation bundle F. We wish to reduce to the case where p is even. For this purpose we briefly consider the multiplicative properties of the topological and analytical indices.

Suppose that X_1 and X_2 are compact foliated spaces as above and V_i, W_i are tangentially smooth Hermitian bundles over X_i. Let $X = X_1 \times X_2$ and define bundles V and W over X by

$$V = (V_1 \otimes V_2) \oplus (W_1 \otimes W_2),$$
$$W = (W_1 \otimes V_2) \oplus (V_1 \otimes W_2).$$

Let D_1, D_2 be tangential, tangentially elliptic pseudodifferential operators of positive order. (If the D_i are nonpositive we modify as in [Atiyah and Singer 1968a, pp. 528–529]). Define $D_1 \# D_2$ by the matrix

$$\begin{pmatrix} D_1 \otimes I_{V_2} & -I_{W_1} \otimes D_2^* \\ I_{V_1} \otimes D_2 & D_1^* \otimes I_{W_2} \end{pmatrix}$$

Then $D_1 \# D_2$ is tangential and tangentially elliptic.

Recall that $\iota_D^{\text{top}} = \operatorname{ch}_\tau(D)\operatorname{Td}_\tau(X)$ denotes the topological index.

Proposition 8.16. *Let ν_1, ν_2 be invariant transverse measures on X_1, X_2, and let $\nu_1 \times \nu_2$ be the product measure. Then*

(a) $\displaystyle\int \iota_{D_1\#D_2}^{\text{top}}\, d(\nu_1 \times \nu_2) = \left(\int \iota_D^{\text{top}}\, d\nu_1\right)\left(\int \iota_{D_2}^{\text{top}}\, d\nu_2\right).$

(b) $\displaystyle\int \iota_{D_1 \# D_2}\, d(\nu_1 \times \nu_2) = \left(\int \iota_{D_1}\, d\nu_1\right)\left(\int \iota_{D_2}\, d\nu_2\right).$

Proof. The multiplicative property of the classical index [Palais 1965, p. 217–228] implies that

$$\iota^{\text{top}}_{D_1 \# D_2|\ell} = \iota^{\text{top}}_{D_1|\ell_1} \times \iota^{\text{top}}_{D_2|\ell_2},$$

where $\ell = \ell_1 \times \ell_2$ is a leaf of $X_1 \times X_2$. Thus

$$\iota^{\text{top}}_{D_1 \# D_2} = \iota^{\text{top}}_{D_1} \times \iota^{\text{top}}_{D_2}.$$

Then

$$\int \iota^{\text{top}}_{D_1 \# D_2}\, d(\nu_1 \times \nu_2) = \int (\iota^{\text{top}}_{D_1} \times \iota^{\text{top}}_{D_2})\, d(\nu_1 \times \nu_2)$$
$$= \left(\int \iota^{\text{top}}_{D_1}\, d\nu_1\right)\left(\int \iota^{\text{top}}_{D_2}\, d\nu_2\right),$$

as required. A similar argument holds for $\iota_{D_1 \# D_2}$. □

We do not claim that the multiplicative property holds at the level of

$$H^{p_1}_\tau(X_1) \times H^{p_2}_\tau(X_2) \to H^{p_1+p_2}_\tau(X_1 \times X_2),$$

since not every invariant transverse measure on $X_1 \times X_2$ is determined by product measures. However this *is* certainly true if $X_2 = M$ (one leaf).

Corollary 8.17. *If the Index Theorem 8.1 holds for all X with p even, it holds for p arbitrary.*

Proof. Suppose that the index theorem holds for all X with p even and suppose given a foliated space X with p odd. Then $X \times S^1$ is foliated with leaves of even dimension $(p+1)$. Let T be the operator on the circle defined by

$$Te^{inx} = \begin{cases} e^{i(n+1)x} & \text{if } n \geq 0, \\ e^{inx} & \text{if } n < 0. \end{cases}$$

Then $T = e^{ix}P + (1-P)$, where $P : L^2(S^1) \to H^2(S^1)$ is the orthogonal projection onto the Hardy space. Thus P and (hence) T are pseudodifferential operators of order zero, and

$$\sigma(T)(x,\xi) = \begin{cases} e^{ix} & \text{if } \xi > 0, \\ 1 & \text{if } \xi < 0, \end{cases}$$

so T is elliptic. A direct check shows $\operatorname{Ker} T = 0$, $\operatorname{Cok} T$ is generated by constant functions, and so $\operatorname{ind}(T) = -1$. The map

$$K^0(F_X) \to K^0(F_{X \times S^1})$$

given by multiplication by the symbol of T is an isomorphism by Bott periodicity. Thus every symbol class in $K^0(F_{X \times S^1})$ may be represented by $\sigma(P)\sigma(T)$ for some pseudodifferential operator P on X. As the topological and analytical indices are multiplicative by Proposition 8.16, the corollary follows. □

Let X be a compact foliated space with leaves of dimension $p = 2q$ and F oriented. Fix an invariant transverse measure ν. The functions

$$D \mapsto \int \iota_D \, d\nu \quad \text{and} \quad D \mapsto \int \mathrm{ch}_\tau(D)\,\mathrm{Td}_\tau(X)\, d\nu$$

depend only upon the class of the tangential principal symbol $\sigma(D)$ and extend to $\mathbb{R}$-linear functions $K^0(F) \otimes \mathbb{R} \to \mathbb{R}$. This is clear for the topological index. For the analytic index we must show that

$$\iota_{D_1 \oplus D_2} = \iota_{D_1} + \iota_{D_2}.$$

This is immediate if one thinks of $D_1 \oplus D_2$ as

$$\begin{pmatrix} D_1 & 0 \\ 0 & D_2 \end{pmatrix}.$$

Further, the two functions agree on the classes of the symbols $[\sigma(A_V)]$ of the twisted signature operators.

We note that Lemma 8.15, Theorem 8.17, and the next result together imply the Index Theorem 8.1.

Proposition 8.18. *Suppose that X is compact foliated space with oriented foliation bundle F of dimension $p = 2q$. Then the classes $[\sigma(A_V)]$ of principal symbols of twisted signature operators span the vector space $K^0(F) \otimes \mathbb{R}$.*

In fact we shall prove the following more general proposition which Atiyah [1975] refers to, in the case of X foliated by a single leaf, as the Global Bott theorem.

Proposition 8.19. *Let X be a compact foliated space with oriented foliation bundle F of dimension $p = 2q$. For any open subset Y of X let F_Y be the restriction of F to Y and define*

$$\theta = \theta_Y : K^0(Y) \otimes \mathbb{R} \to K^0(F_Y) \otimes \mathbb{R}$$

by

$$\theta(V) = [\sigma(A_V)].$$

Then θ is an isomorphism.

We begin by clarifying the map θ.

Proposition 8.20. *If V is a tangentially smooth complex vector bundle over X then*

$$[\sigma(A_V)] = V \cdot [\sigma(A)] \in K^0(F).$$

Thus θ is given by multiplication by the symbol of the signature operator:

$$\theta(V) = V \cdot [\sigma(A)]$$

and hence extends to a transformation

$$\theta : K^*(Y) \otimes \mathbb{R} \to K^*(F_Y) \otimes \mathbb{R}$$

which is natural with respect to inclusions of subspaces and boundary maps.

Proof. The twisted signature complex factors as $\Gamma_\tau(V) \otimes \Lambda^*(F^*_{\mathbb{C}})$. □

Proposition 8.21. *Let X be a compact foliated space with oriented foliation bundle F of dimension $p = 2q$ and let Y be an open subset of X. Suppose that θ_Y is an isomorphism whenever F_Y is a trivial bundle. Then θ_Y is an isomorphism for all Y and Proposition 8.19 holds.*

Proof. Say that Y is *k-trivial* if there is an open cover $\{U_1, \dots U_k\}$ of X such that each $F_{Y\cap U_i}$ is a trivial bundle. Every compact foliated space X is k-trivial for some k over X since X is compact. The property passes to open subsets, and this implies that every open subset $Y \subset X$ is k-trivial for some k.

The proposition holds for all 1-trivial spaces by assumption, since $U_1 = Y$ in that case. We complete the proof by induction on k using the Mayer–Vietoris sequence. □

In order to complete the proof of the Index Theorem 8.1 then, we are reduced to considering the case where $X = \ell^{2q} \times N$ is a product foliated space. A Mayer–Vietoris argument on ℓ shows that we may reduce further to $X = \mathbb{R}^{2q} \times N$. That is, we must show that the map

$$\theta : K^*(\mathbb{R}^{2q} \times N) \otimes \mathbb{R} \to K^*(R^{2q} \times (\mathbb{R}^{2q} \times N)) \otimes \mathbb{R}$$

is an isomorphism.

Next we consider the diagram

$$\begin{array}{ccc} K^*(\mathbb{R}^{2q} \times N) \otimes \mathbb{R} & \xrightarrow{\theta_{\mathbb{R}^{2q}\times N}} & K^*(\mathbb{R}^{2q} \times \mathbb{R}^{2q} \times N) \otimes \mathbb{R} \\ \alpha\otimes 1 \uparrow & & \uparrow \alpha \otimes 1 \\ K^*(\mathbb{R}^{2q}) \otimes K^*(N) \otimes \mathbb{R} & \xrightarrow{\theta_{\mathbb{R}^{2q}} \otimes 1} & K^*(\mathbb{R}^{2q} \times \mathbb{R}^{2q}) \otimes K^*(N) \otimes \mathbb{R} \end{array}$$

where α denotes the Künneth map (an isomorphism over $\mathbb{R}$). The diagram commutes by the naturality of the Künneth pairing and of θ. So it suffices to demonstrate that the map

$$\theta_{\mathbb{R}^{2q}} : K^*(\mathbb{R}^{2q}) \otimes \mathbb{R} \to K^*(\mathbb{R}^{2q} \times \mathbb{R}^{2q}) \otimes \mathbb{R}$$

is an isomorphism. The groups are isomorphic by the Bott periodicity map β.

Theorem 8.22. $\theta_{R^{2q}} = 2^q\beta$, *and hence* $\theta_{\mathbb{R}^{2q}}$ *is an isomorphism.*

The proof of this lemma involves careful consideration of the Dirac operator on $\mathbb{R}^{2q}$ and some classical representation theory. We omit the proof and refer the reader to [Atiyah 1975] for details.

This completes the proof of Proposition 8.19 and hence the proof of the Index Theorem 8.1.

□ □□□□□ □□□□

There have been a variety of applications of Connes' Index theorem, to some extent paralleling the aftermath of the proof of the Atiyah–Singer Index Theorem. For example, Heitsch and Lazarov [1990] and Benameur [1997] established longitudinal Lefschetz theorems. These have been developed further by Deninger and his collaborators; see below.

Hurder's paper [1993] on the topology of covers and the spectral theory of geometric operators uses the full measure theory of this book and has other interesting analytical features in it.

Douglas, Hurder, and Kaminker [Douglas et al. 1991] show that the relative eta invariant for a foliated bundle is the index of a longitudinal operator. They use a direct spectral calculation, going from the longitudinal index to a renormalized transverse index. It was the first result to show that secondary characteristic classes arise naturally in the index pairing. This was later followed by [Moriyoshi 2002] and particularly [Moriyoshi and Natsume 1996] on the Godbillon-Vey class and longitudinal Dirac operators.

The paper of A. L. Carey, K. C. Hannabuss, V. Mathai, and P. McCann [Carey et al. 1998] is part of a general program of studying spectral invariants, generalizing the program of Bellissard. The larger program of spectral invariants started by Gromov and Shubin, and pursued by Lück [2002] and his school is really about the measured index theorem for certain types of groupoids.

Hurder [1990] uses the hull closure of the space of symbols to define a measured space and then calculate the longitudinal index here to obtain the relative eta invariants. This paper is a very general setup for applying the measured index theory in fact, as it defines the general concept of *almost periodic compactification* to general group actions.

Recently the Gap Labeling Conjecture of Jean Bellissard was proved — in three different ways [Bellissard et al. 2005; Benameur and Oyono-Oyono 2003; Kaminker and Putnam 2003] — and the Index Theorem for Foliated Spaces plays a central role. The generalization of Connes' theorem from foliated manifolds to foliated spaces is essential for this application. One of us (Schochet) was asked to do a Featured Review of these papers for *Mathematical Reviews*. We have included that review as Appendix D of this book.

What about bigger and better index theorems? We are firmly convinced that there is no such thing as *the most general* index theorem. Of course we knew that the Connes–Skandalis theorem [1984] was more general than the present result in that it identified the index class in KK and had something to say even in the Type III situation. There was also a parallel (or rather, perpendicular) body of literature that dealt with *transversely elliptic* operators. Here one had to assume that there was a foliated manifold present so that one could differentiate transversely to the leaves and hence form transverse differential operators. When we wrote the first edition the only index theorem available for such operators was (of course) Atiyah's distributional index theorem [1974].

The problem of calculating the index of transversely elliptic operators has been completely solved due to the work of Alain Connes and Henri Moscovici. First [1995] they discovered a general abstract local index formula in the general context of spectral triples. (There is a recent simpler proof of this result by Nigel Higson [2006]). When they tried to apply this result to transverse index theory they faced a wall. They overcame the obstacle in an amazing way [Connes and Moscovici 1998]. Their extraordinary discovery was that there is a natural Hopf algebra $\mathcal{H}(n)$ (depending on the codimension n of the foliation but *not* on the foliation) which acts on the transverse frame bundle of any codimension n foliation and that index computations take place within its Hopf cyclic cohomology, which is computed in terms of the well-known Gelfand–Fuchs cohomology of the Lie algebra of formal vector fields. As Connes puts it: *The entire differentiable transverse structure is captured by the action of the Hopf algebra $\mathcal{H}(n)$, thus reconciling our approach to noncommutative geometry to a more group theoretical one, in the spirit of the Klein program.* The result is a vast generalization of the local form of the Atiyah–Singer Index Theorem. See [Connes 1999] for a survey of this work.

Alain Connes has developed amazing connections between noncommutative geometry and topology and number theory, particularly the Riemann Conjecture. He has written extensively about these connections, for instance in his classic book [Connes 1994] and in [Connes 2000].

Christopher Deninger (see [Deninger 2001] and the references there, as well as [Deitmar and Deninger 2003] for a more recent Lefschetz trace formula) has pioneered the use of foliations and dynamical systems in connection with number-theoretical zeta functions in a different way. In his view: *The two most prominent places in mathematics where laminated spaces occur naturally are in number theory e.g. as adelic points of algebraic groups and in the theory of dynamical systems as attractors* [Deninger 2001, p. 20]. Deninger uses tangential cohomology on the foliations associated with the dynamical systems as well as the index theorem (as it appears, for instance, in Appendix A of this book, written by Steve Hurder). An example: he seeks to relate the compact orbits of a flow with the alternating sum of suitable traces on tangential cohomology.

APPENDIX A

The $\bar{\partial}$-Operator

By Steven Hurder

CONTENTS

The purpose of this Appendix is to discuss the conclusion of the foliation index theorem in the context of foliations whose leaves are two-dimensional. Such foliations provide a class of reasonably concrete examples; while they are certainly not completely representative of the wide range of foliations to which the theorem applies, they are sufficiently complicated to warrant special attention, and possess the smallest leaf dimension for which the leaves have interesting topology. There is another, more fundamental reason for studying these foliations: given any leafwise C^∞-Riemannian metric on a two-dimensional foliation $\mathcal{F}$, there is a corresponding complex-analytic structure on leaves making $\mathcal{F}$ into a leafwise complex analytic foliation. Thus, two-dimensional foliations automatically possess a Teichmüller space, and for each point in this space of complex structures, there is an associated Dirac operator along the leaves. The foliation index theorem then assumes the role of a Riemann–Roch Theorem for these complex structures.

We begin in Section A1 with a discussion of the average Euler characteristic of Phillips–Sullivan, which is the prototype for the topological index character of the foliation index theorems for surfaces. In Section A2, the index theorem is reformulated for the $\bar{\partial}$-operator along the leaves of a leafwise-complex foliation. The Teichmüller spaces for two-dimensional foliations are discussed in Section A3, and a few remarks about their properties are given. In Section A4, some homotopy questions concerning the K-theory of the symbols of leafwise elliptic operators are discussed, with regard to the determination of all possible topological indices for a fixed foliation. Finally Section A5 describes *some* of the "standard" foliations by surfaces, especially of three-manifolds, and the calculation of the foliation indices for them.

The reader will observe that this Appendix concentrates upon topological aspects of the foliation index theorem and serves as an elaboration upon Connes' example of a foliation by complex lines on the four-manifold $\mathbb{C}/\Lambda_1 \times \mathbb{C}/\Lambda_2$ described in Section A3. A key point of this example is that the meaning of the analytic index along the leaves can also be explicitly described in terms of functions with prescribed zeros-and-poles and a growth condition. For the foliations we consider, such an explicit description of the analytic index is much harder to describe, and would take us too far afield, but must be considered an interesting open problem, especially with regards to the Riemann–Roch nature of the foliation index theorem.

A1. Average Euler Characteristic

The index theorem for the de Rham complex of a compact even-dimensional manifold, M, yields the Chern–Gauss–Bonnet formula for its Euler characteristic, which is equal to the alternating sum of the Betti numbers of M. In a likewise fashion, it was shown in Chapter VIII that the foliation index theorem for the tangential de Rham complex of a foliated space yields an alternating sum of "Betti measures". When the transverse measure ν has a special form, i.e., it is defined by an averaging sequence, the d-foliation index can also be interpreted as the ν-average Euler characteristic of the leaves. We examine this latter concept more closely, for it provides a prototype for the calculation of the topological index in the general foliation index theorem. First, recall the integrated form of Theorem 8.7 for the Euler characteristic:

Theorem A1.1 (d-Foliation Index Theorem). *Let ν be a transverse invariant measure for a foliation $\mathcal{F}$ of a foliated space X, with $C_\nu \in H_p^\tau(X)$ the associated Ruelle–Sullivan homology class of ν. Let d be the de Rham operator on the tangential de Rham complex of $\mathcal{F}$. Assume the tangent bundle FX is oriented, with associated Euler form $e^\tau(X)$. Then*

$$\chi(\mathcal{F}, \nu) \equiv \int_X \iota_d \cdot d\nu = \int_X e^\tau(X)\, d\nu = \langle e^\tau(X), C_\nu \rangle. \tag{A1.2}$$

The left-hand side of (A1.2) is interpreted in Chapter VIII as the alternating sum of the ν-dimensions of the L^2-harmonic forms on the leaves of $\mathcal{F}$. To give a geometric interpretation of the right-hand side of (A1.2), we require that ν be the limit of discrete regular measures:

Definition A1.3. An *averaging sequence* [Goodman and Plante 1979] for $\mathcal{F}$ is a sequence of compact subsets $\{L_j \mid j = 1, 2, \dots\}$, where each L_j is a submanifold with boundary of some leaf of $\mathcal{F}$, and

$$\frac{\operatorname{vol} \partial L_j}{\operatorname{vol} L_j} \to 0.$$

(The sets $\{L_j\}$ may belong to differing leaves as j varies, and we are assuming a Riemannian metric on FX has been chosen and fixed.)

The sequence $\{L_j\}$ is *regular* if the submanifolds ∂L_j of X have bounded geometry, meaning that there is a uniform bound on the sectional curvatures, the injectivity radii and the second fundamental forms of the ∂L_j.

For X compact, the measure ν_L associated to an averaging sequence is defined, on a tangential measure λ, by the rule

$$\int_X \lambda \, d\nu_L = \lim_{j\to\infty} \frac{1}{\operatorname{vol} L_j} \int_{L_j} \lambda,$$

where, if necessary, we pass to a subsequence of the $\{L_j\}$ for which the integrals converge in a weak-$*$ topology. The closed current associated to ν_L determines an asymptotic homology class denoted by $C_L \in H_p(X; \mathbb{R})$.

We say a transverse invariant measure ν is *regular* if $\nu = \nu_L$ for some regular averaging sequence $\{L_j \mid j = 1, 2, \dots\}$.

Not all invariant transverse measures arise from averaging sequences, but there are many examples where they do, the primary case being foliations with growth restrictions on the leaves. Choose a Riemannian metric on FX. Its restriction to a leaf $L \subset X$ of $\mathcal{F}$ defines a distance function and volume form on L. Pick a base point $x \in L$ and let $g(r, x)$ be the volume of the ball of radius r centered at x. We say L has

polynomial growth of degree $\le n$ if $\displaystyle\limsup_{r\to\infty} \frac{g(r,x)}{r^n} < \infty$;

subexponential growth if $\displaystyle\limsup_{r\to\infty} \frac{1}{r} \log g(r,x) = 0$;

nonexponential growth if $\displaystyle\liminf_{r\to\infty} \frac{1}{r} \log g(r,x) = 0$;

exponential growth if $\displaystyle\liminf_{r\to\infty} \frac{1}{r} \log g(r,x) > 0$.

For X compact, the growth type of L is independent of the choice of metric on FX and the basepoint x.

For a leaf L with nonexponential growth, there is a sequence of radii $r_j \to \infty$ for which the balls L_j of radius r_j centered at X form an averaging sequence [Plante 1975]. In this case, all of the sets L_j are contained in the same leaf L.

For X compact and the foliation of class C^2, these sets L_j can be modified to make them regular as well.

For a foliation $\mathcal{F}$ with even-dimensional leaves and a regular measure ν, the d-Index Theorem becomes

$$\chi(\mathcal{F},\nu) = \lim_{j\to\infty} \frac{1}{\operatorname{vol} L_j} \int_{L_j} e^{\tau}(X).$$

By the Gauss–Bonnet theorem,

$$\int_{L_j} e^{\tau}(X) = e(L_j) + \int_{\partial L_j} \epsilon_j,$$

where $e(L_j)$ is the Euler characteristic of L_j and ϵ_j is a correction term depending on the Riemannian geometry of ∂L_j. The assumption that the submanifolds $\{\partial L_j\}$ have uniformly bounded geometry implies there is a uniform estimate

$$\left| \int_{\partial L_j} \epsilon_j \right| \leq K \cdot \operatorname{vol} \partial L_j.$$

Therefore, in the limit we have

$$\chi(\mathcal{F},\nu) = \lim_{j\to\infty} \frac{e(L_j)}{\operatorname{vol} L_j} \qquad \text{(A1.4)}$$

and the right side of (A1.4) is called the *average Euler characteristic* of the averaging sequence $\{L_j\}$. Phillips and Sullivan [1981] and Cantwell and Conlon [1977] use this invariant of a noncompact Riemannian manifold to give examples of quasi-isometry types of manifolds which cannot be realized as leaves of foliations of a manifold X with $H_p(X,\mathbb{R}) = 0$.

Consider three examples of open two-manifolds [Phillips and Sullivan 1981] whose metric is defined by the given embedding in E^3. Each of the following, with their quasi-isometry class of metrics, can be realized as leaves of some foliation of some three-manifold, but the first two cannot be realized (with the given quasi-isometry class of metrics) as leaves in S^3.

Jacob's ladder:

(A1.5) $L \sim$ 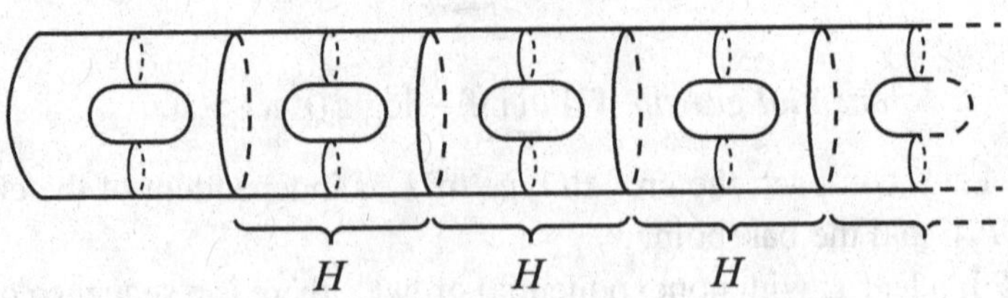

The growth type of L is linear, and the average Euler characteristic of L is $1/\operatorname{vol} H$.

Infinite Jail Cell Window:

(A1.6) $L \sim$ 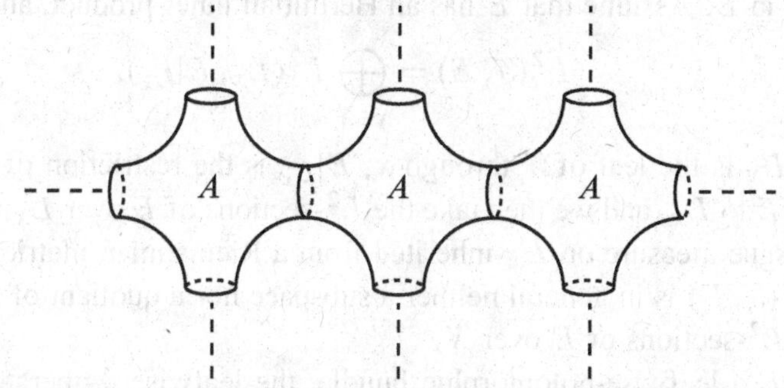

The growth of L is quadratic, and the average Euler characteristic of L is $2/\operatorname{vol} A$.

Infinite Loch Ness Monster:

(A1.7) $L \sim$ 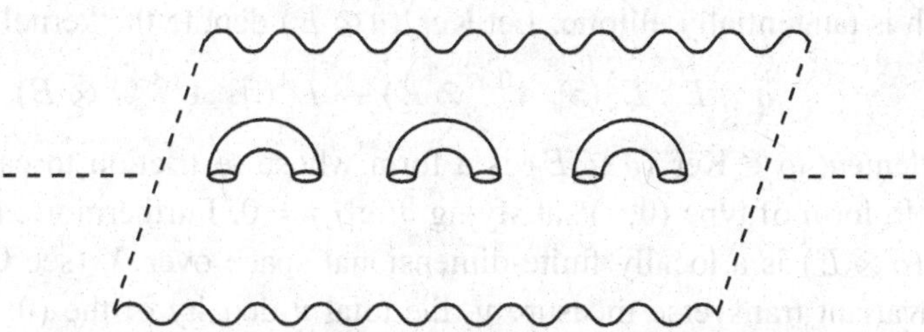

The growth of L is quadratic, but the average Euler characteristic is zero.

The construction of the average Euler characteristic for surfaces suggests that a similar geometric interpretation can be given for the topological index of other differential operators. For the $\bar{\partial}$-operator of complex line foliations, this is indeed true, as discussed further in Section A3.

A2. The $\bar{\partial}$-Index Theorem and Riemann–Roch

We next examine in detail the meaning of the foliation index theorem for the tangential $\bar{\partial}$-operator. Let $\mathcal{F}$ be a foliation of a foliated space X and assume the leaves of $\mathcal{F}$ are complex manifolds whose complex structure varies continuously in X. That is, in Definition 2.1 (page 32), we assume that foliation charts $\{\varphi_x\}$ can be chosen for which the composition $t_y \circ \varphi_x^{-1}(\cdot\,, n)$ is holomorphic for all n, and $n \mapsto t_y \circ \varphi_x^{-1}(\cdot\,, n)$ is continuous in the space of holomorphic maps.

Let k be such that the dimension of the leaves of $\mathcal{F}$ is $p = 2k$.

A continuous vector bundle $E \to X$ is *holomorphic* if for each leaf $L \subset X$ with given complex structure, the restriction $E|_L \longrightarrow L$ is a holomorphic bundle. As before, FX is the tangent bundle to the leaves of $\mathcal{F}$, and this is holomorphic in the above sense. Let $A^{r,s} \to X$ be the bundle of smooth tensors of type (r,s):

$$A^{r,s} = \Lambda^{r,s}(F_{\mathbb{C}}X^*).$$

Given a holomorphic bundle E, let $A^{r,s} \otimes E$ denote the (r,s)-forms with coefficients in E. Assume that E has an Hermitian inner product, and then set

$$L^2(\mathcal{F}, E) = \bigoplus_{x \in X} L^2(L_x, E|_{L_x}),$$

where L_x is the leaf of $\mathcal{F}$ through x, $E|_{L_x}$ is the restriction of the Hermitian bundle E to L_x, and we then take the L^2-sections of E over L_x with respect to a Lebesgue measure on L_x inherited from a Riemannian metric on FX. Note that $L^2(\mathcal{F}, E)$ is in general neither a subspace nor a quotient of $L^2(X, E)$, the global L^2-sections of E over X.

For E a leafwise-holomorphic bundle, the leafwise $\bar{\partial}$-operator for $\mathcal{F}$ has a densely defined extension to

$$\bar{\partial} \otimes E : L^2(\mathcal{F}, A^{r,s} \otimes E) \to L^2(\mathcal{F}, A^{r,s+1} \otimes E)$$

which is tangentially elliptic. Let $\mathrm{Ker}_s(\bar{\partial} \otimes E)$ denote the kernel of

$$\bar{\partial} \otimes E : L^2(\mathcal{F}, A^{0,s} \otimes E) \to L^2(\mathcal{F}, A^{0,s+1} \otimes E).$$

An element $\omega \in \mathrm{Ker}_s(\bar{\partial} \otimes E)$ is a form whose restriction to each leaf L is a smooth form of type $(0,s)$ satisfying $\bar{\partial}(\omega|_L) = 0$. Furthermore, for each $s \geq 0$, $\mathrm{Ker}_s(\bar{\partial} \otimes E)$ is a locally finite-dimensional space over X (see Chapter I). For an invariant transverse measure ν, the total ν-density of the $(0,s)$-solutions ω to the equation $\bar{\partial} \otimes E(\omega) = 0$ is $\dim_\nu ker_s(\bar{\partial} \otimes E)$, and we set

$$\dim_\nu \mathrm{Ker}(\bar{\partial} \otimes E) = \sum_{s=0}^{k} \dim_\nu \mathrm{Ker}_s(\bar{\partial} \otimes E).$$

Similar arguments apply to the adjoint $\bar{\partial}^*$, and with the notation of Chapter IV we have

$$\int_X \iota_{\bar{\partial} \otimes E}\, d\nu = \dim_\nu \mathrm{Ker}(\bar{\partial} \otimes E) - \dim_\nu \mathrm{Ker}(\bar{\partial}^* \otimes E).$$

Theorem A2.1 ($\bar{\partial}$-Index Theorem). *Let* ν *be an invariant transverse measure for a complex foliation* $\mathcal{F}$ *of* X, $C_\nu \in H^\tau_{2\kappa}(X;\mathbb{R})$ *the associated Ruelle–Sullivan homology class, and* $\mathrm{Td}_\tau(X) = \mathrm{Td}(FX \otimes \mathbb{C})$ *the tangential Todd class for* $\mathcal{F}$. *Then*

(A2.2)
$$\int_X \iota_{\bar{\partial} \otimes E}\, d\nu = \langle \mathrm{ch}(\bar{\partial} \otimes E)\, \mathrm{Td}_\tau(X), C_\nu \rangle.$$

The left-hand side of (A2.2) is identified with the *arithmetic genus* of $\mathcal{F}$ with coefficients in E,

$$\chi(\bar{\partial} \otimes E, \nu) = \sum_{i=0}^{\kappa} (-1)^i \dim_\nu H^i(\mathcal{F}; E),$$

where

$$H^i(\mathcal{F}, E) \equiv \mathrm{Ker}_i(\bar{\partial} \otimes E)/\,\mathrm{Ker}_i(\bar{\partial}^* \otimes E)$$

is a locally finite-dimensional space over X. The number $\dim_\nu H^i(\mathcal{F}; E)$ measures the density of this cohomology group in the support of ν, and generalizes the ν-Betti numbers of the operator d.

On the right-hand side of (A2.2), the term $\mathrm{ch}(\bar{\partial} \otimes E)$ is the Chern character of the K-theory class determined by the complex

$$A^{0,*} \otimes E.$$

There is a standard simplification of the cup product

$$\mathrm{ch}(\bar{\partial} \otimes E)\,\mathrm{Td}(FX \otimes \mathbb{C}),$$

which yields:

Corollary A2.3. $\chi(\bar{\partial} \otimes E, \nu) = \big\langle \mathrm{ch}(E)\,\mathrm{Td}_\tau(FX), C_\nu \big\rangle.$

Proof. Use the splitting principle and the multiplicativity of the Chern and Todd characters. For details, see [Shanahan 1978]. □

Corollary A2.3 is exactly the classical Riemann–Roch Theorem in the context of foliations. The arithmetical genus $\chi(\bar{\partial} \otimes E, \nu)$ is the ν-density of the alternating sum of the dimensions of the $\bar{\partial}$-closed L^2-forms on the leaves of $\mathcal{F}$. The right-hand side is a topological invariant of E, FX and C_ν. For a given measure ν, one can hope to choose the bundle E so that $\chi(\bar{\partial} \otimes E, \nu) \neq 0$, guaranteeing the existence for ν-a.e. leaf L of $\mathcal{F}$ of $\bar{\partial}$-closed L^2-forms on L with coefficients in E.

A3. Foliations by Surfaces (Complex Lines or $k = 1$)

Let X be a compact foliated space with foliation $\mathcal{F}$ having leaves of dimension $p = 2$. For example, we may take $X = M$ to be a smooth manifold and assume TM admits a 2-plane subbundle F. Then by [Thurston 1976], F is homotopic to a bundle FM which is tangent to a smooth foliation of M by surfaces.

Lemma A3.1. *Let $\mathcal{F}$ be a two-dimensional foliation of X with FX orientable. Then every Riemannian metric g on FX canonically determines a continuous complex structure on the leaves of $\mathcal{F}$. That is, the pair $(\mathcal{F}, g)$ determines a complex foliation of X.*

Proof. Define a J-operator J_g on FX to be rotation by $+\pi/2$ with respect to the given metric g and the orientation. For each leaf L, the structure $J_g|L$ is integrable as the leaf is two-dimensional hence uniquely defines a complex structure on L. Furthermore, by the parametrized Riemann mapping theorem [Ahlfors 1966], there exist foliation charts for $\mathcal{F}$ with each $t' \circ \varphi_x(\cdot, n)$ holomorphic and continuous in the variable ν. □

We remark that if $\mathcal{F}$ has a given complex structure, J, then a metric g can be defined on FX for which $J_g = J$. Thus, the construction of Lemma A3.1 yields all possible complex structures on $\mathcal{F}$. This suggests the definition of the Teichmüller space of a two-dimensional foliation $\mathcal{F}$ of a space X. We say two metrics g and g' on FX are *holomorphically equivalent* if there is a homeomorphism $\phi : X \to X$ mapping the leaves of $\mathcal{F}$ smoothly onto themselves, and $\phi^* g'$ is conformally equivalent to g. We say that g and g' are *measurably holomorphically equivalent* if there is a measurable automorphism ϕ of X mapping leaves of $\mathcal{F}$ smoothly onto leaves of $\mathcal{F}$, and $\phi^*(g')$ is conformally equivalent to g by a measurable conformal factor on X.

Definition A3.2. *Teichmüller space* $T(X, \mathcal{F})$ is the set of holomorphic equivalence classes of metrics on FX. The *measurable Teichmüller space* $T_m(X, \mathcal{F})$ is the subset of $T(X, \mathcal{F})$ consisting of measurably holomorphic equivalence classes.

When $\mathcal{F}$ consists of one leaf, this reduces to the usual Teichmüller space of a surface. When $\mathcal{F}$ is defined by a fibration $X \to Y$ with fibre a surface Σ, let $T(\Sigma)$ be the Teichmüller space of Σ, then

$$T(X, \mathcal{F}) = C^0(Y, T(\Sigma))$$

is infinite-dimensional. The more interesting question is to study $T(X, \mathcal{F})$ for an ergodic foliation $\mathcal{F}$. There are constructions of foliated manifolds, due to E. Ghys, which show that $T(X, \mathcal{F})$ can be infinite-dimensional, even for $\mathcal{F}$ ergodic [Ghys 1997; 1999].

Related to this is a problem first posed by J. Cantwell and L. Conlon: when does there exist a metric on FX for which every leaf has constant negative curvature? A complete solution is given for codimension-one, proper foliations [Cantwell and Conlon 1989], as well as for leaves in Markov exceptional minimal sets [Cantwell and Conlon 1991]. There is also a more general problem, which is to "uniformize" $\mathcal{F}$—that is, to find a metric on the leaves such that the curvature is constant. This problem was solved by Alberto Candel [1993] in the case all leaves are hyperbolic, or in the case they are spherical. Ghys [1997; 1999] gives a discussion and survey of the more general case of leaves of mixed type. As an analogue of the Phillips–Sullivan Theorem in Section A1, one can ask if given a surface Σ with complex structure J_Σ, and given a compact manifold X, does there exist a foliation $\mathcal{F}$ of X and $[g] \in T(X, \mathcal{F})$ with Σ a leaf of $\mathcal{F}$ so that the complex structure induced on Σ by $[g]$ coincides with J_Σ? The average Euler characteristic of Σ still provides an obstruction to solving this problem, when Σ has nonexponential growth type, but the additional requirement that Σ have a prescribed complex structure should force other obstructions to arise. This would be especially interesting to understand for Σ of exponential growth-type, where no obstructions are presently known.

We now turn to consideration of the $\bar{\partial}$-Index Theorem for a foliation by complex lines, and derive an analogue of the average Euler characteristic.

Lemma A3.3. *Let $\mathcal{F}$ be a complex line foliation of X. Then*

$$\text{(A3.4)} \qquad \chi(\bar{\partial} \otimes E, \nu) = \langle c_1(E), C_\nu \rangle + \tfrac{1}{2}\,\chi(\mathcal{F}, \nu).$$

Proof. The degree-two component of $\mathrm{ch}_\tau(E)\,\mathrm{Td}_\tau(X)$ is

$$c_1(E) + \tfrac{1}{2}\,c_1(FX). \qquad \square$$

Our goal is to give a geometric interpretation of the term $\langle c_1(E), C_\nu \rangle$ in (A3.4) similar to the average Euler characteristic.

Let $\kappa \to \mathbb{C}\mathrm{P}^N$ be the canonical bundle over the complex projective N-space. For large N, there exists a tangentially smooth map

$$f_E : X \to \mathbb{C}\mathrm{P}^N \qquad \text{with} \qquad f_E^*\kappa = E.$$

(We say that f_E classifies E.) Let $H \subset \mathbb{C}\mathrm{P}^N$ be a hypersurface dual to the first Chern class $c_1 \in H^2(\mathbb{C}\mathrm{P}^N)$ of κ. For convenience, we now assume X is a C^1 manifold and $\mathcal{F}$ is also C^1. The complex structure on $\mathcal{F}$ orients its leaves, and the complex structure on $\mathbb{C}P^N$ orients the normal bundle to H. A connection on $\kappa \to \mathbb{C}\mathrm{P}^N$ pulls back under the f_E to a connection on $E \to X$, so $f_E^*(c_1) = c_1(E)$ holds both for cohomology classes and on the level of forms. Furthermore, a C^1-perturbation of f_E results in a C^0-perturbation of the form $c_1(E)$.

Given a regular averaging sequence $\{L_j\}$, for each $j \geq 1$ choose a C^1-perturbation f_j of f_E so that $f_j(L_j)$ is transverse to H, and $f_j^*(c_1)$ converges uniformly to $c_1(E)$. We say a point $x \in L_j \cap f_j^{-1}(H)$ is a *zero* of E if $f_j(L_j)$ is positively oriented at $f_j(x)$, and a *pole* if the orientation is reversed. Let $Z(L_j)$ and $P(L_j)$ denote the corresponding set of zeros and poles in L_j. Then elementary geometry shows that

$$\int_{L_j} c_1(E) = \#Z(L_j) - \#P(L_j) + \epsilon_j,$$

where the error term ϵ_j is proportional to $\mathrm{vol}\,\partial L_j$. This uses that $\{\partial L_j\}$ has uniformly bounded geometry. Combined with Lemma A3.3, we obtain:

Proposition A3.5. *Let X be a C^1 manifold and assume $\mathcal{F}$ is a C^1-holomorphic foliation by surfaces. For $\nu = \nu_L$ given by a regular averaging sequence $\{L_j\}$,*

$$\chi(\bar{\partial} \otimes E, \nu) = \lim_{j\to\infty} \frac{\#Z(L_j)}{\operatorname{vol} L_j} - \lim_{j\to\infty} \frac{\#P(L_j)}{\operatorname{vol} L_j} + \frac{1}{2}\chi(\mathcal{F}, \mu)$$

$$= \text{(average density of zeros of E)}$$
$$-\text{(average density of poles of E)} + \tfrac{1}{2}\text{(average Euler char)}.$$

Consider the case of a foliation of a 3-manifold X by surfaces. Let $\{\gamma_1, \dots, \gamma_d\}$ be a collection of d embedded closed curves in X which are transverse to $\mathcal{F}$, and $\{n_1, \dots, n_d\}$ a collection of nonzero integers. This data defines a complex line bundle $E \to X$, and for a leaf L the restriction $E|_L$ is associated to the divisor

$$\sum_{i=1}^{d} n_i \cdot (\gamma_i \cap L).$$

Let ν be an invariant transverse measure. Then Proposition A3.5 takes on the more precise form:

Proposition A3.6.

$$\dim_\nu H^0(\mathcal{F}; E) - \dim_\nu H^1(\mathcal{F}; E) = \sum_{i=1}^{d} n_i \cdot \nu(\gamma_i) + \frac{1}{2}\chi(\mathcal{F}, \nu).$$

Proof. $c_1(E)$ is dual to the 1-cycle $\sum_{i=1}^{d} n_i \cdot \gamma_i$. □

If $\nu = \nu_L$ is defined by an averaging sequence $\{L_j\}$, then $\nu(\gamma_i)$ is precisely the limit density of $(\gamma_i \cap L_j)$ in L_j, so Proposition A3.6 relates the ν-dimension of L^2-harmonic forms on the leaves of $\mathcal{F}$ with the average density of the zeros and poles of E. This is exactly what a Riemann–Roch Theorem should do. The latitude in choosing E for a given $\mathcal{F}$ means one can often ensure that either $H^0(\mathcal{F}; E)$, the L^2-meromorphic functions on the leaves of $\mathcal{F}$ with order at least $\sum n_i \cdot \gamma_i$, or the corresponding space of meromorphic 1-forms $H^1(\mathcal{F}; E)$ has positive ν-density. This type of result is of greatest interest when the complex structures of the leaves of $\mathcal{F}$ can be prescribed in advance, as in Example A3.7 below.

For a complex line foliation $\mathcal{F}$ of an n-manifold X, given closed oriented submanifolds $\{V_1, \dots, V_d\}$ of codimension 2 in X transverse to $\mathcal{F}$, and integers $\{n_1, \dots, n_d\}$, there is a holomorphic line bundle $E \to X$ corresponding to the divisor $\sum_{i=1}^{d} n_i \cdot V_i$. The existence of such closed transversals V_i to $\mathcal{F}$, and more generally of holomorphic vector bundles $E \to X$, is usually hard to ascertain. However, there is one geometric context in which such V_i always exists in multitude, the foliations given as in (2.2) of Chapter II. We briefly recall their construction.

Let Y be a compact oriented manifold of dimension $n-2$, $\sum_g$ a surface of genus g, and $\rho : \Gamma_g \to \mathrm{Diff}(Y)$ a representation of the fundamental group $\Gamma_g = \kappa_1(\Sigma_g)$. The quotient manifold

$$M = (\tilde{\Sigma} \times Y)/\Gamma_g$$

has a natural 2-dimensional foliation transverse to the fibres of

$$\kappa : M \to \Sigma_g.$$

The leaves of $\mathcal{F}$ are coverings of Σ_g associated to the isotropy groups of ρ, and inherit complex structures from Σ_g. The d-index theorem for $\mathcal{F}$ can be deduced from Atiyah's L^2-index theorem for coverings [Atiyah 1976]. For the $\bar{\partial}$-index theorem, this is no longer the case. Also, note that the Teichmüller spaces of this class of foliations always has dimension at least that of Σ_g, as every metric on $T\Sigma_g$ lifts to a metric on FM. However, they need not have the same dimension, and $T(M, \mathcal{F})$ or $T_m(M, \mathcal{F})$ provide a very interesting geometric "invariant" of the representation ρ of Γ_g on Y.

For each point $x \in \Sigma_g$, the fibre $\pi^{-1}(x) \subset M$ is a closed orientable transversal to $\mathcal{F}$. To obtain further transversals, we assume the fibration $M \to \Sigma_g$ is trivial, so there is a commutative diagram

$$\begin{array}{ccc} M & \xrightarrow{\;\cong\;} & \Sigma_g \times Y \\ & {\scriptstyle \pi}\searrow \quad \swarrow & \\ & \Sigma_g & \end{array}$$

Note that the foliation $\tilde{\mathcal{F}}$ on $\Sigma_g \times Y$ induced from its identification with M will not, in general, be the product foliation. A transversal to $\mathcal{F}$ corresponds to a transversal to $\tilde{\mathcal{F}}$, and the latter can often be found explicitly.

Example A3.7. Consider the example described in [Connes 1982]. Here, $\Sigma_1 = \mathbb{C}/\Gamma_1$ is a complex torus, as is $Y = \mathbb{C}/\Gamma_2$, for lattices Γ_1 and Γ_2 in $\mathbb{C}$. Let Γ_1 act by translations on $\mathbb{C}/\Gamma_2$, and form

$$\begin{array}{c} M = (\mathbb{C} \times \mathbb{C}/\Gamma_2)/\Gamma_1 \cong (\mathbb{C}/\Gamma_1) \times (\mathbb{C}/\Gamma_2) \\ \Big\downarrow {\scriptstyle \kappa} \\ \mathbb{C}/\Gamma_1 \end{array}$$

Connes takes $V_1 = 0 \times \mathbb{C}/\Gamma_2$ and $V_2 = \mathbb{C}/\Gamma_1 \times 0$ as the transversals in $\Sigma_1 \times Y$. Neither V_1 nor V_2 is homotopic to a fibre $\kappa^{-1}(x)$ so the $\bar{\partial}$-index theorem for E associated to the divisor $V_1 - V_2$ is not derivable from the L^2-index theorem for coverings. For ν the Euclidean volume on $\mathbb{C}/\Gamma_2$, Connes remarks that

$$\chi(\bar{\partial} \otimes E, \nu) = \text{density } \Gamma_2 - \text{density } \Gamma_1,$$

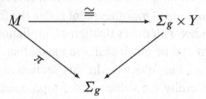

so the dimension of the space of L^2-harmonic functions on almost every leaf $\mathbb{C} \subset M$ with divisor $\mathbb{C} \cap (V_1 - V_2)$ is governed by the density of the lattices Γ_1 and Γ_2. Again, this is exactly the role of a Riemann–Roch Theorem, where for foliations the degree of a divisor is replaced with the average density of the divisor.

A4. Geometric *K*-Theories

The examples described at the end of Section A3 for the $\bar{\partial}$-operator suggest that to obtain analytical results from the foliation index theorem, it is useful to understand the possible topological indices of leafwise elliptic operators. In the examples above, the ν-topological indices are varied by making choices of "divisors" which pair nontrivially with the foliation cycle C_ν. As a consequence, various spaces of meromorphic forms are shown to be nontrivial. To obtain similar results for a general foliation, $\mathcal{F}$, it is useful to determine the range of topological indices of leafwise elliptic operators for $\mathcal{F}$. In this section, we briefly describe the formal "calculation" of these indices in terms of K-groups of foliation groupoids. In some cases, these abstract results can be explicitly calculated, giving very useful information. The reader is referred to the literature for more detailed discussions. One other point is that the foliation index theorem equates the analytic index with the evaluation of a foliation cycle on a K-theory class; these evaluations can be much easier to make, than to fully determine the topological K-theory of the foliation. In this section, and in Section A5, we will examine more carefully the values of the topological index paired with a foliation current for some classes of foliations.

Recall from Definition 2.20 of Chapter II the *holonomy groupoid*, or *graph*, $G(X)$ associated to the foliated space X. A point in $G(X)$ is an equivalence class $[\gamma_{xy}]$ of paths $\gamma : [0,1] \to X$ with $\gamma(0) = x$, $\gamma(1) = y$ and γ remains on the same leaf for all t. Two paths are identified if they have the same holonomy. $G(X)$ is a topological groupoid with the multiplication defined by concatenation of paths.

Also associated to the foliated manifold $(X, \mathcal{F})$ is a groupoid $\Gamma(X)$, constructed in [Haefliger 1984]. The groupoid $\Gamma(X)$ coincides with one of the restricted groupoids $G_N^N(X)$ of Chapter II. Let $\{U_\alpha\}$ be a locally finite open cover of X by foliation charts such that $U_\alpha \cap U_\beta$ is contractible if nonempty. For each α, there is given a diffeomorphism

$$\phi_\alpha : U_\alpha \to \mathbb{R}^p \times \mathbb{R}^q$$

sending the leaves of $\mathcal{F}|_{U_\alpha}$ to $\mathbb{R}^p \times pt$. Define a transversal

$$T_\alpha = \phi_\alpha^{-1}(\{0\} \times \mathbb{R}^q) \subset U_\alpha$$

for each α. By a judicious choice of the $\{U_\alpha\}$, we can assume the $\{T_\alpha\}$ are pairwise disjoint; see [Hilsum and Skandalis 1983]. Then set $N = \bigcup T_\alpha$, an embedded open q-submanifold of X. It is an easy exercise to show $G_N^N(X)$ coincides with the Haefliger groupoid $\Gamma(X)$ constructed from the foliation charts $\{\phi_\alpha : U_\alpha \to \mathbb{R}^{p+q}\}$.

The inclusion $N \times N \subset X \times X$ induces an inclusion of topological groupoids $\Gamma(X) \subset G(X)$. The cofibre of the inclusion is modeled on the trivial groupoid $R^p \times R^p$, where all pairs (x, y) are morphisms. One thus expects the above inclusion to be an equivalence, and Haefliger [1984] shows that this is indeed so:

Theorem A4.1 (Haefliger). *The inclusion $\Gamma(X) \subset G(X)$ is a Morita equivalence of categories.*

For any topological groupoid $\mathcal{G}$, there is a classifying space $B\mathcal{G}$ of $\mathcal{G}$ structures, which is constructed using a modification of the Milnor join construction [Haefliger 1971; Milnor 1956]. Applying this to $G(X)$ yields the space $BG(X)$ which is fundamental for foliation K-theory; see [Connes 1982, Chapter 9]. Applying the B-construction to $\Gamma(X)$, we obtain a space $B\Gamma(X)$ which is fundamental for the characteristic class theory of $\mathcal{F}$.

Corollary. *Let $(X, \mathcal{F})$ be a foliated space. The inclusion $\Gamma(X) \subset G(X)$ induces a homotopy equivalence $B\Gamma(X) \simeq BG(X)$.*

Thus, the topological invariants of $B\Gamma(X)$ and $BG(X)$ agree. Note the open contractible covering $\{U_\alpha\}$ of X defines a natural continuous map $X \to B\Gamma(X)$. If all leaves of $\mathcal{F}$ are contractible, this inclusion is a homotopy equivalence, so that the topological type of $BG(X)$ is the same as X. By placing weaker restrictions on the topological types of the leaves of $\mathcal{F}$, one can more generally deduce that the inclusion is an N-equivalence on homotopy groups; see [Haefliger 1984]. For the generic foliation, however, one expects that the space $BG(X)$ will have a distinct topological type from X, probably more complicated.

The space $B\Gamma(X)$ can be studied from a "universal viewpoint" by introducing the Haefliger classifying spaces. For the class of transversally C^r-differentiable foliations of codimension q, Haefliger defines a space $B\Gamma_q^{(r)}$, and there is a universal map

$$i_X : B\Gamma(X) \to B\Gamma_q^{(r)}.$$

The cohomology groups of $B\Gamma_q^{(r)}$ then define universal classes which pull back to $B\Gamma(X)$ via $(i_X)^*$. The nontriviality of $(i_X)^*$ is then a statement about both the topology of $B\Gamma(X)$ and the inclusion i_X. A short digression will describe the situation for C^∞ foliations.

Let $B\Gamma_q$ be the universal classifying space of codimension q C^∞-foliations. (It is important to specify the transverse differentiability of $\mathcal{F}$, as the topology of $B\Gamma_q$ depends strongly on how much differentiability is required.) The composition

$$f_{\mathcal{F}} : X \to B\Gamma(X) \to B\Gamma_q,$$

or more precisely its homotopy class, was introduced by Haefliger in order to "classify" the C^∞-foliations on a given X. The classification is modulo an equivalence relation which turns out to be *concordance* for X compact, and *integrable homotopy* for X open; see [Haefliger 1971].

For $B\Gamma(X)$, the principal invariants are the characteristic classes. Recall the definition of the differential graded algebra

$$WO_q = \Lambda(h_1, h_3, \ldots, h_{q'}) \otimes \mathbb{R}[c_1, c_2, \ldots, c_q]_{2q},$$

where the subscript $2q$ indicates that this is a truncated polynomial algebra, truncated in degrees greater than $2q$, and q' is the greatest odd integer not exceeding q. The differential is determined by $d(h_i \otimes 1) = 1 \otimes c_i$ and $d(1 \otimes c_i) = 0$. The monomials $\wedge c_J = h_{1_1} \wedge \cdots \wedge h_{i_\ell} \wedge c_1^{j_1} \cdots c_q^{j_q}$, where

(A4.2) $\quad 1_1 < \cdots < i_\ell, \quad |J| = j_1 + 2j_2 + \cdots + q j_q \le q, \quad i_1 + |J| > q$

are closed, and they span the cohomology $H^*(WO_q)$ in degrees greater than $2q$. The *Vey basis* is a subset of these [Bott and Haefliger 1972; Kamber and Tondeur 1974; 1975; Lawson 1974].

A foliation $\mathcal{F}$ on M determines a map of differential algebras into the de Rham complex of M, $\Delta_{\mathcal{F}}$: $WO_q \to \Omega^*(M)$. The induced map in cohomology,

$$\Delta_{\mathcal{F}}^* : H^*(WO_q) \to H^*(M),$$

depends only the integrable homotopy class of $\mathcal{F}$. The secondary classes of $\mathcal{F}$ are spanned by the images $\Delta_{\mathcal{F}}^*(h_I \wedge c_J)$ for $h_I \wedge c_J$ satisfying (A4.2).

The construction of the map $\Delta_{\mathcal{F}}$ is functorial, so there exists a universal map

$$\tilde{\Delta}_* : H^*(WO_q) \to H^*(B\Gamma_q)$$

(see [Lawson 1977]), and for given $\mathcal{F}$ on X we obtain its secondary classes via

$$\Delta_* = f_{\mathcal{F}}^* \circ \tilde{\Delta}_* : H^*(WO_q) \to H^*(X).$$

We next describe how the topology of $BG(X)$ is related to the topological indices of leafwise elliptic operators of $\mathcal{F}$. For $\mathcal{F}$ a C^1-foliation of a manifold X, the groupoid $G(X)$ has a natural map to $\mathrm{GL}(q, \mathbb{R})$ obtained by taking the Jacobian matrix of the holonomy along a path $[\gamma_{xy}]$. This induces a map

$$BG(X) \to B\,\mathrm{GL}(q, \mathbb{R}),$$

which defines a rank q vector bundle $\xi \to BG(X)$ whose pullback to X under $X \to B\Gamma(X) \to BG(X)$ is the normal bundle to $\mathcal{F}$. The ξ-twisted K-theory of

$BG(X)$ is defined as

$$K_*^{\xi}(BG(X)) \equiv K_*(B(\xi), S(\xi)),$$

where $B(\xi)$ is the unit disc subbundle of $\xi \to BG(X)$, and $S(\xi)$ is the unit sphere bundle.

Connes and Skandalis [1984] construct a map

$$\mathrm{Ind}_t : K_*^{\xi}(BG(X)) \to K_*(C_r^*(X)),$$

which they call the topological index map, via an essentially topological procedure that converts a vector bundle or unitary over $BG(X)$ into an idempotent or invertible element over $C_r^*(X)$. Let $F_1^* X$ denote the unit cotangent bundle to $\mathcal{F}$ over X. Then there is a natural map of K-theories,

$$b : K^1(F_1^* X) \to K_0^{\xi}(BG(X)),$$

obtained from the exact sequence for the pair $(B(\xi), S(\xi))$. If $\mathcal{F}$ admits a transverse invariant measure ν, there is a linear functional ϕ_ν on $K_0(C_r^*(X))$ (Proposition 6.23), and the composition $\phi_\nu \circ \mathrm{Ind}_t \circ b = \mathrm{Ind}_\nu^t$, the topological measured index. That is, for D a leafwise operator with symbol class $u = [\sigma_D] \in K^1(F_1^* X)$.

$$\phi_\nu \circ \mathrm{Ind}_t \circ b(u) = \big\langle \mathrm{ch}(D)\, \mathrm{Td}_\tau(X), C_\nu \big\rangle.$$

Connes and Skandalis also construct a direct map,

$$\mathrm{Ind}_a : K^1(F_1^* X) \to K_0(C_r^*(X)),$$

which they call the analytic index homomorphism, by associating to an invertible u the index projection operator over $C_r^*(X)$ of a zero-order leafwise elliptic operator whose symbol class is u. Also,

$$\mathrm{Ind}_\nu^a \equiv \phi_\nu \circ \mathrm{Ind}_a(u)$$

is the analytic index of this operator, calculated using the dimension function associated to ν. They then proved in [Connes and Skandalis 1984]:

Theorem A4.3 (Connes–Skandalis General Foliation Index Theorem). *For any foliation $\mathcal{F}$, there is an equality of maps*

$$\mathrm{Ind}_a = \mathrm{Ind}_t \circ b : K^1(F_1^* X) \to K_0(C_r^*(X)).$$

Note that Theorem A4.3 makes sense even when $\mathcal{F}$ possesses no invariant measures. If there is an invariant measure, ν, then by the above remarks, the theorem implies the ν-measured foliation index theorem proved in Chapters 7 and 8. Note also that this formulation of the index theorem shows that the possible range of the analytic traces of leafwise operators, with respect to a given invariant measure ν, are contained in the image of the map

$$\phi_\nu \circ \mathrm{Ind}_t : K_0^{\xi}(BG(X)) \to \mathbb{R}.$$

This is the meaning of the earlier statement that the topology of $BG(X)$ dictates the possible analytic indices of leafwise operators, and motivates the study of $BG(X)$. In fact, Connes has conjectured that this space has K-theory isomorphic to that of $C_r^*(X)$.

Conjecture A4.4. *Suppose that all holonomy groups of* $\mathcal{F}$ *are torsion-free. Then* Ind_t *is an isomorphism.*[1]

It is known that Conjecture A4.4 is true if $\mathcal{F}$ is defined by a free action of a simply connected solvable Lie group on X; see [Connes 1982]. Also, for flows on the 2-torus and for certain "Reeb foliations" of three-manifolds, the work of Torpe [1985] and Penington [1983] shows that conjecture A4.4 holds.

Given a foliated manifold X with both FX and TX orientable, a natural problem, related to Conjecture A4.4, is to determine to what extent the composition

$$K_*(X) \xrightarrow[\cong]{\text{Thom}} K_*^{\xi}(X) \longrightarrow K_*^{\xi}(BG(X)) \xrightarrow{\operatorname{Ind}_t} K_*(C_r^*(X))$$

is an isomorphism. We describe three quite general results on this, and then show that the $\bar{\partial}$-Index Theorem also sheds some light on this problem in particular cases.

Let G be a connected Lie group. A locally free action of G on X is *almost free* if given $g \in G$ with fixed point $x \in X$, either $g = \mathrm{id}$ or the germ of the action of g near x is nontrivial. If $\mathcal{F}$ is defined by an almost free action of G on X, then $G(X) \cong X \times G$. If G is also contractible, then $X \to BG(X)$ is a homotopy equivalence.

Theorem A4.5 [Connes 1982]. *Let* $\mathcal{F}$ *be defined by an almost free action of a simply connected solvable Lie group* G *on* X*. Then there is a natural isomorphism* $K_*(X) \cong K_*(C_r^*(X))$.

For $B^p = \Gamma \backslash G/K$ a locally symmetric space of rank one with negative sectional curvatures, there is a natural action of the lattice Γ on the sphere at infinity ($\cong S^{p-1}$) of the universal cover G/K. The manifold

$$M = (G/K \times S^{p-1})/\Gamma$$

can be identified with the unit tangent bundle T^1B. The foliation of M of codimension $q = p-1$ defined in Chapter II corresponds here with the Anosov (= weak stable) foliation of T^1B.

Theorem A4.6 [Takai 1986]. *The index yields an isomorphism*

$$K_*(M) \cong K_*(C_r^*(M)).$$

---

[1] We have been told that this conjecture is still open as of 2004.

For B a surface of genus ≥ 2, this result is due to Connes [1982, Chapter 12].

The third result deals with the characteristic classes of C^∞-foliations. Recall from above that each class $[z] \in H^*(WO_q)$ defines a linear functional $\Delta_*[z]$ on $H_*(X)$. Connes [1986] has shown that $[z]$ also defines a linear functional on $K_*(C_r^*(X))$, and these functionals are natural with respect to the map

$$H_*(X) \to K_*(C_r^*(X)).$$

From this one concludes:

Theorem A4.7 [Connes 1986]. *Suppose there exist*

$$[z] \in H^*(WO_n) \quad \text{and} \quad [u] \in H_*(X)$$

such that $\Delta_*[z]([u])$ does not vanish. Then $[u]$ is mapped to a nontrivial class in $K_*(C_r^*(X))$.

Theorem A4.7 shows that the characteristic classes of $\mathcal{F}$ can be used to prove certain classes in $H_*(X)$ inject into $K_*(C_r^*(X))$.

After these generalities, we consider foliations of three-manifolds with an invariant measure ν given, and study the ν-topological index, $\mathrm{Ind}_\nu^t(u)$, for $u \in K_1(X)$, which calculates the composition

$$K_1(X) \to K_0^\xi(X) \cong K^1(F_1^*X) \xrightarrow{\mathrm{Ind}_\nu^a} \mathbb{R}.$$

First, here is a general statement for such foliations. Recall that a simple closed curve in γ in X transverse to $\mathcal{F}$ determines a complex line bundle E_γ over $\mathcal{F}$ with divisor $[\gamma]$. Take $\bar\partial$ along leaves and form $\bar\partial \otimes E_\gamma$; this gives a map

$$H_1(X;Z) \to K^1(F_1^*X)$$
$$[\gamma] \mapsto [\bar\partial \otimes E_\gamma]$$

and composing with Ind_a yields a map

$$\mathrm{Ind} : H_1(X;Z) \to K_0(C_r^*(X)).$$

Proposition A4.8. *Let $\mathcal{F}$ be a codimension-one C^1-foliation of a compact three-manifold X. Assume both TX and FX are orientable.*

(a) *Suppose ν is an invariant transverse measure with $C_\nu \neq 0$ in $H_2(X;\mathbb{R})$, and the support of ν does not consist of isolated toral leaves. (A toral leaf L is isolated if no closed transverse curve to $\mathcal{F}$ intersects L.) Then there exists a holomorphic line bundle $E \to X$ such that* $\mathrm{Ind}_\nu(\bar\partial \otimes E)$, *and thus* $\mathrm{Ind}(\bar\partial \otimes E) \in K_0(C_r^*(X))$, *are nonzero.*

(b) *Let $\{\nu_1, \ldots, \nu_d\}$ be a collection of invariant transverse measures such that the associated currents $\{C_1, \ldots, C_d\} \subset H_2(X;\mathbb{R})$ are linearly independent when evaluated on closed transversals to $\mathcal{F}$. Then there exist* *holomorphic line bundles $E_1, \ldots, E_d$ over X such that the elements*

$$\{\mathrm{Ind}(\bar{\partial} \otimes E_i) \mid i = 1, \ldots, d\} \subset K_0(C_r^*(X))$$

are linearly independent.

For example, it is not hard to show that if $\mathcal{F}$ has a dense leaf and the currents $\{C_1, \ldots, C_d\} \subset H_2(X; \mathbb{R})$ of part (b) are independent, then they are independent on closed transversals. Define $H(\Lambda) \subset H_2(X; \mathbb{R})$ to be the subspace spanned by the currents associated to the invariant measures for $\mathcal{F}$.

Corollary A4.9. *If $\mathcal{F}$ has a dense leaf, there is an inclusion*

$$H(\Lambda) \subset K_0(C_r^*(X)) \otimes \mathbb{R}.$$

Proof of Proposition A4.8. First assume there is a closed transverse curve γ to $\mathcal{F}$ which intersects the support of ν. Then $\nu(\gamma) \neq 0$, and we define $E = E_{n \cdot \gamma}$ and use (A3.4) to calculate

$$\mathrm{Ind}_\nu(\bar{\partial} \otimes E_{n \cdot \gamma}) \neq 0$$

for all but at most one value of n. If no such curve γ exists, then the support of ν must consist of compact leaves. One can show these leaves must be tori which are isolated and this contradicts the hypothesis that there is a nonisolated toral leaf in the support of ν. This proves (a). The proof of (b) is similar. □

A5. Examples of Complex Foliations of Three-Manifolds

The geometry of foliations on three-manifolds has been intensively studied. In this section, we select four classes of these foliations for study, and consider the $\bar{\partial}$-index theorem for each. Let M be a compact oriented Riemannian three-manifold. Then M admits a nonvanishing vector field, and this vector field is homotopic to the normal field of some codimension one foliation of M. Moreover, M even has uncountably many codimension one foliations which are distinct up to diffeomorphism and concordance; see [Thurston 1974]. This abundance of foliations on three-manifolds makes their study especially appealing.

There are exactly two simply connected solvable Lie groups of dimension two, the abelian group R^2 and the solvable affine group on the line.

$$A^2 = \left\{ \begin{pmatrix} x & y \\ 0 & x^{-1} \end{pmatrix} \middle| \; x > 0 \right\} \subset \mathrm{SL}(2, \mathbb{R}).$$

A locally free action of R^2 or A^2 on a three-manifold M defines a codimension one foliation with very special properties. The foliations defined by an action of R^2 have been completely classified: see the next two pages. For $\pi_1 M$ solvable, the locally free actions of A^2 on M have been classified in [Ghys and Sergiescu 1980] and [Plante 1975]; see pages 245–247. For $\pi_1 M$ not solvable, some restrictions on the possible A^2-actions are known.

Note that Connes' Theorem A4.5 applies only when $\mathcal{F}$ is defined by an almost free action of R^2 or A^2. This assumption does not always hold in the following examples, so we must use the geometry of $\mathcal{F}$ to help calculate the image of the index map.

Throughout, M will denote a closed, oriented Riemannian three-manifold and $\mathcal{F}$ an oriented two-dimensional foliation of M.

Locally free $\mathbb{R}^2$-actions. Let $a \in \mathrm{SL}(2, \mathbb{Z})$, which defines a diffeomorphism $\phi_a : T^2 \to T^2$, and a torus bundle over S^1 by setting

$$M_a = T^2 \times \mathbb{R}/(x,t) \sim (\phi_a(x), t+1).$$

Theorem A5.1 [Rosenberg et al. 1970]. *Suppose M admits a locally free action of R^2. Then M is diffeomorphic to M_a for some $a \in \mathrm{SL}(2, \mathbb{Z})$.*

For $\mathcal{F}$ defined by an R^2-action. $\pi_1 M$ is solvable by Theorem A5.1 and $\mathcal{F}$ has no Reeb components. The foliated three-manifolds with $\pi_1 M$ solvable and no Reeb components have been completely classified by Plante [1979, 4.1]: note that only his cases II, III or V are possible for an R^2-action).

For $\pi_1 M$ solvable, there is also a classification of the invariant measures for any $\mathcal{F}$ on M:

Theorem A5.2 (Plante–Thurston). *If $\pi_1 M$ is solvable and $\mathcal{F}$ is transversally oriented, the space $H(\Lambda) \subset H_2(M)$ of foliation cycles has real dimension* 1.

For $\mathcal{F}$ defined by an R^2-action, this implies there is a unique nontrivial projective class of cycles in $H_2(M)$ which arise from invariant transverse measures. Fix such an invariant measure ν.

For the d-index theorem, evaluation on C_ν yields the average Euler characteristic of the leaves in the support of ν. These leaves are covered by R^2, hence have average Euler characteristics zero, and T_ν annihilates the class $\mathrm{Ind}(d)$.

For the operator $\bar{\partial}$, we use formula (A3.4) to construct holomorphic bundles over M for which $T_\nu \circ \mathrm{Ind}(\bar{\partial} \otimes E) \neq 0$. The number of such bundles is controlled by the *period mapping* of ν. This is a homomorphism $P_\nu : H_1(M; \mathbb{Z}) \to \mathbb{R}$ defined as $P_\nu(\alpha) = \nu(\gamma)$, where γ is a simple closed curve representing the homology class α. The rank of its image is called the *rank* of $(\mathcal{F}, \nu)$, denoted by $r(\mathcal{F})$. Note that $1 \le r(\mathcal{F}) \le 3$.

Proposition A5.3. *The elements $\mathrm{Ind}(\bar{\partial} \otimes E) \in K_0(C_r^*(X))$, for $E \to M$ a holomorphic line bundle, generate a subgroup with rank at least $r(\mathcal{F})$.*

Proof. For each $\alpha \in \pi_1 M$ with $P_\nu(\alpha) \neq 0$, choose a simple closed curve γ in M representing α and transverse to $\mathcal{F}$. This is possible by Theorem A5.1 and the known structure of R^2-actions. Then take $E = E_\gamma$ as in Section A3 to obtain

$$T_\nu \circ \mathrm{Ind}(\bar{\partial} \otimes E) = \langle \mathrm{ch}(E), C_\nu \rangle = \nu(\gamma) = P_\nu(\gamma).$$

This shows the map T_ν is onto the image of P_ν. □

It is easy to see that $r(\mathcal{F}) = 3$ if and only if $\mathcal{F}$ is a foliation by planes. This coincides with the R^2-action being free, and then one knows by Theorem A4.5 that

$$\alpha \mapsto \operatorname{Ind}(\bar{\partial} \otimes E_\gamma)$$

is an isomorphism from $H_2(M; Z)$ onto the summand of $K_0(C_r^*(M))$ corresponding to the image of $H_2(M; \mathbb{Z}) \subset K_0(M) \cong K_0(C_r^*(M))$.

An $\mathbb{R}^2$-action on a nilmanifold. Let N_3 be the nilpotent group of strictly triangular matrices in $\mathrm{GL}(3, \mathbb{R})$:

$$N_3 = \left\{ \begin{pmatrix} 1 & a & b \\ 0 & 1 & c \\ 0 & 0 & 1 \end{pmatrix} \text{ such that } a, b, c \in \mathbb{R} \right\}.$$

For each integer $n > 0$, define a lattice subgroup

$$\Gamma_n = \left\{ \begin{pmatrix} 1 & p & r/n \\ 0 & 1 & q \\ 0 & 0 & 1 \end{pmatrix} \text{ such that } p, q, r \in \mathbb{Z} \right\}.$$

Then $M = N_3/\Gamma_n$ is a compact oriented three-manifold, and the subgroup

$$R^2 = \left\{ \begin{pmatrix} 1 & a & b \\ 0 & 1 & 0 \\ 0 & 0 & 1 \end{pmatrix} \right\}$$

acts almost freely on M via left translations. Also note M is a circle bundle over T^2, and $H_2(M; \mathbb{R}) \cong \mathbb{R}^2$. By Theorem A4.5, the index map is an isomorphism, so $K_0(C_r^*(M)) \cong \mathbb{Z}^3$. The curve representing the homology class of

$$\alpha = \begin{pmatrix} 1 & 0 & 0 \\ 0 & 1 & 1 \\ 0 & 0 & 1 \end{pmatrix} \in \pi_1 M$$

is transverse to $\mathcal{F}$ and $P_\nu(\alpha) \neq 0$ for a transverse measure ν with $C_\nu \neq 0$. However, $\operatorname{Ind}(\bar{\partial} \otimes E_\gamma)$ cannot detect the contribution to $K_0(C_r^*(M))$ from the curve defined by a fibre of $M \to T^2$.

Foliations without holonomy. If for every leaf L of a foliation, $\mathcal{F}$, the holonomy along each closed loop in L is trivial, then we say $\mathcal{F}$ is without holonomy. In codimension-one, such foliations can be effectively classified up to topological equivalence. We discuss this for the case of C^2-foliations. By Sacksteder's Theorem [Lawson 1977], a codimension-one, C^2-foliation without holonomy of a compact manifold admits a transverse invariant measure ν whose support is all of M. Moreover, there is foliation-preserving homeomorphism between M and a model foliated space,

$$X = (\widetilde{B} \times S^1)/\Gamma,$$

where Γ is the fundamental group of a compact manifold B, $\widetilde{B}$ is its universal cover with Γ acting via deck translations, and Γ acts on S^1 via a representation

$$\exp(2\pi i \rho) : \Gamma \to \mathrm{SO}(2),$$

for $\rho : \Gamma \to \mathbb{R}$. The foliation of X by sheets $\widetilde{B} \times \{\theta\}$ has a canonical invariant measure, $d\theta$, and ν corresponds to $d\theta$ under the homeomorphism. Since the index invariants are topological, in this case we can assume that M is one of these models. For a three-manifold this implies $B = \Sigma_g$ for Σ_g a surface of genus $g \geq 1$. The case $g = 1$ is a special case of examples (A5.1) above.

Let Λ denote the abelian subgroup of $\mathbb{R}$ which is the image of ρ. Denote by $r(\mathcal{F})$ the rank of Λ. It is an easy geometrical exercise to see that the group Λ agrees with the image of the evaluation map

$$[d\theta] : H_1(M; Z) \to \mathbb{R}.$$

Moreover, there exists simple closed curves $\{\gamma_1, \ldots, \gamma_r\}$ in M transverse to $\mathcal{F}$ for which $\{P_\nu(\gamma_i)\}$ yields a $\mathbb{Z}$-basis for Γ. Form the holomorphic bundles $\{E_i\}$ corresponding to the $\{\gamma_i\}$, then the set $\{\mathrm{Ind}(\bar{\partial} \otimes E_i)\}$ generates a free subgroup of rank r in $K_0(C_r^*(M))$. Since $H_2(BG(M); \mathbb{R})$ has rank r, this implies

Proposition A5.4. *The index map*

$$K_0^\tau(BG(M)) \to K_0(C_r^*(M))$$

is a monomorphism.

These foliations have been analyzed in further detail by Natsume [1985], where he shows that this map is also a surjection.

Solvable group actions. The locally free actions of A^2 on three-manifolds has been studied by many authors; see in particular [Ghys and Sergiescu 1980; Ghys 1984; 1985; 1993]:

Theorem A5.5. *Let $\pi_1 M$ be solvable and suppose A^2 acts on M. Then M is diffeomorphic to a torus bundle M_a over S^1, and the monodromy map $a \in$ $\mathrm{SL}(2, \mathbb{R})$ has two distinct real eigenvalues.*

Theorem A5.6 [Ghys 1985]. *Suppose that A^2 acts locally free on M and preserves a smooth volume form. Then M is diffeomorphic to $\mathrm{SL}(2, \mathbb{R})/\Gamma$ for some cocompact lattice in the universal covering group*

$$\widetilde{\mathrm{SL}(2, \mathbb{R})},$$

and the action of A^2 on M is via left translations.

Proposition A5.7. *Suppose $H_1(M) = 0$ and A^2 acts locally freely on M. Then the action preserves a smooth volume form on M.*

Let us describe the foliation on $M_0 = T^2 \times \mathbb{R}/\phi_a$. Let $\bar{v} \in \mathbb{R}^2$ be an eigenvalue with eigenvalue $\lambda > 0$. The foliation of $\mathbb{R}^3$ by planes parallel to the span of $\{(\bar{v} \times 0), (\bar{0} \times 1)\}$ is invariant under the covering transformations of $\mathbb{R}^3 \to M_a$, so descends to a foliation $\mathcal{F}_\lambda$ on M_a. When $\lambda = 1$, the R^2-action on $\mathbb{R}^3$ defining the foliation there descends to an $\mathbb{R}^2$ action on M_a, defining $\mathcal{F}_\lambda$. When $\lambda \neq 1$, the leaves of $\mathcal{F}_\lambda$ are defined by an action of A^2 on M_a.

For A^2-actions on M with $\pi_1 M$ not solvable, it seems reasonable to conjecture they must have this form given in Theorem A5.6.

If the action of A^2 preserves a volume form on M^3, then $\mathcal{F}$ is transversally affine [Ghys and Sergiescu 1980], so there can be no invariant measures for $\mathcal{F}$. In this case Theorem 8.7 of Chapter VIII reveals no information about $K_0(C_r^*(M))$. However, one has Connes' Theorem A4.5 since the A^2-action is almost free. To give an illustration, let $\Gamma \subset \mathrm{SL}(2,\mathbb{R})$ be a cocompact lattice, and set $M = \mathrm{SL}(2,\mathbb{R})/\Gamma$. The group A^2 acts via left translations and preserves a smooth volume form on M. Then

$$G(M) \cong M \times A^2,$$

$$K_0^\tau(BG(M)) \cong K^0(M),$$

and

$$\mathrm{Ind} : K_0^\tau(BG(M)) \to K_0(C_r^*(M))$$

is an isomorphism. Note the foliation on M admits $2g$ closed transversals $\{\gamma_1, \dots, \gamma_{2g}\}$ which span $H_1(M)$. Form the corresponding bundles $E_i \to M$, and consider the classes $\{\mathrm{Ind}(\bar{\partial} \otimes E_i)\} \subset K_0(C_r^*(M))$. It is natural to ask whether these classes are linearly independent, and for a geometric proof if so.

Foliations with all leaves proper. A leaf $L \subset M$ is *proper* if it is locally closed in M. $\mathcal{F}$ is proper if every leaf is proper. The geometric theory of codimension-one proper foliations is highly developed [Cantwell and Conlon 1981; Hector and Hirsch 1986]. We recall a few general facts relevant to our discussion.

Theorem A5.8. *Let $\mathcal{F}$ be a proper foliation of arbitrary codimension. Then the quotient measure space $M/\mathcal{F}$, endowed with the Lebesgue measure from M, is a standard Borel space.*

Corollary A5.9. *Let $\mathcal{F}$ be a proper foliation of arbitrary codimension. Then any ergodic invariant transverse measure for $\mathcal{F}$ with finite total mass is supported on a compact leaf.*

Theorem A5.10. *For a codimension one proper foliation $\mathcal{F}$, all leaves of $\mathcal{F}$ have polynomial growth, and the closure of each leaf of $\mathcal{F}$ contains a compact leaf.*

Let $\mathcal{F}$ be a proper codimension-one foliation of M^3. Given a transverse invariant measure ν, we can assume without loss of generality that the support of ν is a compact leaf L. If L has genus at least 2, then there exists a closed transversal γ which intersects L, so $T_\nu \circ \mathrm{Ind}(\bar\partial \otimes E_{n\cdot\gamma}) \neq 0$ for all but at most one value of n. Thus, the class

$$[L] \in H_2(M; Z)$$

corresponds to a nontrivial class

$$\mathrm{Ind}(\bar\partial \otimes E_{n\cdot\gamma}) \in K_0(C_r^*(M)).$$

If L is a 2-torus, then it is difficult to tell whether the homology class of L is nonzero, and if so, whether it generates a nonzero class in $K_0(C_r^*(M))$. There is a geometric criterion which yields an answer.

Theorem A5.11 (Rummler–Sullivan). *Suppose M admits a metric for which each leaf of $\mathcal{F}$ is a minimal surface. Then every compact leaf of $\mathcal{F}$ has a closed transversal which intersects it.*

Corollary A5.12. *Suppose $\mathcal{F}$ is a proper and minimal foliation. For each ergodic invariant transverse measure ν, there is a holomorphic bundle $E_\nu \to M$ such that* $\mathrm{Ind}(\bar\partial \otimes E_\nu) \in K_0(C_r^*(M))$ *is nonzero, and* $\mathrm{Ind}_\nu(\bar\partial \otimes E_\nu) \neq 0$.

We cannot conclude from Corollary A5.12 that the elements

$$\{\mathrm{Ind}(\bar\partial \otimes E_\nu) \mid \nu \text{ ergodic}\}$$

are independent. (Consider the product foliation $\Sigma_g \times S^1$.) However, if M has a metric for which every leaf is geodesic submanifold, then there are as many independent classes in $K_0(C_r^*(M))$ as there are independent currents $C_\nu \in H_2(M; \mathbb{R})$.

The Reeb foliation of S^3 is another relevant example of a proper foliation. It is not minimal, and $K_0(C_r^*(M)) \cong \mathbb{Z}$ so the toral leaf does not contribute; see [Penington 1983; Torpe 1985].

Foliations with nonzero Godbillon–Vey class. There is exactly one characteristic class for codimension-one foliations (of differentiability at least C^2), the Godbillon–Vey class $GV \in H^3(M; \mathbb{R})$. Recall from Section A4 that GV defines linear functionals, also denoted by GV, on $K_*(M)$ and (noncanonically) on $K_*(C_r^*(M))$,[2] and these functionals agree under the map

$$K_*(M) \to K_*(C_r^*(M)).$$

If $GV \neq 0$ in $H^3(M)$, then there is a class $[u] \in K_*(C_r^*(M))$ on which GV is nontrivial. From this we conclude that the composition

$$H_3(M; Z) \to K_1^{\xi}(BG(M)) \to K_0(C_r^*(M))$$

is injective.

[2]The map $GV : K_*(C_r^*(M)) \to \mathbb{R}$ depends upon the choice of a smooth dense subalgebra of $C_r^*(M)$.

The information on $K_1(C_r^*(M))$ obtained from GV is about all one knows for these foliations $\mathcal{F}_\alpha$ on M, which underlines the need for better understanding of how the geometry of a foliation is related to the analytic invariants in $K_0(C_r^*(M))$.

□ □□□□□ □□□□

Since the first edition of this book, there have been great advances in understanding the relationship between the foliation indices and the geometry of $\mathcal{F}$. We mention in particular the works of Hitoshi Moriyoshi, who has given a very explicit description of the Godbillon–Vey invariant as an analytic invariant [Moriyoshi 1994a; 1994b; 2002, Moriyoshi and Natsume 1996].

APPENDIX B

L^2 Harmonic Forms on Noncompact Manifolds

By Calvin C. Moore, Claude Schochet, and Robert J. Zimmer

If M is a compact oriented manifold then the Hodge theorem supplies a unique harmonic form associated to each de Rham cohomology class of M. If the compactness assumption is dropped the situation becomes considerably more sensitive. In this appendix we demonstrate how to use the index theorem for foliated spaces to produce L^2 harmonic forms on the leaves of certain foliated spaces.

We begin by recalling the Hirzebruch signature theorem. If M is a compact oriented manifold of dimension $4r$ then its signature is defined to be the signature of the bilinear form on $H^{2r}(M)$ given by

$$(x, y) = \int_M x \wedge y.$$

Recall that there is a signature operator A (Chapter VIII), and the signature of the manifold, Sign M, is the Fredholm index of this operator. If M has positive signature then $H^{2r}(M)$ must be nontrivial and must contain classes represented by harmonic forms, by Hodge theory. (An easy special case: take $M^{4r} = \mathbb{C}P^{2r}$. Then Sign $M = 1$, $H^{2r}(M) = \mathbb{R}$ and so $\mathbb{C}P^{2r}$ has harmonic forms in its middle dimension $2r$.)

Let X denote a compact metrizable foliated space with leaves of dimension $4r$ and oriented foliation bundle F. Then there is a signature operator $A = \{A_\ell\}$ with local trace denoted here by $a = \{a_\ell\}$ and associated partial Chern character

$$c(a) = [a] \in \bar{H}^{4r}_\tau(X).$$

For each invariant transverse measure ν we define the signature of X by

$$\mathrm{Sign}(X, \nu) = \langle [a], [C_\nu] \rangle = \int_X a_\ell \, d\nu,$$

where C_ν is the Ruelle–Sullivan current associated to ν. This is independent of the metric chosen but of course does depend upon ν. The foliated space version of the signature theorem states that $[a] = [L_r]$, where L_r is the Hirzebruch L-polynomial in the tangential Pontryagin classes of F. If $\mathrm{Sign}(X, \nu) > 0$ then there are ν-nontrivial L^2 harmonic $2r$-forms on X (that is to say, there are nonzero L^2 harmonic $2r$-forms on some of the leaves of X, and the support of ν is positive on the union of these leaves).

Here is our first result.

Theorem B.1. *Suppose that X is a compact oriented foliated space with leaves of dimension 4. Assume that X has a tangential Riemannian structure so that each leaf is isometric to the complex 2-disk B^2 (with its Poincaré metric). Let ν be an invariant transverse measure on X. Then* $\mathrm{Sign}(X, \nu) > 0$.

Corollary B.2. *The space X cannot be written as a product of foliated spaces.*

This also follows from the (significantly more general) assertions of [Zimmer 1983].

Corollary B.3. *The space B^2 has nontrivial L^2 harmonic 2-forms.*

Remark. This is actually a corollary of the proof that follows. It may be enough to assume that each leaf of X is quasi-isometric to B^2.

Our proof of B.1 is somewhat roundabout. First we prove B.1 in a very special case in the setting of automorphic forms. Then we prove the corollaries. Finally we deduce the general case of B.1 from Corollary B.3. The foliated spaces index theorem is used twice, in different directions.

Proof. Consider the following special case. Let G be a group of holomorphic automorphisms of B^2, let Γ be a cocompact torsionfree lattice in G, and let K be a maximal compact subgroup of G. Then B^2 is isometric to the homogeneous space G/K. The quotient space B^2/Γ is a compact complex manifold of real dimension 4. We assume that it is oriented. The lattice Γ may be chosen so that $\mathrm{Sign}(B^2/\Gamma)$ is strictly positive; we assume this to be the case.

Let S be a smooth manifold upon which Γ acts without fixed points and suppose that S has a finite Γ-invariant measure μ. (For instance, take $S = G/\Gamma'$ for some suitable lattice Γ'.) Define an action of Γ on $B^2 \times S$ by

$$(b, s)\gamma = (b\gamma, s\gamma)$$

and let

$$X = (B^2 \times S)/\Gamma$$

denote the resulting orbit space. Then X is a compact space foliated by the images of the various maps

$$B^2 \times \{s\} \to B^2 \times S \to X$$

so each leaf is isometric to B^2. There is a natural projection

$$\pi : X \to B^2/\Gamma$$

given by sending (b, s) to the image of b under the map $B^2 \to B^2/\Gamma$. The restriction of π to each leaf ℓ is a covering map $\ell \to B^2/\Gamma$. The tangent bundle

F to the foliated space is simply the pullback of the tangent bundle of (the manifold) B^2/Γ by π.

Let us compare the signature theorems on X and on B^2/Γ. The Hirzebruch signature theorem (in this low-dimensional situation) reads

$$\operatorname{Sign}(B^2/\Gamma) = \int \tfrac{1}{3} p_1(T(B^2/\Gamma)^*)\,\mathrm{dvol}$$

where dvol is the volume form on B^2/Γ and p_1 is the first Pontryagin class. The Connes signature theorem applied to the signature operator A with respect to the invariant transverse measure ν corresponding to the invariant measure μ on S reads

$$\operatorname{Sign}(X, \nu) = \int \tfrac{1}{3} p_1^\tau(F^*)\,d\nu.$$

As $F = \pi^*(T(B^2/\Gamma))$ and p_1 projects to p_1^τ under the map from de Rham to tangential cohomology, we have

$$\operatorname{Sign}(B^2/\Gamma) = \int \tfrac{1}{3}\pi_1(T(B^2/\Gamma)^*)\,\mathrm{dvol} = \int \tfrac{1}{3} p_1^\tau(F^*)\,d\nu = \operatorname{Sign}(X, \nu),$$

so that

$$\operatorname{Sign}(X, \nu) = \operatorname{Sign}(B^2/\Gamma) > 0.$$

Thus $\operatorname{Sign}(X, \nu)$ is strictly positive, and in fact is a positive integer (if we properly normalize μ originally). This proves the theorem for this particular class of foliated spaces.

Next we establish Corollary B.3. By the definition of $\operatorname{Sign}(X, \nu)$ we see that

$$\int a_\ell\,d\nu > 0$$

in our example above. Now each leaf ℓ is isometric to B^2 and the measure a_ℓ is the local trace of the signature operator on B^2, so that in this example the measure a_ℓ really does not depend upon ℓ. As

$$a_\ell = \operatorname{Ker}(A_\ell) - \operatorname{Ker}(A_\ell^*)$$

as signed measures, we see that $\operatorname{Ker}(A_\ell)$ must be nontrivial for some leaves ℓ; thus the space B^2 must have nontrivial L^2 harmonic 2-forms. This proves Corollary B.3.

We turn next to the general case of Theorem B.1. Let X be a compact foliated space as in the statement of the theorem. Then the local trace $a = \{a_\ell\}$ of the signature operator is independent of the leaf ℓ. Thus

$$\operatorname{Sign}(X, \nu) = \int a_\ell\,d\nu > 0$$

by our earlier argument. Apply the foliation index theorem again (in the opposite direction) and we see that

$$\int \tfrac{1}{3} p_1^\tau(F^*)\, dv > 0$$

which implies that the class $[p_1^\tau(F^*)] \neq 0$ in $\overline{H}_\tau^4(X)$.

Finally, X cannot split as a product of foliated spaces since that would imply that $\mathrm{Sign}(X, \nu) = 0$. This completes the proof of B.1, B.2, and B.3. □

In order to generalize, one need only look at those properties of B^2 which were actually used in the proof. The key fact was that there was a lattice group Γ such that $B^2 \to B^2/\Gamma$ was well-behaved, and such that B^2/Γ was a compact manifold with positive signature.

Definition B.4. A *Clifford–Klein form* of a connected and simply connected Riemannian manifold B is a Riemannian manifold B' whose universal Riemannian covering is isomorphic to B.

A. Borel [1963] has shown that a simply connected Riemannian symmetric space B always has a compact Clifford–Klein form. Let $\mathbb{B}$ be the collection of spaces which are finite products of irreducible symmetric domains whose compact counterparts are

$$\frac{U(p+2r)}{U(p)\times U(2r)}, \quad \frac{\mathrm{SO}(4k+2)}{\mathrm{SO}(4k)\times \mathrm{SO}(2)}, \quad \text{or} \quad \frac{E_6}{\mathrm{Spin}(10)\times T^1}.$$

The space B^2 is in $\mathbb{B}$ since B^2 is associated to the space

$$\frac{U(3)}{U(1)\times U(2)} \cong \mathbb{C}\mathrm{P}^2.$$

If B is a simply connected Riemannian symmetric space then there are two possibilities:

(1) If B is not an element of $\mathbb{B}$ then $\mathrm{Sign}(B') = 0$.

(2) If $B \in \mathbb{B}$ then $\mathrm{Sign}(B') \geq 1$, by [Borel 1963, §3].

This is all that we need.

Theorem B.5. *Let X be a compact oriented foliated space with leaves of dimension p. Suppose that X has a tangential Riemannian structure such that each leaf is isometric to some fixed $B \in \mathbb{B}$. Then* $\mathrm{Sign}(X, \nu) > 0$ *for each invariant transverse measure ν.*

Corollary B.6. *If $B \in \mathbb{B}$ is a manifold of dimension $4r$, then B has nontrivial L^2 harmonic $2r$-forms.*

We omit the proof, which is essentially the same as the special case $B = B^2$.

We turn next to the use of the Chern–Gauss–Bonnet theorem. Recall that if X is a compact oriented foliated space with leaves of dimension $2q$ then the Index Theorem applied to the de Rham operator yields

$$[\chi] = [K_\tau]/2\pi$$

in $\bar{H}^*_\tau(X)$, where χ is the alternating sum of the Betti measures 8.7. Given an invariant transverse measure ν, the theorem reads

$$\chi(X,\nu) = \int K_\tau/2\pi \, d\nu,$$

where

$$\chi(X,\nu) = \int \chi \, d\nu$$

is the tangential Euler characteristic of (X,ν).

Suppose that G is a semisimple Lie group with maximal compact subgroup K and torsionfree lattice Γ. Let S be some compact smooth manifold upon which Γ acts without fixed points and let μ be a finite Γ-invariant measure on S. Let $B = G/K$ and define

$$X = (B \times S)/\Gamma$$

where Γ acts diagonally. Then X is a foliated manifold with leaves corresponding to the image of $B \times \{s\}$. The space B/Γ is a compact smooth manifold and each leaf ℓ is a covering space for B/Γ. The space X has an invariant transverse measure ν corresponding to the measure μ on the global transversal S. For instance, if $G = \mathrm{PSL}(2,\mathbb{R})$ then B is the upper half plane H and X is foliated by copies of H. (Note that H has constant negative curvature — it is homeomorphic but not isometric to $\mathbb{C}$.)

The Euler characteristic of B/Γ is given by the classical Chern–Gauss–Bonnet theorem:

$$\chi(B/\Gamma) = \int K/2\pi \, \mathrm{dvol},$$

where K is the curvature form on B/Γ and dvol is the volume form on B/Γ.

Specialize to the case where each leaf has dimension 2. The Betti measure β_0 is always zero since there are no L^2 harmonic functions on noncompact manifolds. Duality implies that $\beta_2 = 0$. Thus the foliation Chern–Gauss–Bonnet theorem reduces to

$$\int -\beta_1 \, d\nu = \int K_\tau/2\pi \, d\nu$$

where K_τ is the Gauss curvature along the leaves. Arguing just as in the proof of the special case of Theorem B.1, we see that

$$\chi(B/\Gamma) = \int K/2\pi \, \mathrm{dvol} = \int K_\tau/2\pi \, d\nu = \int -\beta_1 \, d\nu.$$

Assume that the surface B/Γ has genus greater than 2. Then $\chi(B/\Gamma)$ is negative and hence the Betti measure β_1 is strictly positive. Since leaves have dimension 2, we see that

$$\int \operatorname{Ker}(d \oplus d^*)_{(1-\text{forms})} > 0$$

In our example we are again integrating a constant function. Thus on the generic leaf $\ell = G/K$ there are nontrivial L^2 harmonic 1-forms.

If we continue as in the study of the signature operator, we can obtain the following theorem.

Theorem B.7. *Let X be a compact oriented foliated space with tangential Riemannian structure such that each leaf is isometric to the upper half plane. Let ν be an invariant transverse measure. Then the tangential Euler characteristic $\chi(X, \nu)$ is strictly positive and X has nontrivial L^2 harmonic 1-forms.*

Remark. If the leaves have dimension greater than 2 then β_1 does not correspond so neatly to the Euler characteristic. For example, if the leaves have dimension 4 and $\chi(B/\Gamma) \leq 0$ then

$$\int (-\beta_1 + \beta_2 - \beta_3)\, d\nu < 0$$

so that

$$\int \beta_2\, d\nu < \int (\beta_1 + \beta_3)\, d\nu.$$

As the left hand side is nonnegative, this implies that the integral of either β_1 or β_3 (and hence both of them, by duality) must be strictly positive. Thus there are L^2 harmonic 1 and 3-forms.

APPENDIX C

Positive Scalar Curvature Along the Leaves

By Robert J. Zimmer

Mikhael Gromov and Blaine Lawson, in their classic paper [1980], use Dirac operators with coefficients in appropriate bundles and associated topological invariants to investigate whether or not a given compact nonsimply connected manifold can support a metric of positive scalar curvature. In this appendix we consider the analogous problem for foliated spaces. We use appropriate tangential Dirac operators to investigate the existence of a tangential Riemannian metric with positive scalar curvature along the leaves of a compact foliated space. Gromov and Lawson use the $\hat{A}$-genus and the Atiyah–Singer index theorem; we shall use the tangential $\hat{A}$-genus and the Connes index theorem.

Let M be a compact oriented manifold of dimension $p = 2d$ with associated Hirzebruch $\hat{A}$-class, $\hat{A}(M) \in H^{\text{even}}(M, \mathbb{R})$, a polynomial in the Pontryagin classes. If M is a spin manifold, then there are the associated bundles of half-spinors $S^{\pm}(M)$, and an associated Dirac operator

$$D^{+} : \Gamma^{\infty}(S^{+}) \to \Gamma^{\infty}(S^{-}).$$

The Atiyah–Singer theorem implies that index (D^{+}) vanishes unless p is divisible by 4, and in that case

$$\text{index } (D^{+}) = \hat{A}[M],$$

where $\hat{A}[M]$ is the $\hat{A}$-genus of M, i.e., $\hat{A}[M] = \langle \hat{A}(M), [M] \rangle$. If E is any Hermitian bundle over M (with a unitary connection) then, following [Gromov and Lawson 1980], $S(M) \otimes E$ is called a *twisted spin bundle* over M. Associated to this bundle there is also an elliptic operator called the *twisted Dirac operator* D^{+}. The Atiyah–Singer theorem now implies that

$$\text{index } (D^{+}) = (-1)^{d} \langle \text{ch}(E)\hat{A}(M), [M] \rangle.$$

Suppose now that X is a compact foliated space with oriented foliation bundle F and invariant transverse measure ν. Suppose further that F is a spin foliation, i.e., F has a spin structure. Then there is an associated bundle of spinors and for each leaf ℓ an associated Dirac operator D_{ℓ}^{+} on the leaf and hence a tangentially elliptic operator $D^+ = \{D_\ell^+\}$. Then, by Connes' theorem,

$$\mathrm{Index}_\nu(D^+) = (-1)^d \langle \hat{A}_\tau(F), [C_\nu]\rangle,$$

where $[C_\nu]$ is the homology class of the Ruelle–Sullivan current associated to ν. Define

$$\hat{A}_\nu[X] = \langle \hat{A}_\tau(F), [C_\nu]\rangle,$$

the *tangential $\hat{A}$-genus* of X with respect to the invariant transverse measure ν. Note that if Ker $D_\ell = 0$ as an unbounded operator on $L^2(\ell)$ for ν-almost every ℓ, then $\hat{A}_\nu[X] = 0$.

Choose some tangential Riemannian metric on X and let κ denote the scalar curvature along the leaves. We say that the metric has *positive scalar curvature on the leaf* ℓ if $\kappa \geq 0$ on ℓ and if $\kappa > 0$ at some point ℓ. If this is so, then by Lichnerowicz's computations, Ker $D_\ell^2 = 0$, and since we are in L^2 and D_ℓ is formally self-adjoint, Ker $D_\ell = 0$. Thus:

Proposition C.1. *Let X be a compact foliated space with foliation bundle F with a given spin structure, and let ν be an invariant transverse measure. If there exists a metric on X which has positive scalar curvature along ν-almost every leaf, then $\hat{A}_\nu[X] = 0$.*

Now suppose that E is an Hermitian bundle on X with a unitary tangential connection. For any leaf ℓ, let E_ℓ be the restriction of E to ℓ. Then there is a twisted spin bundle $S(F) \otimes E$ on X, and a twisted Dirac operator $D^+ = \{D_\ell^+\}$. Once again, Connes' theorem implies:

Proposition C.2. $\mathrm{Ind}_\nu(D^+) = \langle \mathrm{ch}_\tau(E)\hat{A}_\tau(F), [C_\nu]\rangle$.

Thus if $\mathrm{Ker}(D^+) = 0$, then $\langle \mathrm{ch}_\tau(E)\hat{A}_\tau(F), [C_\nu]\rangle = 0$.

For each leaf ℓ, the equation

$$D_\ell^2 = \nabla_\ell^* \nabla_\ell + \kappa/4 + (R_0)_\ell$$

holds where ∇ is a certain first order tangential operator, and R_0 is described in [Gromov and Lawson 1980, Theorem 1.3], in terms of the Clifford multiplication and the tangential curvature tensor of E_ℓ. An argument as in this same reference yields the following proposition.

Proposition C.3. *If $\kappa \geq 4(R_0)_\ell$ and $\kappa > r(R_0)_\ell$ at some point, then* Ker $D_\ell = 0$.

In particular, this would yield vanishing of $\langle \mathrm{ch}_\tau(E)\hat{A}_\tau(F), [C_\nu]\rangle$.

Definition C.4. Call a manifold M *expandable* if for each r, there is a smooth embedding of the Euclidean ball

$$e_r : B_r \to \widetilde{M}$$

(where $\widetilde{M}$ is the universal cover of M) such that

$$ae_r(v) \geq v \quad \text{for all } v \in TB_r.$$

Example C.5. The torus T^n is expandable.

Proposition C.6 (Gromov and Lawson).

(1) *A compact solvmanifold is expandable.*

(2) *A manifold of nonpositive curvature is expandable.*

Definition C.7 (slight modification of [Gromov and Lawson 1980]). We call a compact manifold M of dimension n *enlargeable* if for each $c > 0$ there is a finite covering $M' \to M$ and a c-contracting map $M' \to S^n$ of nonzero degree.

Proposition C.8. *Let M be a compact expandable manifold and suppose that $\pi_1(M)$ is residually finite. Then M is enlargeable.*

Theorem C.9 (Gromov and Lawson). *Suppose that M is an enlargeable manifold of even dimension and suppose that some finite cover of M is a spin manifold. Then M has no metric of positive scalar curvature.*

Corollary C.10. *No compact solvmanifold and no manifold of nonpositive curvature with a finite spin covering supports a metric of positive scalar curvature.*

We move to the context of foliated spaces.

Theorem C.11. *Let M be a compact enlargeable manifold of even dimension with a finite spin covering M'. Let $\pi_1(M)$ act on a space Y with an invariant measure ν (not necessarily smooth). Form the associated foliated bundle over M*

$$Y \to X = \tilde{M} \times_{\pi_1(M)} Y \to M$$

so that each leaf is the form $\tilde{M}/(\text{subgroup of } \pi_1(M))$. Then there is no tangential Riemannian metric on the foliated space X such that every leaf has everywhere positive scalar curvature.

Corollary C.12. *For a foliated bundle over any compact solvmanifold or over any manifold of nonpositive curvature with a finite spin cover, the result holds.*

Proof. For the solvmanifold case in odd dimension, cross with S^1 with the foliation (leaf) $\times S^1$ over solvmanifolds. □

Proof of Theorem C.11. Suppose that there were such a metric. Let $0 < \kappa_0 \leq \min \kappa$ on almost all leaves. Passing to finite covers yields the diagram

$$\begin{array}{ccccc} Y & \longrightarrow & X' & \longrightarrow & X \\ & & {\scriptstyle\rho}\downarrow & & \downarrow \\ & & M' & \longrightarrow & M \end{array}$$

with c-contracting map $f : M' \to S^{2n}$ of nonzero degree, where

$$c^2 < \kappa_0/\alpha$$

and α depends upon the dimension of M and data on a fixed Hermitian bundle $E_0 \to S^{2n}$ with $c_n(E_0) \neq 0$. Proposition C.3 and computation as in [Gromov and Lawson 1980, Proposition 3.1] imply that

$$\langle \mathrm{ch}_\tau(\rho^* f^* E_0)\hat{A}_\nu(F), [C_\nu]\rangle = 0.$$

Since

$$\mathrm{ch}_\tau(\rho^* f^* E_0) = \frac{1}{(n-1)!}\rho^* f^*(c_n^\tau(E_0)) + 1$$

and $\hat{A}_\nu[X] = 0$ by Proposition C.1, it follows that

$$\langle \rho^* f^* c_n^\tau(E_0), [C_\nu]\rangle = 0.$$

Since

$$\int_{S^{2n}} f^*(c_n^\tau(E_0)) \neq 0,$$

we use the basic computation that $\langle \rho^*\omega, [C_\nu]\rangle \neq 0$ for foliated bundles, where $\int \omega \neq 0$. This is a contradiction. □

Gromov and Lawson show in their Corollary A that any metric of nonnegative scalar curvature on the torus T^n is flat. That suggests the following conjectures.

Conjectures C.13.

(1) For foliations over T^n, $\kappa \geq 0$ along the leaves implies that $\kappa = 0$ along the leaves.

(2) (stronger) If $\kappa \geq 0$ then the leaves are Ricci flat, or even

(3) (still stronger) If $\kappa \geq 0$ then the leaves are flat.

Remark C.14. Kazdan and Warner [1975] have shown that, if M is a manifold with nonnegative scalar curvature and with $\kappa > 0$ at one point of M, then there is a conformal change in the metric of M such that $\kappa > 0$ everywhere on M. Suppose that X is a compact foliated space and suppose that X has positive scalar curvature along the leaves. Is it true that the metric on X may be altered so that $\kappa > 0$ everywhere? This may be done one leaf at a time; the difficulty lies in making the change continuous tranversely.

APPENDIX D

Gap Labeling

Featured Review, *Mathematical Reviews*, 2005f:46121

Note: This is a review of three articles: [Bellissard et al. 2005] (Jean Bellissard, Riccardo Benedetti and Jean-Marc Gambaudo, "Spaces of tilings, finite telescopic approximations, and gap-labeling", to appear in *Communications in Mathematical Physics*), [Benameur and Oyono-Oyono 2003] ("Gap-labelling for quasi-crystals", pp. 11–22 in *Operator algebras and mathematical physics*, Theta Foundation, Bucharest, 2003), and [Kaminker and Putnam 2003] ("A proof of the gap labeling conjecture", *Michigan Mathematical Journal* **51** (2003), 537–546). It first appeared as a Featured Review in *Mathematical Reviews*, and is reprinted here by permission, with slight modifications. The three reviewed articles are herein referred to as BBG, BO and KP.

The Gap Labeling Theorem was originally conjectured in [Bellissard et al. 2000]. The problem arises in a mathematical version of solid state physics in the context of aperiodic tilings. Its three proofs, discovered independently by the authors above, all lie in K-theory. Here is the core result of these papers:

Theorem D.1. *Let Σ be a Cantor set and let*

$$\Sigma \times \mathbb{Z}^d \longrightarrow \Sigma$$

be a free and minimal action of $\mathbb{Z}^d$ on Σ with invariant probability measure μ. Let

$$\mu : C(\Sigma) \longrightarrow \mathbb{C}$$

and

$$\tau_\mu : C(\Sigma) \rtimes \mathbb{Z}^d \longrightarrow \mathbb{C}$$

be the traces induced by μ and denote likewise their induced maps in K-theory. Then

$$\mu\big(K_0(C(\Sigma))\big) = \tau_\mu\big(K_0(C(\Sigma) \times \mathbb{Z}^d)\big)$$

as subsets of $\mathbb{R}$.

We shall try to explain why this core result has anything to do with something called gap labeling.

1. The Origin of the Problem. We model the motion of a particle in a solid via the tight binding approximation as follows. The solid is modeled by a tiling, where the tiles represent the locations of the atoms, and the particle hops from tile to tile. The (simplified!) quantum mechanical model of this motion is a certain self-adjoint Schrödinger operator on the space of square summable functions on the set of tiles. So the position of the particle is represented by a tile and momentum corresponds to translation. We are interested in the spectrum of this operator. In the crystal context, Bloch theory shows that the periodic structure of the atoms leads to a spectrum consisting of bands — i.e., a union of closed intervals, and hence there are gaps in the spectrum. The challenge in the present problem is to determine the gaps in the spectrum of the Schrödinger operator in a solid which is not periodic but is *almost* periodic.

More formally, a *tiling* T of $\mathbb{R}^d$ is a collection of subsets $\{t_1, t_2, \dots\}$ called tiles, such that their union is $\mathbb{R}^d$ and their interiors are pairwise disjoint. We assume that each tile is homeomorphic to a closed ball. Any translate $T + x$ of T by some $x \in \mathbb{R}^d$ is again a tiling. Take the set $T + \mathbb{R}^d$ of all translates and endow it with a metric: for $0 < \epsilon < 1$ say the distance between T_1 and T_2 in $T + \mathbb{R}^d$ is less than ϵ if there are vectors x_1, x_2 of length less than ϵ such that $T_1 + x_1$ and $T_2 + x_2$ coincide on the open ball $B(0, 1/\epsilon)$. Let Ω denote the closure of $T + \mathbb{R}^d$ in this metric. Then $\mathbb{R}^d$ acts on Ω; the action is denoted ω. The space Ω is the *continuous hull* of the tiling. This is the quick and dirty definition of the metric and Ω: there are much better and more natural definitions (see BBG).

We assume that for any $R > 0$ there are only finitely many subsets of T whose union has diameter less than R (the so-called *finite pattern condition*), which ensures that Ω is compact. The orbit of T is obviously dense. We assume that *every* orbit is dense: in other words, that the $\mathbb{R}^d$ action on Ω is minimal. This is the case if and only if for every finite patch P in T there is some $R > 0$ such that for each $x \in \mathbb{R}^d$ there is a translate of P contained in $T \cap B(x, R)$. This is called the *repetitivity* condition.

There is an equivalent version of this construction using the notion of repetitive Delone sets of finite type due to Lagarias. Bellissard, Zarrouati, and Hermann [Bellissard et al. 2000] replace a discrete point set by the sum of mass one Dirac measures at each site. The compactness of the hull is then a trivial consequence of well-known theorems in measure theory. This way of doing things is more natural from the point of view of the hull topology.

A tiling T is *aperiodic* if $T + x \neq T$ for all $x \in \mathbb{R}^d - \{0\}$, and a tiling is *strongly aperiodic* if Ω contains no periodic tilings. Assume henceforth that T is strongly aperiodic and satisfies the finite pattern and repetitivity conditions; thus Ω is compact with a free and minimal $\mathbb{R}^d$-action ω. There is a natural C^*-algebra to model the situation, namely $C(\Omega) \rtimes \mathbb{R}^d$, referred to by Bellissard as the *noncommutative Brillouin zone*. Bellissard's deep insight was to regard the dynamical system via this C^*-algebra as a *noncommutative* space, in the sense introduced by Alain Connes, and to show that the resolvents of the Schrödinger operator lie in it. Gaps in the spectrum will yield projections in $C(\Omega) \rtimes \mathbb{R}^d$ and the classes of those projections lie in $K_0(C(\Omega) \rtimes \mathbb{R}^d)$. Any trace on the C^*-algebra yields a homomorphism $K_0(C(\Omega) \rtimes \mathbb{R}^d) \to \mathbb{R}$ whose image is a countable subgroup of $\mathbb{R}$. For natural choices of the trace, these numbers have physical and mathematical meaning. They are related to the integrated density of states and also can be obtained experimentally. Thus it is worthwhile to try to determine this subgroup of $\mathbb{R}$.

Sadun and Williams [2003] show that the hull Ω contains a Cantor set Σ with a minimal $\mathbb{Z}^d$-action such that there is a homeomorphism

$$\Sigma \times_{\mathbb{Z}^d} \mathbb{R}^d \cong \Omega.$$

(The set Σ can be constructed as a canonical transversal. To do so, each prototile is associated with a point in its interior; then take Σ to be the union of the tilings having one tile with point at the origin. Then Σ is defined modulo the choice of a point in each prototile. In the description via a Delone set there is no choice, since the position of atoms is already fixed and therefore the transversal becomes "canonical.") This homeomorphism does not conjugate the $\mathbb{R}^d$-actions. However, KP show that there is a strong Morita equivalence of associated C^*-algebras

$$C(\Sigma) \rtimes \mathbb{Z}^d \approx C(\Omega) \rtimes \mathbb{R}^d$$

and so these two C^*-algebras have isomorphic K-theory groups. We regard Σ with its $\mathbb{Z}^d$-action as a discrete model for the foliated space Ω.

2. Foliated Spaces. Every point in Ω has an open neighborhood of the form $U \times N$, where U is open in $\mathbb{R}^d$ and N is a Borel subset of Ω. If N were an open subset of Euclidean space then this would be the local picture of a foliated manifold. This is not the case generally. Instead, this is the local picture of a *foliated space*.

A side note on terminology. In ancient times a *lamination* was a space obtained by deleting some leaves of a foliated manifold. The first edition of this book introduced *foliated space* to describe a space whose local picture was $U \times N$ as above. This included laminations as well as other situations such as the continuous hull. This usage is found, for example, in [Candel and Conlon 2000]. More recently, Ghys [1999] and others have taken to using *lamination* for this more general concept. We will stick with the *foliated space* terminology.

Suppose given a $\mathbb{Z}^d$-invariant probability measure $\mu : C(\Sigma) \to \mathbb{C}$. This gives rise to an invariant transverse measure on Ω with corresponding Ruelle–Sullivan current C_μ and associated homology class

$$[C_\mu] \in H_d^\tau(\Omega).$$

Here H_*^τ denotes tangential homology (see Chapter III of this book). This gives rise to traces

$$\mu : C(\Sigma) \longrightarrow \mathbb{C} \qquad \text{and} \qquad \tau_\mu : C(\Sigma) \rtimes \mathbb{Z}^d \longrightarrow \mathbb{C}$$

and associated homomorphisms

$$\mu : K_0(C(\Sigma)) \longrightarrow \mathbb{R} \qquad \text{and} \qquad \tau_\mu : K_0(C(\Sigma) \rtimes \mathbb{Z}^d) \longrightarrow \mathbb{R}.$$

The group $K_0(C(\Sigma))$ is isomorphic to $C(\Sigma, \mathbb{Z})$, the group of continuous, integer-valued functions on Σ, and we may describe its image under the trace $\mu(K_0(C(\Sigma)))$ as the subgroup of $\mathbb{R}$ generated by the measures of the clopen sets of Σ. It is not very hard to prove that

$$\mu\big(K_0(C(\Sigma))\big) \subseteq \tau_\mu\big(K_0(C(\Sigma) \rtimes \mathbb{Z}^d)\big).$$

The deepest part of the Gap Labeling Theorem is to demonstrate that this inclusion is actually an equality of sets.

Note that each gap in the spectrum of the self-adjoint operator associated to the motion of the particle in the initial tiling corresponds to a projection in the C^*-algebra $C(\Omega) \rtimes \mathbb{R}^d$ of the foliated space Ω and hence to a class in

$$K_0(C(\Omega) \rtimes \mathbb{R}^d) \cong K_0(C(\Sigma) \rtimes \mathbb{Z}^d).$$

Bellissard, Herrmann, and Zarrouati [Bellissard et al. 2000] prove that the integrated density of the states of the operator depend only upon the noncommutative space Ω itself, and not upon the operator. Thus the possible values of the gap labeling are independent of the choice of operator; they depend only upon the noncommutative topology of Ω.

All three proofs of the Gap Labeling Theorem proceed by translating the gap labeling problem to tangential cohomology via some version of the Chern character and then by a combination of direct computation and deep general results.

3. The BBG Proof. BBG consider a somewhat more general situation than described above. As this review focuses upon the K-theory result, we must omit details. We urge the reader to study the paper as it has interesting applications beyond the immediate K-theoretic concern of the Gap Labeling Theorem. BBG provide a geometric analysis of the foliated space itself. They represent Ω as topologically conjugate to the inverse limit of expanding flattening sequences of branched oriented flat manifolds of dimension d (*BOF d-manifolds*) with $\mathbb{R}^d$ action by parallel transport under constant vector fields. The cohomology of the

BOF manifolds is analyzed combinatorially via cellular cohomology and a spectral sequence is used to calculate the K-theory of the associated C^*-algebras. Taking direct limits then yields a very concrete description of $K_*(C(\Omega \rtimes \mathbb{R}^d)$. The associated Ruelle–Sullivan maps are then explicitly calculated. They use a partial Chern character map c and then must deal with the diagram

$$\begin{array}{ccc}
K_0(C(\Omega) \rtimes \mathbb{R}^d) & \xrightarrow{\ c\ } & H_\tau^d(C(\Omega) \rtimes \mathbb{R}^d) \\
\downarrow{\scriptstyle \tau_\mu} & & \downarrow{\scriptstyle (-)\cap C_\mu} \\
\mathbb{R} & \xrightarrow{\ \cong\ } & \mathbb{R}
\end{array}$$

where $\cap C_\mu$ is the cap product by the class $[C_\mu] \in H_d^\tau(\Omega)$ of the Ruelle–Sullivan current induced by the trace. Their proof requires the use of Connes' Thom Isomorphism theorem [Connes 1981a] as well as cyclic cohomology [Connes 1986].

4. Common Features of the BO and the KP Proofs. Consider the diagram

$$\begin{array}{ccc}
K_0(C(\Sigma)) & \xrightarrow{\ \mu\ } & \mathbb{R} \\
\downarrow{\scriptstyle i_*} & & \downarrow{\scriptstyle \cong} \\
K_0(C(\Sigma \rtimes \mathbb{Z}^d)) & \xrightarrow{\ \tau_\mu\ } & \mathbb{R} \\
\downarrow{\scriptstyle m.e.} & & \downarrow{\scriptstyle \equiv} \\
K_0(C(\Omega \rtimes \mathbb{R}^d)) & \xrightarrow{\ \bar{\tau}_\mu\ } & \mathbb{R} \\
\uparrow{\scriptstyle \cong\, \phi_c} & & \uparrow{\scriptstyle \equiv} \\
K_d(C(\Omega)) & & \mathbb{R} \\
\downarrow{\scriptstyle \mathrm{ch}^d} & & \downarrow{\scriptstyle \equiv} \\
H_\tau^d(\Omega; \mathbb{R}) & \xrightarrow{\ \cap C_\mu\ } & \mathbb{R}
\end{array}$$

where Σ is the given Cantor set with the given $\mathbb{Z}^d$ action,

$$\Omega = \Sigma \times_{\mathbb{Z}^d} \mathbb{R}^d$$

is the suspension of the action, ϕ_c is Connes' Thom Isomorphism, i_* is the map induced by the inclusion of C^*-algebras, $m.e.$ is the isomorphism induced by the Morita equivalence of the C^*-algebras, and (this is a result from [Fack and Skandalis 1981])

$$\phi_c([E]) = \mathrm{ind}_a[D_E] \in K_0(C(\Omega \rtimes \mathbb{R}^d))$$

where $\operatorname{ind}_a[D_E]$ is the analytic index of the Dirac D operator twisted by the bundle E. The top square commutes by the definition of the traces. The middle square is shown to commute by looking carefully at properties of the Morita equivalence.

The bottom rectangle commutes by the Index Theorem for Foliated Spaces. KP prove this as KP 2.4, and BO prove it as BO 4.2. (Since Ω is a foliated space but not a foliated manifold, one needs the version of the Index Theorem established by C. C. Moore and the reviewer (in this book).) The analogous result in BBG is Theorem 6.1, which they prove by reduction to a result in cyclic cohomology [Connes 1986].

5. The BO proof. BO filter the leaves of Ω and obtain a pair of spectral sequences

$$E^2 = H_*(\mathbb{Z}^d; C(\Omega, \mathbb{Z})) \Longrightarrow K_*(C^*(C(\Omega) \rtimes \mathbb{R}^d))$$

and

$$\widetilde{E}^2 = H_*(\mathbb{Z}^d; C(\Omega, \mathbb{R})) \Longrightarrow H^*_\tau(C(\Omega) \rtimes \mathbb{R}^d).$$

The Chern character induces a natural transformation $\mathrm{ch} : E^r \to \widetilde{E}^r$. Both spectral sequences collapse at the E^2 level, essentially because $\mathrm{ch} \otimes \mathbb{Q}$ is an isomorphism. This makes it possible to explicitly identify the image of

$$\mathrm{ch} : K_*\big(C^*(C(\Omega) \rtimes \mathbb{R}^d))\big) \to H^*_\tau(C(\Omega) \rtimes \mathbb{R}^d)$$

as $H_*(\mathbb{Z}^d; C(\Omega, \mathbb{Z}))$. This integrality result leads to an identification of the top component of the Chern character and implies the Gap Labeling Theorem.

6. The KP Proof. KP rely on a less commutative approach. Let

$$\pi : \Sigma \times \mathbb{R}^d \to \Omega$$

be the quotient map, let L denote the union of the hyperplanes parallel to the coordinate axis and going through the points of $\mathbb{Z}^d$, let $Y = \pi(\Sigma \times L)$ and $j : \Omega - Y \to \Omega$ the inclusion, and let

$$\alpha : K_0(C(\Sigma)) \to K_0(C(\Omega) \rtimes \mathbb{R}^d)$$

be the map described in [Connes 1994, p. 120], modified for foliated spaces, that associates — to a clopen set in a transversal to a foliation — a projection in its foliation algebra. They show (KP 3.2) that the natural diagram

$$\begin{array}{ccc}
K_0(C(\Sigma)) & \xrightarrow{\ \alpha\ } & K_0(C(\Omega) \rtimes \mathbb{R}^d) \\
\Big\downarrow{\scriptstyle \beta} & & \Big\uparrow{\scriptstyle \phi_c} \\
K_d(C_0(\Omega - Y)) & \xrightarrow{\ j_*\ } & K_d(C(\Omega))
\end{array}$$

commutes, where β is Bott periodicity. Then an explicit study of the partial Chern character ch_n implies the Gap Labeling Theorem.

7. Earlier Results. To complete the report, we note that there were previous partial results on the problem. The conjecture was first established in the case $d = 1$ by Bellissard [1992] using the Pimsner–Voiculescu long exact sequence, and the case $d = 2$ was done by van Elst [1994] using similar technique. The $d = 2$ result was re-established using the Kasparov spectral sequence in [Bellissard et al. 1998]. In the case where the hull is given by an action of $\mathbb{Z}^d$ on a Cantor set Σ, Forrest and Hunton [1999] used spectral sequence techniques to prove that the K-theory group is isomorphic to group cohomology — $H^*(\mathbb{Z}^d; C(\Sigma, \mathbb{Z}))$, which made calculation possible in many practical situations that occur in physics, as well as the case $d = 3$.

References

[Ahlfors 1966] L. V. Ahlfors, *Lectures on quasiconformal mappings*, Van Nostrand Mathematical Studies **10**, Van Nostrand, Toronto, 1966. With the assistance of Clifford J. Earle, Jr.

[Anantharaman-Delaroche and Renault 2000] C. Anantharaman-Delaroche and J. Renault, *Amenable groupoids*, Monographies de L'Ens. Math. **36**, L'Enseignement Mathématique, Geneva, 2000.

[Arveson 1976] W. Arveson, *An invitation to C^*-algebras*, Springer, New York, 1976.

[Atiyah 1967] M. F. Atiyah, *K-theory*, W. A. Benjamin, New York, 1967. Lecture notes by D. W. Anderson.

[Atiyah 1970] M. F. Atiyah, "Global theory of elliptic operators", pp. 21–30 in *Proc. Internat. Conf. on Functional Analysis and Related Topics* (Tokyo, 1969), Univ. of Tokyo Press, Tokyo, 1970.

[Atiyah 1974] M. F. Atiyah, *Elliptic operators and compact groups*, Lecture notes in mathematics **401**, Springer, Berlin, 1974.

[Atiyah 1975] M. F. Atiyah, "Classical groups and classical differential operators on manifolds", pp. 5–48 in *Differential operators on manifolds* (Varenna, 1975), edited by E. Vensentini, Cremonese, Rome, 1975.

[Atiyah 1976] M. F. Atiyah, "Elliptic operators, discrete groups and von Neumann algebras", pp. 43–72 in *Colloque "Analyse et Topologie" en l'Honneur de Henri Cartan* (Orsay, 1974), Astérisque **32-33**, Soc. Math. France, Paris, 1976.

[Atiyah and Hirzebruch 1961] M. F. Atiyah and F. Hirzebruch, "Vector bundles and homogeneous spaces", pp. 7–38 in *Differential geometry*, Proc. Sympos. Pure Math. **3**, Amer. Math. Soc., Providence, R.I., 1961.

[Atiyah and Segal 1968] M. F. Atiyah and G. B. Segal, "The index of elliptic operators, II", *Ann. of Math.* (2) **87** (1968), 531–545.

[Atiyah and Singer 1968a] M. F. Atiyah and I. M. Singer, "The index of elliptic operators, I", *Ann. of Math.* (2) **87** (1968), 484–530.

[Atiyah and Singer 1968b] M. F. Atiyah and I. M. Singer, "The index of elliptic operators, III", *Ann. of Math.* (2) **87** (1968), 546–604.

[Atiyah and Singer 1971] M. F. Atiyah and I. M. Singer, "The index of elliptic operators, IV", *Ann. of Math.* (2) **93** (1971), 119–138.

[Atiyah et al. 1964] M. F. Atiyah, R. Bott, and A. Shapiro, "Clifford modules", *Topology* **3**:suppl. 1 (1964), 3–38.

[Atiyah et al. 1973] M. Atiyah, R. Bott, and V. K. Patodi, "On the heat equation and the index theorem", *Invent. Math.* **19** (1973), 279–330. Errata in *Invent. Math.* **28** (1975), 277–280.

[Auslander and Moore 1966] L. Auslander and C. C. Moore, *Unitary representations of solvable Lie groups*, Mem. Amer. Math. Soc. **62**, Amer. Math. Soc., Providence, R.I., 1966.

[Baum and Connes 2000] P. Baum and A. Connes, "Geometric K-theory for Lie groups and foliations", *Enseign. Math.* (2) **46**:1-2 (2000), 3–42.

[Bedford and Smillie 1999] E. Bedford and J. Smillie, "Polynomial diffeomorphisms of $\mathbb{C}^2$, VII: Hyperbolicity and external rays", *Ann. Sci. École Norm. Sup.* (4) **32**:4 (1999), 455–497.

[Bellissard 1992] J. Bellissard, "Gap labelling theorems for Schrödinger operators", pp. 538–630 in *From number theory to physics* (Les Houches, 1989), edited by M. Waldschmidt et al., Springer, Berlin, 1992.

[Bellissard et al. 1998] J. Bellissard, E. Contensou, and A. Legrand, "K-théorie des quasi-cristaux, image par la trace: le cas du réseau octogonal", *C. R. Acad. Sci. Paris Sér. I Math.* **326**:2 (1998), 197–200.

[Bellissard et al. 2000] J. Bellissard, D. J. L. Herrmann, and M. Zarrouati, "Hulls of aperiodic solids and gap labeling theorems", pp. 207–258 in *Directions in mathematical quasicrystals*, edited by M. Baake and R. V. Moody, CRM Monogr. Ser. **13**, Amer. Math. Soc., Providence, RI, 2000.

[Bellissard et al. 2005] J. Bellissard, R. Benedetti, and J.-M. Gambaudo, "Spaces of tilings, finite telescopic approximations, and gap-labeling", *Comm. Math. Phys.* (2005). Available at http:/arxiv.org/abs/math/0109062. to appear.

[Benameur 1997] M.-T. Benameur, "A longitudinal Lefschetz theorem in K-theory", *K-Theory* **12**:3 (1997), 227–257.

[Benameur and Oyono-Oyono 2003] M.-T. Benameur and H. Oyono-Oyono, "Gap-labelling for quasi-crystals (proving a conjecture by J. Bellissard)", pp. 11–22 in *Operator algebras and mathematical physics* (Constanţa, 2001), edited by J.-M. Combes, Theta, Bucharest, 2003.

[Blackadar 1998] B. Blackadar, *K-theory for operator algebras*, 2nd ed., Mathematical Sciences Research Institute Publications **5**, Cambridge University Press, Cambridge, 1998.

[Borel 1963] A. Borel, "Compact Clifford–Klein forms of symmetric spaces", *Topology* **2** (1963), 111–122.

[Bott 1969] R. Bott, *Lectures on $K(X)$*, W. A. Benjamin, New York, 1969.

[Bott and Haefliger 1972] R. Bott and A. Haefliger, "On characteristic classes of Γ-foliations", *Bull. Amer. Math. Soc.* **78** (1972), 1039–1044.

[Bott and Tu 1982] R. Bott and L. W. Tu, *Differential forms in algebraic topology*, Graduate Texts in Mathematics **82**, Springer, New York, 1982.

[Bourbaki 1958] N. Bourbaki, *Éléments de mathématique: Topologie générale, chapitre 9: Utilisation des nombres réels en topologie générale*, deuxième ed., Actualités Scientifiques et Industrielles **1045**, Hermann, Paris, 1958.

[Bowen 1978] R. Bowen, *On Axiom A diffeomorphisms*, CBMS Regional Conf. Ser. Math. **35**, Amer. Math. Soc., Providence, R.I., 1978.

[Breuer 1968] M. Breuer, "Fredholm theories in von Neumann algebras, I", *Math. Ann.* **178** (1968), 243–254.

[Brown et al. 1977] L. G. Brown, P. Green, and M. A. Rieffel, "Stable isomorphism and strong Morita equivalence of C^*-algebras", *Pacific J. Math.* **71**:2 (1977), 349–363.

[Brylinski and Nistor 1994] J.-L. Brylinski and V. Nistor, "Cyclic cohomology of étale groupoids", *K-Theory* **8**:4 (1994), 341–365.

[Calegari 2003] D. Calegari, "Problems in foliations and laminations of 3-manifolds", pp. 297–335 in *Topology and geometry of manifolds* (Athens, GA, 2001), edited by G. Matic and C. McCrory, Proc. Sympos. Pure Math. **71**, Amer. Math. Soc., Providence, RI, 2003.

[Candel 1993] A. Candel, "Uniformization of surface laminations", *Ann. Sci. École Norm. Sup.* (4) **26**:4 (1993), 489–516.

[Candel and Conlon 2000] A. Candel and L. Conlon, *Foliations, I*, Graduate Studies in Mathematics **23**, Amer. Math. Soc., Providence, RI, 2000.

[Candel and Conlon 2003] A. Candel and L. Conlon, *Foliations, II*, Graduate Studies in Mathematics **60**, Amer. Math. Soc., Providence, RI, 2003.

[Cannas da Silva and Weinstein 1999] A. Cannas da Silva and A. Weinstein, *Geometric models for noncommutative algebras*, Berkeley Mathematics Lecture Notes **10**, Amer. Math. Soc., Providence, RI, 1999.

[Cantwell and Conlon 1977] J. Cantwell and L. Conlon, "Leaves with isolated ends in foliated 3-manifolds", *Topology* **16**:4 (1977), 311–322.

[Cantwell and Conlon 1981] J. Cantwell and L. Conlon, "Poincaré–Bendixson theory for leaves of codimension one", *Trans. Amer. Math. Soc.* **265**:1 (1981), 181–209.

[Cantwell and Conlon 1989] J. Cantwell and L. Conlon, "Leafwise hyperbolicity of proper foliations", *Comment. Math. Helv.* **64**:2 (1989), 329–337.

[Cantwell and Conlon 1991] J. Cantwell and L. Conlon, "Markov minimal sets have hyperbolic leaves", *Ann. Global Anal. Geom.* **9**:1 (1991), 13–25.

[Carey et al. 1998] A. L. Carey, K. C. Hannabuss, V. Mathai, and P. McCann, "Quantum Hall effect on the hyperbolic plane", *Comm. Math. Phys.* **190**:3 (1998), 629–673.

[Cheeger et al. 1982] J. Cheeger, M. Gromov, and M. Taylor, "Finite propagation speed, kernel estimates for functions of the Laplace operator, and the geometry of complete Riemannian manifolds", *J. Differential Geom.* **17**:1 (1982), 15–53.

[Chernoff 1973] P. R. Chernoff, "Essential self-adjointness of powers of generators of hyperbolic equations", *J. Functional Analysis* **12** (1973), 401–414.

[Connes 1973] A. Connes, "Une classification des facteurs de type III", *Ann. Sci. École Norm. Sup.* (4) **6** (1973), 133–252.

[Connes 1978] A. Connes, "The von Neumann algebra of a foliation", pp. 145–151 in *Mathematical problems in theoretical physics* (Rome, 1977), edited by G. D. to nio et al., Lecture Notes in Phys. **80**, Springer, Berlin, 1978.

[Connes 1979] A. Connes, "Sur la théorie non commutative de l'intégration", pp. 19–143 in *Algèbres d'opérateurs* (Les Plans-sur-Bex, 1978), edited by P. de la Harpe, Lecture Notes in Math. **725**, Springer, Berlin, 1979.

[Connes 1981a] A. Connes, "An analogue of the Thom isomorphism for crossed products of a C^*-algebra by an action of **R**", *Adv. in Math.* **39**:1 (1981), 31–55.

[Connes 1981b] A. Connes, "Feuilletages et algèbres d'opérateurs", pp. 139–155 in *Séminaire Bourbaki* 1979/80, Lecture Notes in Math. **842**, Springer, Berlin, 1981.

[Connes 1982] A. Connes, "A survey of foliations and operator algebras", pp. 521–628 in *Operator algebras and applications* (Kingston, Ont., 1980), Part I, Proc. Sympos. Pure Math. **38**, Amer. Math. Soc., Providence, R.I., 1982.

[Connes 1985a] A. Connes, "Noncommutative differential geometry, I: The Chern character in K-homology", *Inst. Hautes Études Sci. Publ. Math.* **62** (1985), 257–309.

[Connes 1985b] A. Connes, "Noncommutative differential geometry, II: de Rham homology and noncommutative algebra", *Inst. Hautes Études Sci. Publ. Math.* **62** (1985), 310–360.

[Connes 1986] A. Connes, "Cyclic cohomology and the transverse fundamental class of a foliation", pp. 52–144 in *Geometric methods in operator algebras* (Kyoto, 1983), edited by H. Araki and E. G. Effros, Pitman Res. Notes Math. Ser. **123**, Longman Sci. Tech., Harlow, 1986.

[Connes 1994] A. Connes, *Noncommutative geometry*, Academic Press, San Diego, CA, 1994.

[Connes 1999] A. Connes, "Hypoelliptic operators, Hopf algebras and cyclic cohomology", pp. 164–205 in *Algebraic K-theory and its applications* (Trieste, 1997), edited by H. Bass et al., World Sci. Publishing, River Edge, NJ, 1999.

[Connes 2000] A. Connes, "Noncommutative geometry—year 2000", pp. 481–559 in *Visions in mathematics: towards 2000*, vol. II, edited by N. Alon et al., Birkhäuser, Basel, 2000. Special Volume of *Geometric and Functional Analysis*.

[Connes 2002] A. Connes, "Noncommutative geometry year 2000", pp. 49–110 in *Highlights of mathematical physics* (London, 2000), edited by A. Fokas et al., Amer. Math. Soc., Providence, RI, 2002.

[Connes and Moscovici 1995] A. Connes and H. Moscovici, "The local index formula in noncommutative geometry", *Geom. Funct. Anal.* **5** (1995), 174–243.

[Connes and Moscovici 1998] A. Connes and H. Moscovici, "Hopf algebras, cyclic cohomology and the transverse index theorem", *Comm. Math. Phys.* **198** (1998), 199–246.

[Connes and Skandalis 1981] A. Connes and G. Skandalis, "Théorème de l'indice pour les feuilletages", *C. R. Acad. Sci. Paris Sér. I Math.* **292**:18 (1981), 871–876.

[Connes and Skandalis 1984] A. Connes and G. Skandalis, "The longitudinal index theorem for foliations", *Publ. Res. Inst. Math. Sci.* **20**:6 (1984), 1139–1183.

[Connes and Takesaki 1977] A. Connes and M. Takesaki, "The flow of weights on factors of type III", *Tôhoku Math. J.* (2) **29**:4 (1977), 473–575.

[Crainic and Moerdijk 2000] M. Crainic and I. Moerdijk, "A homology theory for étale groupoids", *J. Reine Angew. Math.* **521** (2000), 25–46.

[Crainic and Moerdijk 2001] M. Crainic and I. Moerdijk, "Foliation groupoids and their cyclic homology", *Adv. Math.* **157**:2 (2001), 177–197.

[Davidson 1996] K. R. Davidson, *C^*-algebras by example*, Fields Institute Monographs **6**, Amer. Math. Soc., Providence, RI, 1996.

[Davis 1983] M. W. Davis, "Groups generated by reflections and aspherical manifolds not covered by Euclidean space", *Ann. of Math.* (2) **117**:2 (1983), 293–324.

[Deitmar and Deninger 2003] A. Deitmar and C. Deninger, "A dynamical Lefschetz trace formula for algebraic Anosov diffeomorphisms", *Abh. Math. Sem. Univ. Hamburg* **73** (2003), 81–98.

[Deninger 2001] C. Deninger, "Number theory and dynamical systems on foliated spaces", *Jahresber. Deutsch. Math.-Verein.* **103**:3 (2001), 79–100.

[Dixmier 1969a] J. Dixmier, *Les algèbres d'opérateurs dans l'espace hilbertien (algèbres de von Neumann)*, deuxième ed., Cahiers scientifiques **25**, Gauthier-Villars, Paris, 1969.

[Dixmier 1969b] J. Dixmier, *Les C^*-algèbres et leurs représentations*, deuxième ed., Cahiers scientifiques **24**, Gauthier-Villars, Paris, 1969.

[Dixmier and Douady 1963] J. Dixmier and A. Douady, "Champs continus d'espaces hilbertiens et de C^*-algèbres", *Bull. Soc. Math. France* **91** (1963), 227–284.

[Douglas et al. 1991] R. G. Douglas, S. Hurder, and J. Kaminker, "Cyclic cocycles, renormalization and eta-invariants", *Invent. Math.* **103**:1 (1991), 101–179.

[Duflo and Moore 1976] M. Duflo and C. C. Moore, "On the regular representation of a nonunimodular locally compact group", *J. Functional Analysis* **21**:2 (1976), 209–243.

[Dugundji 1965] J. Dugundji, *Topology*, Allyn and Bacon, Boston, 1965.

[Dunford and Schwartz 1958] N. Dunford and J. T. Schwartz, *Linear operators, I: General theory*, Pure and Applied Mathematics, Interscience, New York, 1958. With the assistance of William G. Bade and Robert G. Bartle.

[Dunford and Schwartz 1963] N. Dunford and J. T. Schwartz, *Linear operators, II: Spectral theory; self adjoint operators in Hilbert space*, Pure and Applied Mathematics, Interscience, New York, 1963. With the assistance of William G. Bade and Robert G. Bartle.

[Dunford and Schwartz 1971] N. Dunford and J. T. Schwartz, *Linear operators, III: Spectral operators*, Interscience, New York, 1971.

[Dupont 1978] J. L. Dupont, *Curvature and characteristic classes*, vol. 640, Lecture Notes in Math., Springer, Berlin, 1978.

[Ehresmann 1963] C. Ehresmann, "Structures feuilletées", pp. 109–172 in *Proceedings of the Fifth Canadian Mathematical Congress* (Montreal, 1961), edited by E. M. Rosenthall, University of Toronto Press, Toronto, 1963.

[Eilenberg and Steenrod 1952] S. Eilenberg and N. Steenrod, *Foundations of algebraic topology*, Princeton Univ. Press, Princeton, NJ, 1952.

[El Kacimi-Alaoui 1983] A. El Kacimi-Alaoui, "Sur la cohomologie feuilletée", *Compositio Math.* **49**:2 (1983), 195–215.

[Epstein et al. 1977] D. B. A. Epstein, K. C. Millett, and D. Tischler, "Leaves without holonomy", *J. London Math. Soc.* (2) **16**:3 (1977), 548–552.

[Fack and Skandalis 1981] T. Fack and G. Skandalis, "Connes' analogue of the Thom isomorphism for the Kasparov groups", *Invent. Math.* **64**:1 (1981), 7–14.

[Fack and Skandalis 1982] T. Fack and G. Skandalis, "Sur les représentations et idéaux de la C^*-algèbre d'un feuilletage", *J. Operator Theory* **8**:1 (1982), 95–129.

[Feldman and Moore 1977] J. Feldman and C. C. Moore, "Ergodic equivalence relations, cohomology, and von Neumann algebras, I and II", *Trans. Amer. Math. Soc.* **234**:2 (1977), 289–324 and 325–359.

[Feldman et al. 1978] J. Feldman, P. Hahn, and C. C. Moore, "Orbit structure and countable sections for actions of continuous groups", *Adv. in Math.* **28**:3 (1978), 186–230.

[Fillmore 1996] P. A. Fillmore, *A user's guide to operator algebras*, CMS Monographs and Advanced Texts, Wiley, New York, 1996.

[Forrest and Hunton 1999] A. H. Forrest and J. Hunton, "The cohomology and K-theory of commuting homeomorphisms of the Cantor set", *Ergodic Theory Dynam. Systems* **19**:3 (1999), 611–625.

[Friedrichs 1954] K. O. Friedrichs, "Symmetric hyperbolic linear differential equations", *Comm. Pure Appl. Math.* **7** (1954), 345–392.

[Furstenberg 1961] H. Furstenberg, "Strict ergodicity and transformation of the torus", *Amer. J. Math.* **83** (1961), 573–601.

[Gabai 2001] D. Gabai, "3 lectures on foliations and laminations on 3-manifolds", pp. 87–109 in *Laminations and foliations in dynamics, geometry and topology* (Stony Brook, NY, 1998), edited by M. Lyubich et al., Contemp. Math. **269**, Amer. Math. Soc., Providence, RI, 2001.

[Gabai and Oertel 1989] D. Gabai and U. Oertel, "Essential laminations in 3-manifolds", *Ann. of Math.* (2) **130**:1 (1989), 41–73.

[Ghys 1984] É. Ghys, "Flots d'Anosov sur les 3-variétés fibrées en cercles", *Ergodic Theory Dynam. Systems* **4**:1 (1984), 67–80.

[Ghys 1985] É. Ghys, "Actions localement libres du groupe affine", *Invent. Math.* **82**:3 (1985), 479–526.

[Ghys 1993] É. Ghys, "Rigidité différentiable des groupes fuchsiens", *Inst. Hautes Études Sci. Publ. Math.* **78** (1993), 163–185.

[Ghys 1997] É. Ghys, "Sur l'uniformisation des laminations paraboliques", pp. 73–91 in *Integrable systems and foliations = Feuilletages et systèmes intégrables* (Montpellier, 1995), edited by C. Albert et al., Progr. Math. **145**, Birkhäuser, Boston, 1997.

[Ghys 1999] É. Ghys, "Laminations par surfaces de Riemann", pp. 49–95 in *Dynamique et géométrie complexes* (Lyon, 1997), Panor. Synthèses **8**, Soc. Math. France, Paris, 1999.

[Ghys and Sergiescu 1980] E. Ghys and V. Sergiescu, "Stabilité et conjugaison différentiable pour certains feuilletages", *Topology* **19**:2 (1980), 179–197.

[Gilkey 1974] P. B. Gilkey, *The index theorem and the heat equation*, Mathematics Lecture Series **4**, Publish or Perish, Boston, 1974.

[Gilkey 1984] P. B. Gilkey, *Invariance theory, the heat equation, and the Atiyah–Singer index theorem*, Mathematics Lecture Series **11**, Publish or Perish, Wilmington, DE, 1984.

[Godement 1973] R. Godement, *Topologie algébrique et théorie des faisceaux*, troisième ed., Actualités Scientifiques et Industrielles **1252**, Hermann, Paris, 1973.

[Goodman and Plante 1979] S. E. Goodman and J. F. Plante, "Holonomy and averaging in foliated sets", *J. Differential Geom.* **14**:3 (1979), 401–407.

[Gromov and Lawson 1980] M. Gromov and H. B. Lawson, Jr., "Spin and scalar curvature in the presence of a fundamental group. I", *Ann. of Math.* (2) **111**:2 (1980), 209–230.

[Gunning 1966] R. C. Gunning, *Lectures on Riemann surfaces*, Princeton Mathematical Notes, Princeton Univ. Press, Princeton, 1966.

[Haagerup 1979] U. Haagerup, "Operator-valued weights in von Neumann algebras, I and II", *J. Funct. Anal.* **32** (1979), 175–206 and 339–361.

[Haagerup 1987] U. Haagerup, "Connes' bicentralizer problem and uniqueness of the injective factor of type III_1", *Acta Math.* **158**:1-2 (1987), 95–148.

[Haefliger 1962] A. Haefliger, "Variétés feuilletées", *Ann. Scuola Norm. Sup. Pisa* (3) **16** (1962), 367–397.

[Haefliger 1971] A. Haefliger, "Homotopy and integrability", pp. 133–163 in *Manifolds* (Amsterdam 1970), edited by N. H. Kuiper, Lecture Notes in Mathematics **197**, Springer, Berlin, 1971.

[Haefliger 1980] A. Haefliger, "Some remarks on foliations with minimal leaves", *J. Differential Geom.* **15**:2 (1980), 269–284.

[Haefliger 1984] A. Haefliger, "Groupoïdes d'holonomie et classifiants", *Astérisque* no. 116 (1984), 70–97.

[Hahn 1932] H. Hahn, *Reelle Funktionen, 1: Punktfunktionen*, Mathematik und ihre Anwendungen in Monographien und Lehrbuchern **13**, Akademische Verlagsgesellschaft, Leipzig, 1932. Reprinted by Chelsea, New York.

[Hahn 1978] P. Hahn, "The regular representations of measure groupoids", *Trans. Amer. Math. Soc.* **242** (1978), 35–72.

[Hector and Hirsch 1986] G. Hector and U. Hirsch, *Introduction to the geometry of foliations, Part A: Foliations on compact surfaces, fundamentals for arbitrary codimension, and holonomy*, Second ed., Aspects of Mathematics **1**, Vieweg, Braunschweig, 1986.

[Heitsch 1975] J. L. Heitsch, "A cohomology for foliated manifolds", *Comment. Math. Helv.* **50** (1975), 197–218.

[Heitsch and Hurder 1984] J. Heitsch and S. Hurder, "Secondary classes, Weil measures and the geometry of foliations", *J. Differential Geom.* **20**:2 (1984), 291–309.

[Heitsch and Hurder 2001] J. L. Heitsch and S. Hurder, "Coarse cohomology for families", *Illinois J. Math.* **45**:2 (2001), 323–360.

[Heitsch and Lazarov 1990] J. L. Heitsch and C. Lazarov, "A Lefschetz theorem for foliated manifolds", *Topology* **29**:2 (1990), 127–162.

[Higson 2006] N. Higson, "The residue index theorem of Connes and Moscovici", in *Surveys in noncommutative geometry*, edited by J. Roe and N. Higson, Clay Math. Proc. **6**, 2006.

[Higson and Roe 2000] N. Higson and J. Roe, *Analytic K-homology*, Oxford Univ. Press, Oxford, 2000.

[Higson et al. 1997] N. Higson, E. K. Pedersen, and J. Roe, "C^*-algebras and controlled topology", *K-Theory* **11**:3 (1997), 209–239.

[Higson et al. 2002] N. Higson, V. Lafforgue, and G. Skandalis, "Counterexamples to the Baum–Connes conjecture", *Geom. Funct. Anal.* **12**:2 (2002), 330–354.

[Hilsum and Skandalis 1983] M. Hilsum and G. Skandalis, "Stabilité des C^*-algèbres de feuilletages", *Ann. Inst. Fourier (Grenoble)* **33**:3 (1983), 201–208.

[Hirsch 1976] M. W. Hirsch, *Differential topology*, Springer, New York, 1976.

[Hjorth 2000] G. Hjorth, *Classification and orbit equivalence relations*, Mathematical Surveys and Monographs **75**, Amer. Math. Soc., Providence, RI, 2000.

[Hurder 1990] S. Hurder, "Eta invariants and the odd index theorem for coverings", pp. 47–82 in *Geometric and topological invariants of elliptic operators* (Brunswick, ME, 1988), edited by J. Kaminker, Contemp. Math. **105**, Amer. Math. Soc., Providence, RI, 1990.

[Hurder 1993] S. Hurder, "Topology of covers and the spectral theory of geometric operators", pp. 87–119 in *Index theory and operator algebras* (Boulder, CO, 1991), edited by J. Fox and P. Haskell, Contemp. Math. **148**, Amer. Math. Soc., Providence, RI, 1993.

[Husemoller 1975] D. Husemoller, *Fibre bundles*, second ed., Graduate Texts in Mathematics **20**, Springer, New York, 1975.

[Kamber and Tondeur 1974] F. W. Kamber and P. Tondeur, "Characteristic invariants of foliated bundles", *Manuscripta Math.* **11** (1974), 51–89.

[Kamber and Tondeur 1975] F. W. Kamber and P. Tondeur, *Foliated bundles and characteristic classes*, Lecture Notes in Mathematics **493**, Springer, Berlin, 1975.

[Kaminker and Putnam 2003] J. Kaminker and I. Putnam, "A proof of the gap labeling conjecture", *Michigan Math. J.* **51**:3 (2003), 537–546.

[Karoubi 1978] M. Karoubi, *K-theory: An introduction*, Grundlehren der Mathematischen Wissenschaften **226**, Springer, Berlin, 1978.

[Kasparov 1980] G. G. Kasparov, "Hilbert C^*-modules: theorems of Stinespring and Voiculescu", *J. Operator Theory* **4**:1 (1980), 133–150.

[Kazdan and Warner 1975] J. L. Kazdan and F. W. Warner, "Scalar curvature and conformal deformation of Riemannian structure", *J. Differential Geometry* **10** (1975), 113–134.

[Khalkhali 2004] M. Khalkhali, "Very basic noncommutative geometry", Technical report, 2004. Available at arXiv:math.KT/0408416.

[Krieger 1976] W. Krieger, "On ergodic flows and the isomorphism of factors", *Math. Ann.* **223**:1 (1976), 19–70.

[Kumjian 1986] A. Kumjian, "On C^*-diagonals", *Canad. J. Math.* **38**:4 (1986), 969–1008.

[Kumjian and Pask 1999] A. Kumjian and D. Pask, "C^*-algebras of directed graphs and group actions", *Ergodic Theory Dynam. Systems* **19**:6 (1999), 1503–1519.

[Kumjian et al. 1997] A. Kumjian, D. Pask, I. Raeburn, and J. Renault, "Graphs, groupoids, and Cuntz–Krieger algebras", *J. Funct. Anal.* **144**:2 (1997), 505–541.

[Kumjian et al. 1998] A. Kumjian, D. Pask, and I. Raeburn, "Cuntz–Krieger algebras of directed graphs", *Pacific J. Math.* **184**:1 (1998), 161–174.

[Kuratowski 1966] K. Kuratowski, *Topology*, vol. 1, New ed., Academic Press, New York, 1966.

[Lawson 1974] H. B. Lawson, Jr., "Foliations", *Bull. Amer. Math. Soc.* **80** (1974), 369–418.

[Lawson 1977] J. Lawson, H. Blaine, *The quantitative theory of foliations* (St. Louis, MO, 1975), CBMS Regional Conference Series in Mathematics **27**, Amer. Math. Soc., Providence, RI, 1977.

[Lawson and Michelsohn 1989] H. B. Lawson, Jr. and M.-L. Michelsohn, *Spin geometry*, Princeton Mathematical Series **38**, Princeton Univ. Press, Princeton, 1989.

[Loday 1998] J.-L. Loday, *Cyclic homology*, Grundlehren der Mathematischen Wissenschaften **301**, Springer, Berlin, 1998.

[Lück 2002] W. Lück, *L^2-invariants: theory and applications to geometry and K-theory*, Ergebnisse der Math., 3. Folge **44**, Springer, Berlin, 2002.

[Mac Lane 1963] S. Mac Lane, *Homology*, Die Grundlehren der mathematischen Wissenschaften **114**, Springer, Berlin, 1963.

[Mackey 1962] G. W. Mackey, "Point realizations of transformation groups", *Illinois J. Math.* **6** (1962), 327–335.

[Mackey 1963] G. W. Mackey, "Ergodic theory, group theory, and differential geometry", *Proc. Nat. Acad. Sci. USA* **50** (1963), 1184–1191.

[Mackey 1966] G. W. Mackey, "Ergodic theory and virtual groups", *Math. Ann.* **166** (1966), 187–207.

[Mackey 1976] G. W. Mackey, *The theory of unitary group representations*, Univ. of Chicago Press, Chicago, 1976.

[May 1999] J. P. May, *A concise course in algebraic topology*, Chicago Lectures in Mathematics, Univ. of Chicago Press, Chicago, 1999.

[Milnor 1956] J. Milnor, "Construction of universal bundles, I", *Ann. of Math.* (2) **63** (1956), 272–284.

[Milnor and Stasheff 1974] J. W. Milnor and J. D. Stasheff, *Characteristic classes*, Princeton Univ. Press, Princeton, 1974.

[Moerdijk 1997] I. Moerdijk, "On the weak homotopy type of étale groupoids", pp. 147–156 in *Integrable systems and foliations = Feuilletages et systèmes intégrables* (Montpellier, 1995), edited by C. Albert et al., Progr. Math. **145**, Birkhäuser, Boston, 1997.

[Moerdijk 2003] I. Moerdijk, "Lie groupoids, gerbes, and non-abelian cohomology", *K-Theory* **28**:3 (2003), 207–258.

[Moerdijk and Mrčun 2003] I. Moerdijk and J. Mrčun, *Introduction to foliations and Lie groupoids*, Cambridge Studies in Advanced Mathematics **91**, Cambridge University Press, Cambridge, 2003.

[Molino 1973] P. Molino, "Propriétés cohomologiques et propriétés topologiques des feuilletages à connexion transverse projetable", *Topology* **12** (1973), 317–325.

[Boutet de Monvel 1976] L. Boutet de Monvel, *A course on pseudo differential operators and their applications*, Mathematics Department, Duke University, Durham, NC, 1976.

[Moore 1977] C. C. Moore, "Square integrable primary representations", *Pacific J. Math.* **70**:2 (1977), 413–427.

[Moore 1982] C. C. Moore, "Ergodic theory and von Neumann algebras", pp. 179–226 in *Operator algebras and applications* (Kingston, Ont., 1980), vol. 2, edited by R. V. Kadison, Proc. Sympos. Pure Math. **38**, Amer. Math. Soc., Providence, 1982.

[Moriyoshi 1994a] H. Moriyoshi, "The Euler and Godbillon–Vey forms and symplectic structures on $\mathrm{Diff}_+^\infty(S^1)/\mathrm{SO}(2)$", pp. 193–203 in *Symplectic geometry and quantization* (Sanda and Yokohama, 1993), edited by Y. Maeda et al., Contemp. Math. **179**, Amer. Math. Soc., Providence, RI, 1994.

[Moriyoshi 1994b] H. Moriyoshi, "On cyclic cocycles associated with the Godbillon–Vey classes", pp. 411–423 in *Geometric study of foliations* (Tokyo, 1993), edited by T. Mizutani et al., World Sci. Publishing, River Edge, NJ, 1994.

[Moriyoshi 2002] H. Moriyoshi, "Operator algebras and the index theorem on foliated manifolds", pp. 127–155 in *Foliations: geometry and dynamics* (Warsaw, 2000), edited by P. Walczak et al., World Sci. Publishing, River Edge, NJ, 2002.

[Moriyoshi and Natsume 1996] H. Moriyoshi and T. Natsume, "The Godbillon–Vey cyclic cocycle and longitudinal Dirac operators", *Pacific J. Math.* **172**:2 (1996), 483–539.

[Muhly et al. 1987] P. S. Muhly, J. N. Renault, and D. P. Williams, "Equivalence and isomorphism for groupoid C^*-algebras", *J. Operator Theory* **17**:1 (1987), 3–22.

[Natsume 1985] T. Natsume, "The C^*-algebras of codimension one foliations without holonomy", *Math. Scand.* **56**:1 (1985), 96–104.

[Palais 1965] R. S. Palais, *Seminar on the Atiyah-Singer index theorem*, Annals of Mathematics Studies **57**, Princeton University Press, Princeton, NJ, 1965. With contributions by M. F. Atiyah, A. Borel, E. E. Floyd, R. T. Seeley, W. Shih, and R. Solovay.

[Paterson 1999] A. L. T. Paterson, *Groupoids, inverse semigroups, and their operator algebras*, Progress in Mathematics **170**, Birkhäuser, Boston, 1999.

[Pedersen 1979] G. K. Pedersen, *C^*-algebras and their automorphism groups*, London Mathematical Society Monographs **14**, Academic Press, London, 1979.

[Pedersen and Takesaki 1973] G. K. Pedersen and M. Takesaki, "The Radon–Nikodym theorem for von Neumann algebras", *Acta Math.* **130** (1973), 53–87.

[Penington 1983] M. Penington, *K-theory and C^*-algebras of Lie groups and foliations*, Ph.D. thesis, Oxford University, 1983.

[Phillips 1987] J. Phillips, "The holonomic imperative and the homotopy groupoid of a foliated manifold", *Rocky Mountain J. Math.* **17**:1 (1987), 151–165.

[Phillips and Sullivan 1981] A. Phillips and D. Sullivan, "Geometry of leaves", *Topology* **20**:2 (1981), 209–218.

[Plante 1975] J. F. Plante, "Foliations with measure preserving holonomy", *Ann. of Math.* (2) **102**:2 (1975), 327–361.

[Plante 1979] J. F. Plante, "Foliations of 3-manifolds with solvable fundamental group", *Invent. Math.* **51**:3 (1979), 219–230.

[Pukanszky 1971] L. Pukanszky, "Unitary representations of solvable Lie groups", *Ann. Sci. École Norm. Sup.* (4) **4** (1971), 457–608.

[Purves 1966] R. Purves, "Bimeasurable functions", *Fund. Math.* **58** (1966), 149–157.

[Ramsay 1971] A. Ramsay, "Virtual groups and group actions", *Advances in Math.* **6** (1971), 253–322.

[Ramsay 1982] A. Ramsay, "Topologies on measured groupoids", *J. Funct. Anal.* **47**:3 (1982), 314–343.

[Reinhart 1983] B. L. Reinhart, *Differential geometry of foliations*, Ergebnisse der Mathematik und ihrer Grenzgebiete **99**, Springer, Berlin, 1983.

[Renault 1980] J. Renault, *A groupoid approach to C^*-algebras*, Lecture Notes in Mathematics **793**, Springer, Berlin, 1980.

[Renault 1982] J. N. Renault, "C^*-algebras of groupoids and foliations", pp. 339–350 in *Operator algebras and applications* (Kingston, Ont., 1980), Part 2, edited by R. V. Kadison, Proc. Sympos. Pure Math. **38**, Amer. Math. Soc., Providence, 1982.

[Renault 1987] J. Renault, "Représentation des produits croisés d'algèbres de groupoïdes", *J. Operator Theory* **18**:1 (1987), 67–97.

[de Rham 1955] G. de Rham, *Variétés différentiables: formes, courants, formes harmoniques*, Actualités Scientifiques et Industrielles **1222**, Hermann, Paris, 1955.

[Rieffel 1976] M. A. Rieffel, "Strong Morita equivalence of certain transformation group C^*-algebras", *Math. Ann.* **222**:1 (1976), 7–22.

[Roe 1985] J. Roe, *Analysis on manifolds*, Ph.D. thesis, Oxford University, 1985.

[Roe 1987] J. Roe, "Finite propagation speed and Connes' foliation algebra", *Math. Proc. Cambridge Philos. Soc.* **102**:3 (1987), 459–466.

[Roe 1988a] J. Roe, "An index theorem on open manifolds, I", *J. Differential Geom.* **27**:1 (1988), 87–113.

[Roe 1988b] J. Roe, "An index theorem on open manifolds, II", *J. Differential Geom.* **27**:1 (1988), 115–136.

[Roe 1993] J. Roe, *Coarse cohomology and index theory on complete Riemannian manifolds*, Mem. Amer. Math. Soc. **497**, Amer. Math. Soc., Providence, 1993.

[Roe 1996] J. Roe, *Index theory, coarse geometry, and topology of manifolds*, CBMS Regional Conference Series in Mathematics **90**, Amer. Math. Soc., Providence, 1996.

[Roe 1998] J. Roe, *Elliptic operators, topology and asymptotic methods*, second ed., Pitman Research Notes in Mathematics Series **395**, Longman, Harlow, 1998.

[Rosenberg et al. 1970] H. Rosenberg, R. Roussarie, and D. Weil, "A classification of closed orientable 3-manifolds of rank two", *Ann. of Math.* (2) **91** (1970), 449–464.

[Ruelle and Sullivan 1975] D. Ruelle and D. Sullivan, "Currents, flows and diffeomorphisms", *Topology* **14**:4 (1975), 319–327.

[Sadun and Williams 2003] L. Sadun and R. F. Williams, "Tiling spaces are Cantor set fiber bundles", *Ergodic Theory Dynam. Systems* **23**:1 (2003), 307–316.

[Sarkaria 1978] K. S. Sarkaria, *The de Rham cohomology of foliated manifolds*, Ph.D. thesis, SUNY, Stony Brook, NY, 1978.

[Segal 1968] G. Segal, "Equivariant K-theory", *Inst. Hautes Études Sci. Publ. Math.* **34** (1968), 129–151.

[Shanahan 1978] P. Shanahan, *The Atiyah–Singer index theorem*, Lecture Notes in Mathematics **638**, Springer, Berlin, 1978.

[Steenrod 1940] N. E. Steenrod, "Regular cycles of compact metric spaces", *Ann. of Math.* (2) **41** (1940), 833–851.

[Steenrod 1951] N. Steenrod, *The topology of fibre bundles*, Princeton Mathematical Series **14**, Princeton Univ. Press, Princeton, 1951.

[Sullivan 1976] D. Sullivan, "Cycles for the dynamical study of foliated manifolds and complex manifolds", *Invent. Math.* **36** (1976), 225–255.

[Takai 1986] H. Takai, "KK-theory for the C^*-algebras of Anosov foliations", pp. 387–399 in *Geometric methods in operator algebras* (Kyoto, 1983), edited by H. Araki and E. G. Effros, Pitman Res. Notes Math. Ser. **123**, Longman Sci. Tech., Harlow, 1986.

[Takesaki 1979] M. Takesaki, *Theory of operator algebras, I*, Springer, New York, 1979.

[Takesaki 1983] M. Takesaki, *Structure of factors and automorphism groups*, CBMS Regional Conference Series in Mathematics **51**, Amer. Math. Soc., Providence, 1983.

[Taylor 1979] M. E. Taylor, "Fourier integral operators and harmonic analysis on compact manifolds", pp. 115–136 in *Harmonic analysis in Euclidean spaces* (Williamstown, MA, 1978), Part 2, edited by G. L. Weiss and S. Wainger, Proc. Sympos. Pure Math. **35**, Amer. Math. Soc., Providence, 1979.

[Taylor 1981] M. E. Taylor, *Pseudodifferential operators*, Princeton Mathematical Series **34**, Princeton Univ. Press, Princeton, 1981.

[Thom 1964] R. Thom, "Généralisation de la théorie de Morse aux variétés feuilletées", *Ann. Inst. Fourier* (*Grenoble*) **14**:1 (1964), 173–189.

[Thurston 1974] W. Thurston, "The theory of foliations of codimension greater than one", *Comment. Math. Helv.* **49** (1974), 214–231.

[Thurston 1976] W. P. Thurston, "Existence of codimension-one foliations", *Ann. of Math.* (2) **104**:2 (1976), 249–268.

[Torpe 1985] A. M. Torpe, "K-theory for the leaf space of foliations by Reeb components", *J. Funct. Anal.* **61**:1 (1985), 15–71.

[Tu 1999] J.-L. Tu, "La conjecture de Baum–Connes pour les feuilletages moyennables", *K-Theory* **17**:3 (1999), 215–264.

[Tu 2004] J.-L. Tu, "Non-Hausdorff groupoids, proper actions and K-theory", *Doc. Math.* **9** (2004), 565–597.

[Vaisman 1973] I. Vaisman, *Cohomology and differential forms*, Pure and Applied Mathematics **21**, Marcel Dekker, New York, 1973.

[Valette 2002] A. Valette, *Introduction to the Baum–Connes conjecture*, Lectures in Mathematics ETH Zürich, Birkhäuser, Basel, 2002.

[Van Elst 1994] A. Van Elst, "Gap-labelling theorems for Schrödinger operators on the square and cubic lattice", *Rev. Math. Phys.* **6**:2 (1994), 319–342.

[Varadarajan 1963] V. S. Varadarajan, "Groups of automorphisms of Borel spaces", *Trans. Amer. Math. Soc.* **109** (1963), 191–220.

[Wells 1973] R. O. Wells, Jr., *Differential analysis on complex manifolds*, Prentice-Hall, Englewood Cliffs, NJ, 1973.

[Whitehead 1978] G. W. Whitehead, *Elements of homotopy theory*, Graduate Texts in Mathematics **61**, Springer, New York, 1978.

[Winkelnkemper 1983] H. E. Winkelnkemper, "The graph of a foliation", *Ann. Global Anal. Geom.* **1**:3 (1983), 51–75.

[Zimmer 1983] R. J. Zimmer, "Ergodic actions of semisimple groups and product relations", *Ann. of Math.* (2) **118**:1 (1983), 9–19.

[Zimmer 1984] R. J. Zimmer, *Ergodic theory and semisimple groups*, Monographs in Mathematics **81**, Birkhäuser, Basel, 1984.

Notation

Index

Printed in the United States
by Baker & Taylor Publisher Services